Gerhard Goebel
(Editor)

Tinnitus —

Psychosomatic Aspects of Complex Chronic Tinnitus

Occurrence, Effects, Diagnosis and Treatment

Gerhard Goebel
Editor

Tinnitus —

Psychosomatic Aspects of Complex Chronic Tinnitus

Occurrence, Effects, Diagnosis and Treatment

Quintessence

Editor:
Dr. Gerhard Goebel
Medizinisch-psychosomatische Klinik Roseneck
(Medical-psychosomatic Clinic Roseneck)
im Verbund mit der Medizinischen Fakultät der Ludwig
Maximilians-Universität München
(in association with the Medical Faculty of the Ludwig
Maximilian University Munich)
Am Roseneck 6
83209 Prien am Chiemsee
Germany

British Library Cataloguing in Publication Data

Tinnitus : psychosomatic aspects of complex chronic
tinnitus : occurrence, effects, diagnosis and treatment
1. Tinnitus – Psychosomatic aspects
I. Goebel, Gerhard
617.8'042'8

ISBN 1850970424

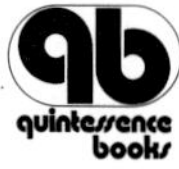

Typeset by Alacrity, Banwell Castle, Somerset
Printed and bound by Bartels & Wernitz, Munich
Lithography by JuP Industire- und Presseklischee, Berlin
Printed in Germany

Foreword

Dr Jonathan W.P. Hazell

It is only 10 years since the first modern textbook on tinnitus appeared. During this time a number of authors involved in the field of tinnitus research have contributed volumes on this important subject with varying degrees of success. Part of the blame for the lack of success in finding solutions to tinnitus must rest with the ENT doctors who "took over" the symptom from psychologists and psychiatrists at the beginning of this century. A largely oto-centric approach to tinnitus has resulted in numerous treatments and claims for cure, all of which have proved ineffective with the passage of time. The reason for this became clear to Richard Hallam, one of the contributors to this book, in his fundamental paper on the habitation of tinnitus, identifying the importance of psychology in the generation of tinnitus complaint, and proposing a model from which others have grown. The main difficulties in finding a solution to tinnitus are made clear in this book. There is no "quick fix". Tinnitus is a complex symptom involving all levels of the auditory system, and at this moment in time, the best way of helping the patient is a cognitive one combining various psychological approaches with "sound therapies". The success of Dr Goebel's treatment concept is in sharp contrast to the constant failures experienced by otolaryngologists using the concept of tinnitus as a cochlear disorder which can be cured by improving its blood supply. Of course the cochlea plays a part in the pathogenesis of tinnitus, deafness is often a risk factor, but it is not the cause of tinnitus distress. 27% of those with total deafness awaiting cochlear implantation have no tinnitus experience whatsoever.

Dr Goebel's recommendations for a multi-disciplinary approach to tinnitus management strongly support the experience and development of our own tinnitus clinics in London (UK) and Baltimore (USA) based on the neurophysiological model proposed by Jastreboff. Distress from any sensory phenomenon must involve other parts of the brain separate from the sensory cortex, in particular the limbic system. Extreme forms of tinnitus distress seen so often in a clinical environment may be viewed as a phobic phenomenon which will require prolonged retraining with appropriate cognitive intervention in order to produce relief. Of course it is not appropriate to "hand back" tinnitus to psychology and psychiatry, we must work together as a team if we are going to help the tinnitus patient with distress.

Dr Goebel's book makes clear how important this approach is, although we still have a long way to go in understanding the interaction between the various symptoms which can coexist with tinnitus, and whether they represent a real part of the tinnitus aetiology or are simply coexistent in a general stress state. Understanding tinnitus involves understanding the whole of the auditory system, the peripheral end organ, the various levels of auditory processing occurring in the sub-cortical pathways, the interaction with the limbic system, the prefrontal cortex, and the way in which the final perception of tinnitus is configured in the temporal lobe of the brain at a conscious level. We have not yet arrived at this point, but Dr Goebel's book makes a most valuable contribution in pointing us in the right direction.

Preface

Dr. Gerhard Goebel

Tinnitus is one of the most frequent diagnoses made in otorhinolaryngological practice. As an acute symptom accompanying hearing loss or dizziness, it helps the physician to establish a diagnosis. On the other hand chronic tinnitus, often the principal cause of the patient's suffering, is among the most difficult, and thus most challenging, tasks of therapy. Considering this fact, it is surprising that chronic tinnitus is a neglected topic in medical school. This deficit is often recognized only in medical practice. A considerable number of different medical and psychological disciplines (i.e. dentistry, orthopedic surgery, internal medicine, neurology, psychiatry and clinical psychology) are involved in the search for possible causes of chronic tinnitus. Specialists often do not know that the cause of the tinnitus lies in their own field and thus many important treatment modalities remain unapplied. Clinical psychologists, who also deal increasingly with therapeutic possibilities for chronic tinnitus, have inadequate clinical training to do so. To be successful in the psychotherapy of chronic tinnitus, the psychologist/psychotherapist must be familiar with treatment requirements and regimes for tinnitus. Finally, the therapist must gain knowledge of specific medical problems and their medical definitions.

This book attempts to be a milestone in the recognition of these problems and intends to overcome the artificial barriers between medicine and psychology, as well as the barriers between different medical specialties.

The book is also an introduction to the treatment of complex chronic tinnitus. Practice-oriented techniques for the various psychotherapeutic concepts are described for the psychotherapist, together with comprehensive information about medical problems.

The physician can thereby develop a deeper understanding of the psychological problems of patients and becomes familiar with the achievements of psychotherapy in this field. This enables greater empathy with the patient over the protracted course of treatment and, where appropriate, facilitates cooperation with other disciplines, including psychotherapy, for the benefit of the patient.

The first chapter is written by an expert in the medical problems of tinnitus, T. Lenartz, who describes the etiological, diagnostic, audiological and therapeutic aspects of tinnitus comprehensively from the point of view of the otorhinolaryngologist. The chapters by B. Scott/P. Lindberg, H. Kurth/R. Gefken, and W. Hiller/G. Goebel deal with tinnitus incidence, psychological effects, and comorbidity of psychological disturbance associated with chronic tinnitus, on the basis of their own studies.

G. Goebel begins the section dealing with therapy with a critical evaluation of published scientific studies concerning the psychological treatment of chronic tinnitus. Subsequent chapters introduce intervention models that have become established and are effective. B. Rabaioli-Fischer describes the course of a type of motivation-guided cognitive behavioral therapy on the basis of a detailed case report. G. Goebel et al introduce in detail an in-patient integrative behavioral-medicine treatment concept and discuss the results of the, at present, most extensive treatment evaluation, including the long-term effects of their therapeutic concept. The internationally recognized psychologists R. S. Hallam, P. Lindberg and B. Scott describe their behavioural therapy approaches and their results, partly using case reports. Stress immunization and its efficiency in overcoming tinnitus, together with an extensive description of hypnotherapy in the treatment of chronic tinnitus are discussed by E. de Camp, U. de Camp and H. Joisten respectively. On the basis of drawings made by a tinnitus patient, C. Palm and G. Goebel describe the concept and treatment methods of art therapy as an integral component of a behavioral therapy treatment concept. The reader is able to develop a deeper understanding of the agonies suffered by tinnitus patients when S. Goebel analyses "dialogues" addressed to the tinnitus in letter form by the patient. An experimental study by H. Milz/G. Goebel deals with anxiety and tinnitus in relation to a specific body perception exercise, as described by G. Alexander.

Disturbances caused by the temporomandibular joint and the cervical spine are frequent, but little recognized, psychosomatic aspects of tinnitus, and therefore undestanding them is an indispensable part of psychotherapeutic and medical knowledge. The chapter dealing with "Tinnitus as a dental problem" by W. Neuhauser, an expert in this complicated field, adds significantly to the material collected in this book. The same is true of the chapter by E. Biesinger, who, as an otorhinolaryngologist and manual-therapist, discusses the frequently noted relationship between tinnitus and syndromes of the cervical spine and describes appropriate therapeutic aids.

The book closes with a treat for the medically or psychologically oriented reader: a comprehensive inter-disciplinary glossary facilitates a mutual understanding of the different concepts.

This book is the result of 20 years of medical and 10 years of psychotherapeutic training and practice. Relying on experience in the psychotherapeutic management of chronic pain, I have been largely responsible for the development of an in-patient treatment concept for the most serious cases of chronic tinnitus. During the course of this development, I have spoken with hundreds of patients. In addition, I have had discussions with many otorhinolaryngologists and psychotherapists who have dealt with the most seriously affected tinnitus patients. I am greatly indebted to the knowledge and experience of my colleagues who have contributed significantly to this book. I also thank all who have contributed to this book by providing chapters or critical evaluation (W. Hiller and B. Kronschnabl).

Special thanks are owed to Manfred Fichter who, as medical director of the Roseneck Clinic, has wholeheartedly supported the treatment and research of chronic tinnitus. His scientific dedication and his progressive understanding of comprehensive psychotherapy are the fertile soil in which it was possible to bring my ideas to fruition. I would also like to thank my teacher and training therapist, Peter Borst. Last but not least, I would like to thank Dr. Christopher Kober who, as an expatriate Canadian and experienced colleague at the Clinic Roseneck, translated the German contributions to this book.

It is my hope that this book will contribute to a greater recognition of the problems of patients with complex chronic tinnitus, that the sterile and unproductive dichotomy between a somatic and psychological approach to tinnitus will be reduced and that in this way a greater public acceptance of psychological treatment will result. My sincere wish is that the various psychotherapeutic techniques will thus be available to as many patients as possible.

Prien am Chiemsee, March 1998

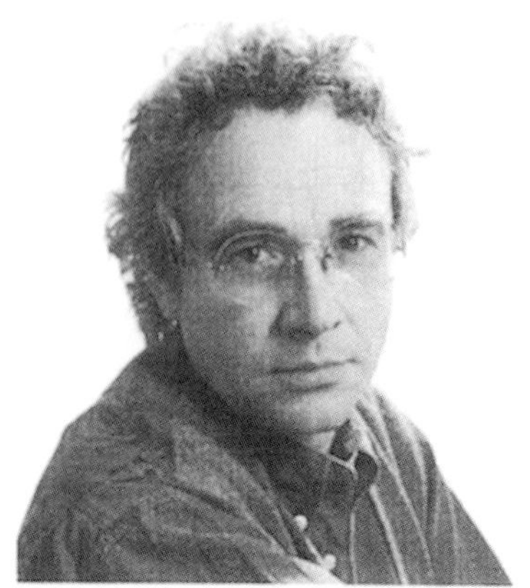

The Editor

Gerhard Goebel, born May 12, 1946 in Giessen, studied medicine in Wurzburg, Innsbruck and Grenoble before completing his medical degree at the Munich Technical University in 1972. After 4 years of research and clinical work at the German Heart Center in Munich, 2 years of training in angiology and radiology in Augsburg and 5 years in the department of Histology/Oncology at the Schwabinger Hospital in Munich, he became senior staff physician at the Medical-Psychosomatic Clinic Roseneck in Prien am Chiemsee in 1985. He has completed psychotherapeutic training with emphasis on psychodrama, gestalt psychology and behavioral therapy. In 1986, together with Wolfgang Keeser, Manfred Fichter, Christine Wildgruber and Bernd Köstler, he established a ward for patients with chronic pain, in which the treatment concept for in-patients with complex chronic tinnitus has developed under his leadership since 1987. He has been a supporting member of the German Tinnitus League since 1987 and, within this framework, founded an interdisciplinary study group for doctors and psychologists in 1990. He is a member of the German Otorhinolaryngological Society, German Audiology Society, Professional Associate of the American Tinnitus Association (ATA) and has been a lecturer at the Lindauer Therapiewochen psychotherapy workshops. Since 1988, he has been teaching behavioral medicine at the Munich Medical Training Institute for Psychotherapy and Psychoanalysis. In addition to editing a book about anorexia and bulimia, he has published numerous scientific articles about behavioral medicine aspects of chronic pain and complex chronic tinnitus and the German Tinnitus-Questionnaire (TQ).

Contributors

Eberhard Biesinger, MD
Otorhinolaryngologist
Chirotherapy, plastic surgery
Maxplatz 5, 83278 Traunstein, Germany

Dipl-Psych, Dipl-Sozialpädagogin
Evelyn de Camp-Schmidt
Psychotherapeutic Practice
Sattlerstraße 30, 12355 Berlin, Germany

Dipl-Psych, Dipl-Ing Ulf de Camp
Psychotherapeutic Practice
Sattlerstraße 30, 12355 Berlin, Germany

Prof, Dipl-Psych Manfred M. Fichter, MD
Medical-Psychosomatic Clinic Roseneck
Affiliated to the Medical Faculty of the University of Munich
Medical Director
Neurologist, Psychiatrist, Psychotherapist
Am Roseneck 6, 83209 Prien am Chiemsee, Germany

Dipl-Psych Reinhard Gefken
Psychology Institute I of the University of Hamburg
Von-Melle-Park 11, 20146 Hamburg 13, Germany

Gerhard Goebel, MD
Medical-Psychosomatic Clinical Roseneck
Affiliated to the Medical Faculty of the University of Munich
Senior Staff Physician, Doctor of Internal Medicine, Doctor of Psychotherapeutic Medicine
Am Roseneck 6, 83209 Prien am Chiemsee, Germany

Richard S. Hallam, PhD
Senior Lecturer, Department of Psychology,
University College, London
Gower Street, London WC1E 6BT,
Great Britain

Dr Dipl-Psych Wolfgang Hiller
Medical-Psychosomatic Clinic Roseneck
Affiliated to the Medical Faculty of the
Ludwig-Maximilians-University of Munich
Am Roseneck 6, 83209 Prien am Chiemsee,
Germany

Dr Dipl-Psych Heribert Joisten
Psychotherapeutic Practice
Robert-Koch-Straße 29,
W-4200 Oberhausen, Germany

Dipl-Psych Heike Kurth
Psychology Institute I of the University of
Hamburg
Von-Melle-Park 11, 20146 Hamburg,
Germany

Priv-Doz Thomas Lenarz
Supervising Senior Physician
Otorhinolaryngological Clinic, University of
Tübingen
Silcherstraße 5, 72076 Tübingen, Germany

Per Lindberg, PhD
Center for Caring Sciences
Uppsala University
S-731, 85 Uppsala, Sweden

Dean Marson
Physical Therapist
Esalen Institute
Big Sur, CA 93920, USA

Helmut Milz, MD
Medical-Psychosomatic Clinic Roseneck
Affiliated to the Medical Faculty of the
Ludwig-Maximilians-University of Munich
Senior Staff Physician,
Doctor of General Practice
Am Roseneck 6, 83209 Prien am Chiemsee,
Germany

Werner Neuhauser, DMD
Commissioner for Psychosomatics of the
Bavarian Chamber of Dentists
Ellharterstr. 49, 87435 Kempten, Germany

Christine Palm
Behavioral Therapist
Medical-Psychosomatic Clinic Roseneck
Affiliated to the Medical Faculty of the
Ludwig-Maximilians-University of Munich
Am Roseneck 6, 83209 Prien am Chiemsee,
Germany

Dipl-Psych Barbara Rabaioli-Fischer
Psychotherapeutic Practice
Ickstattstraße 2b, 80469 Munich,
Germany

Dr Dipl-Psych Winfried Rief
Senior Staff Psychologist
Medical-Psychosomatic Clinic Roseneck
Affiliated to the Medical Faculty of the
Ludwig-Maximilians-University of Munich
Am Roseneck 6, 83209 Prien am Chiemsee,
Germany

Berit Scott, PhD
Department of Clinical Psychology
Uppsala University
S-751 42 Uppsala, Sweden

Contents

Introduction

Dr. Gerhard Goebel

The term "complex chronic tinnitus" defines a condition experienced by 600,000–800,000 individuals in Germany alone. They hear noises (ringing, buzzing, tinkling, etc) which appear to arise in the ear or the head and which cannot be ascribed to any recognizable external source of sound. Only the affected persons themselves can describe the phenomenon which, in the majority of cases, is heard continuously. A minority of cases, however, report significant variations in tinnitus intensity during the course of a day or week. Finally, some subjects experience it episodically, with days of agony interspersed with days during which the tinnitus disappears completely. Most of those affected hear the tinnitus in both ears. Approximately one-third of the subjects hear the tinnitus only in one ear; here, the left side, as in headache patients, appears to predominate. Tinnitus is experienced as a transitory phenomenon by more than a third of the adult population and is per se a physiological phenomenon. When placed in a soundproof room (camera silentia), nine out of ten subjects claim to hear sounds that arise in the ear or the head.

If we compare the rate of occurrence of complex chronic tinnitus (1%–2%) with that of diabetes mellitus (2%), the medical significance of the former is impressive because we are dealing with a symptom far more widespread than is recognized. Externally not audible, shamefully concealed by those affected, medically impossible to master, this symptom and its frequently harsh effects are usually unknown to those not afflicted. Nonetheless, tinnitus is one of the most frequently mentioned symptoms in otorhinolaryngological practice. Rarely is curative treatment successful.

The numerous causes of tinnitus include injuries from long-term exposure to noise, from an acute acoustic trauma to the ear, sudden deafness, and from other diseases that affect hearing. Approximately 70% of those with hearing loss experience tinnitus, but most manage to live with it. Tinnitus also occurs in children and may coexist with normal hearing levels. As a rule, tinnitus is not a symptom of a malignant disease. It may be an early indication of a brain tumor only in very rare instances, and then usually it is an indication of the slowly growing, relatively easily operable acoustic neurinoma.

Tinnitus also occurs in conditions that do not affect otorhinolaryngology primarily. Instead, the disciplines of neurology and internal medicine may be involved, with disease of the central nervous system or disturbances in circulation related to hypertension or metabolic disturbances. Dentistry and orthopedics also are confronted with tinnitus as a symptom. Temporomandibular joint disease and bruxism are associated with tinnitus and may deteriorate an existing case. Traumatic or degenerative changes of the cervical spine caused by chronic muscle tension also elicit various types of tinnitus.

Unfortunately, complete or partial relief through the use of drugs, technical aids (hearing aids, maskers, etc), or surgery is limited to only a small percentage of tinnitus "victims". This fact finds expression in a pessimistic statement of the treating physician, such as: "Nothing can be done for you, you will have to become accustomed to it." That, in turn, elicits a belief in the patient that he has become a burden to the physician and that the complaints are not being taken seriously. Thus the patient does not mention the tinnitus at the next appointment. Finally, he gives up, or is treated by persons who exploit him by making unattainable promises.

The ordinary doctor's appointment leaves little time for an explanation of causal relationships or instruction about the possibilities afforded by dentistry or orthopedics. As a rule, explanations about psychological relationships or the opportunities in psychological therapy are not mentioned at all, because little interest exists in this field on the part of either the doctor or the patient. This is based on the somatic therapeutic approach to tinnitus, in which the thoughts or feelings of the patient towards their tinnitus have no place. An understanding of body and psyche reduced to mechanistic relations makes it difficult to tolerate relationships between the sensory experience of tinnitus and psychosocial factors or factors relevant to personality. Only when the affected person obviously requires psychiatric help are psychological aspects included in the differential diagnosis. Because neuroses and psychoses frequently are equated with "craziness", the affected patients understandably reject being placed in this category and vehemently deny all psychic causes. If psychological treatment is nevertheless suggested, the patient frequently seeks another expert who is expected to find an organic cause of the tinnitus, thereby contributing to the patient's "rehabilitation". In other words, both physicians and patients consider psychological associations with tinnitus as "abnormal". Such relationships are associated with the taint of simulation, unwarranted profiteering from illness, and mental illness.

A purely somatically oriented medicine concentrates inherently on understanding a disease in terms of organ pathology and thus will consider only those procedures that comply with this concept. Thus, it makes it more difficult for both the physician and the patient to find other possibilities that exist in the form of psychological methods to overcome the problem.

The editor of and the contributors to this book want to provide an impetus to understanding health and disease not only from the point of view of technical failure, but also to understanding thoughts and feelings as an important factor in somatic disturbances. Tinnitus caused by an accident may be compensated by psychological intervention; tinnitus caused, for example, by psychogenic bruxism may be alleviated by purely technical dental measures. Both treatment methods can have an additive effect if the patient no longer perceives the illness as something unfamiliar which they want nothing to do with. Body, psyche and soul are not isolated factors in our organism. Illness can be the result of countless forms of behavior, thoughts and perceptions. Frequently illness is also an expression of our lives that must be mastered, just as the wanderer must find his way to reach an unknown destination. Medicine, psychology and the patient can contribute jointly to find the solution to the crisis presented by the illness, by including the patient as a responsible part of the process of overcoming it.

This means considering how tinnitus developed, accepting its existence, and chanelling thoughts and feelings in a direction which will lead to an accpetable solution. The disease itself leads to conclusions that may be applied constructively for the future. Tinnitus should not be perceived only as a disturbance to be uprooted once and for all, but also as a reminder to cope with aspects of life that have been ignored in the past. Medicine then no longer treats tinnitus in the chronic state as a repair job, but accompanies the patient psychologically in the effort to find himself. The goal of treatment defined in this manner is to reintegrate body and soul, to provide a context for the existing tinnitus, and to accept it.

The solution that lies in the integration of tinnitus frequently means understanding tinnitus as a message, the meaning of which is to be learned. There is a sense to what is perceived at first as senseless. There is no answer to the question: "Why me?" because the question implies a comparison with others who appear to be happier, and arises from the demand that justice and health can be forced upon fate. The converse question in this case must be: "Why not?" The questions: "What does tinnitus have to do with my life?" and "What can I do to adjust to tinnitus better and simultaneously to get as much psychic gain from this crisis for my present and future life as possible?" will initiate concrete and productive considerations. These include listening to oneself instead of ignoring inner voices, and ceasing to perceive tinnitus as something foreign, thus finally coming to the realization that "I am my tinnitus (too)."

Many patients have already taken this path. The editor and contributors to this book have met these people and have worked out various methods to overcome tinnitus mutually. The purpose of the book is to contribute to the cooperation necessary between medicine and psychology. The variety of views and treatments proposed is occasionally confusing but all unite to contribute to an interdisciplinary management of complex tinnitus.

In addition, this book intends to bridge the gap that exists between psychoanalysis and behavioral therapy, as well as body oriented therapy on the one hand and psychoanalysis and cognitive therapy on the other. For this reason the selection of the chapter subjects is a subjective choice. Nonetheless, it is intended to provide a comprehensive review for physicians, psychologists, behavioral therapists, and body-oriented therapists, as well as for students of these disciplines.

Chapter 1

Problems in the diagnosis and treatment of chronic tinnitus (from an otorhinolaryngological point of view)

Thomas Lenarz

1.1 Summary

Chronic tinnitus is among the most frequent symptoms encountered in otology. This usually subjectively experienced symptom is characterized by the lack of specific knowledge about its pathophysiology and the very limited medical treatment available. Pathophysiological hypotheses based on the knowledge of hearing research are nonetheless of great value for the development of new therapeutic approaches as well as for patient education. The primary pathophysiological mechanisms are disturbances of the hair cells, the spontaneous discharge pattern of the auditory nerve fibers, rotating stimuli of the central auditory centers and disturbances in the efferent auditory system. The patient's history and individualized diagnostic steps provide the most important elements for clarification. They also provide the basis for the fundamental step in treatment: advising the patient about the cause and nature of the tinnitus. While objective ringing in the ear can usually be referred to surgery, treatment of tinnitus is far more difficult. Acute forms should be approached as sudden deafness and treated rheologically, with good chances for success. Advising the patient by introducing pathological models is part of the cognitive therapy. Drugs and technical methods may be considered in decompensated tinnitus. Behavioral therapy and psychotherapy are indicated in refractory cases, to achieve a state of compensated tinnitus.

1.2 Definitions and epidemiological data

Tinnitus is a hearing disturbance that has neither signal nor information character. Instead, it is caused by a functional disturbance within the auditory system. Thus, it is not produced by external acoustic events. It must be differentiated from auditory hallucinations related to psychoses or neuroses, which point to a disturbance of a conscious perception of auditory phenomena. The functional disturbance may be located at various places of the *auditory system.*

The auditory system includes all anatomic structures that make hearing possible, beginning with the external ear (auricle (ear lobe and the external auditory meatus), the middle ear and the eardrum, the auditory ossicles, the auditory sensory cells (Fig. 1.1), the auditory nerves and the auditory path in the brain stem and the diencephalon, and finally the auditory cortex of the temporal lobe (Fig. 1.2).

Tinnitus occurs frequently in the general population. According to epidemiological studies in Great Britain, 15% of the population report having experienced tinnitus of several minutes' duration at some time in their lives. Sleep disturbances or other symptoms, such as loss of concentration or reduced level of functioning, occur in 8%; 0.5% suffer from tinnitus of such severity as to make a normal lifestyle impossible (Coles, 1984). Based on similar living conditions, similar percentages may be assumed for Germany.

Tinnitus does not initially constitute an independent disease. Rather, it is a *symptom* of a functional disturbance of varying cause and etiology in the auditory system. For that reason, two distinct forms can be identified. An internal source of sound exists in the rare patient with *objective noises* in the ear, i.e., there is no external sound source, as in the normal hearing process. The acoustic signals arise, for example, from acute vascular processes such as stenosis of the carotid artery, arteriovenous shunts, or through muscular disturbances such as spasms, contractions or myoclonus of muscles of the middle ear or of the otopharynx which participate in opening the eustachian tubes (Table 1.1). Acoustic signals are led by air conduction or via the interposed tissue structures and bone to the ear of the patient. There they lead, like external acoustic signals, to stimulation of the internal ear and thus to the normal hearing process. They may be made audible to an observer via a stethoscope or microphone placed near the patient's external ear, i.e., they become objective.

Subjective ear sounds (tinnitus) are much more frequent. They are not caused by an acoustic signal. No means exist as yet for an observer to hear them, because the pathophysiological correlates involved are not understood with certainty and the course of the electrophysiological events is demonstrable only through invasive diagnostic procedures. Thus, the sounds are recognized only by the affected person. They can be characterized only indirectly through psychoacoustic comparative procedures ("tinnitus-matching", see section 1.5.4) and by the frequently accompanying hearing loss. As a rule, functional disturbances of the hair cells of the inner ear are present. Injuries to the middle ear, the auditory nerves, the auditory path and the auditory cortex are less frequent. The large variety of possible causes (Table 1.1.2) emphasises the fact that there is no such condition as tinnitus *per se*. Tinnitus is a

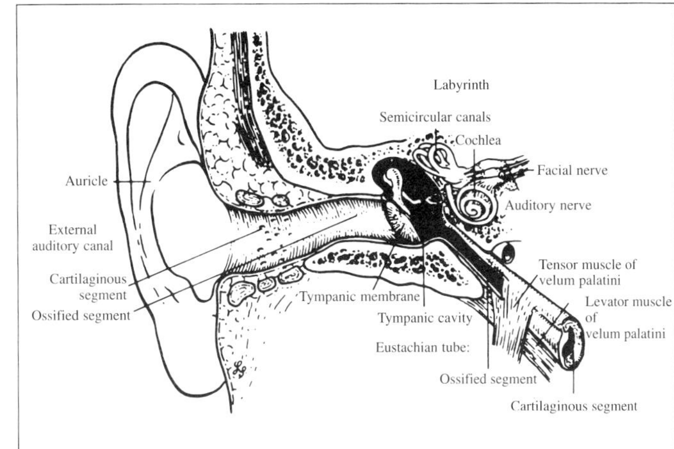

Fig. 1.1 Anatomy of the hearing system, consisting of the external ear, middle ear and auditory nerve (from Boenninghaus, 1990).

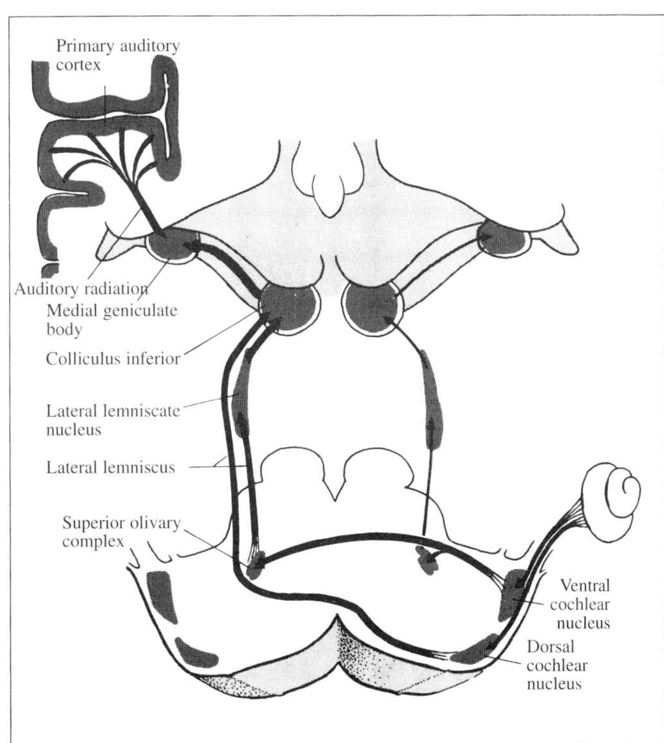

Fig. 1.2 Auditory path: afferent paths from the right cochlea (from Boenninghaus, 1990).

Table 1.1 Possible causes of objective ear sounds

1	Vascular causes
	Extracranial localization
	Carotid stenosis
	Vertebral stenosis
	Carotid glomus tumor
	Hemangioma
	Cardiac defects
	Intracranial localization
	Arteriovenous fistula
	Hemangioma
	Arteriosclerosis of the cerebral arteries
	Tympanic glomus tumor
	Jugular glomus tumor
	Elevation of the jugular vein bulbus
	Altered rheology
	Anemia
	Polycythemia
2	Muscular causes
	Tensor muscles of the middle ear
	Spasm, rarely myoclonus of the tensor tympani muscle
	Spasm, rarely myoclonus of the tensor stapes muscle
	Palate muscles
	Palatomyoclonus of the tensor or levator veli palatini muscles
3	Disturbance of function of the Eustachian tube
	Gaping or open tube

symptom of injury; usually it is accompanied by auditory damage such as hearing loss or loss of clarity of hearing speech or music. The actual causes can be quite varied, ranging from sudden deafness or acoustic trauma to slowly developing damage such as occupational loss of hearing, age related physiological hearing loss (presbycusis) and degenerative or tumorous processes.

It is important to differentiate between patients with *compensated* tinnitus, in which the patients continue to function without significant decrease of the quality of life, and *decompensated* tinnitus, an independent disease, characterized by the development of secondary illness such as disturbances of sleep or psychological abnormalities. Many cases of complex chronic tinnitus fall into this category.

1.3 Symptoms and course of tinnitus

The incidence of tinnitus is highest among those aged 40-60 years. Increased occurrence during the second phase of occupational activity indicates the possible effects of living and working conditions. Aging processes of the auditory system and occupational and non-occupational exposure to noise may interact with specific occupational

Table 1.2 Possible causes of subjective ear sounds (tinnitus aurium)

1	Sudden deafness
2	Menière's disease
3	Acoustic trauma (detonation, explosion trauma)
4	Loss of hearing caused by chronic noise exposure (occupational hearing loss)
5	Presbycusis
6	Hereditary sensorineural loss of hearing
7	Cerebral trauma with or without petrosal bone fracture
8	Acoustic neuroma
9	Quinine, aspirin, diuretic/aminoglycoside antibiotic/cisplatine intoxication
10	Immunogenic inner ear loss of hearing
11	Sensorineural loss of hearing of unknown etiology
12	Otosclerosis
13	Heart diseases, disease of the circulatory system
14	Metabolic diseases
15	Kidney diseases
16	Central nervous system diseases
17	Degenerative changes and functional blockage of the cervical spine
16	Myoarthropathy of the temporomandibular joint

stressors (Coles, 1984). Anxiety and fear of failure may also play a role.

Following sudden onset, often in relation to an external event such as respiratory disease, sudden deafness, or very loud noise, subjects frequently describe a gradual increase in the subjective noise level of the tinnitus. The undulating course of loudness of the tinnitus coincides directly with typical professional and private stress situations. Most patients slowly become accustomed to a slight decrease in the subjective loudness of the tinnitus. Certain conditions such as Ménière's disease are characterized by attacks of recurrent prostrating vertigo, sensorineural hearing loss and an intermittent appearance or increased severity of tinnitus. In most cases, an irreversible functional disturbance of the auditory system is the cause and for this reason the tinnitus persists (Fig. 1.3). *Chronic* tinnitus is therefore defined as a tinnitus which persists for more than 3 months.

Those affected rapidly develop feelings of being at the mercy of this unpleasant, unpredictable, and not consciously alterable and continuously present auditory sensation. Thus, a vicious circle of tinnitus with the development of anxiety leading to increased stress and disturbance of sleep to increased loudness of the tinnitus and psychosomatic sequelae may develop. The tinnitus thus gains an increasing influence on the patient's life and, in this decompensated form, becomes a medico–psychological problem (Fig. 1.4). Additional influences are present in the form of reduced subjective loudness due to ambient noise during the day, and increased subjective loudness in quieter surroundings during the evening and at night.

Tinnitus is experienced subjectively in a variety of forms. Each patient can describe "his" tinnitus extensively and uniquely. Qualitative comparisons are made best with accepted acoustic phenomena. Depending on the frequency of the perceived

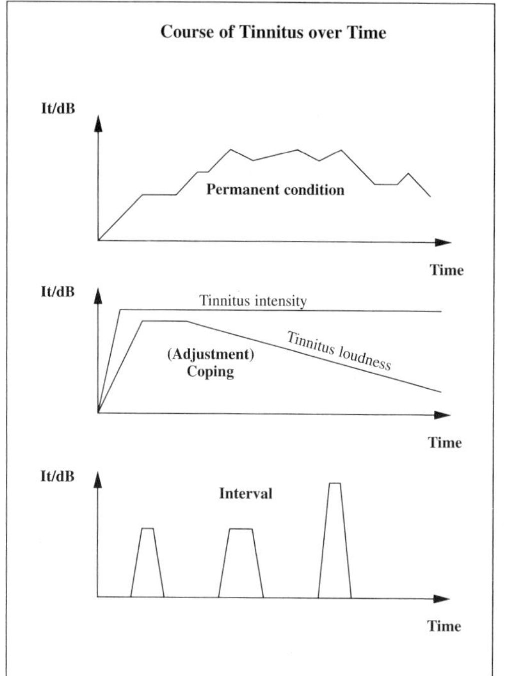

Fig. 1.3 Various courses of tinnitus over time. Depicted is intensity of tinnitus in dB above the hearing threshold (It/dB).

sounds, high frequency whistling and broad band roaring/rustling and humming are mentioned. The *quality* of the tinnitus indicates the type of hearing loss, as may be determined in an audiogram (see section 1.5.3). Thus, high frequency whistling is associated with

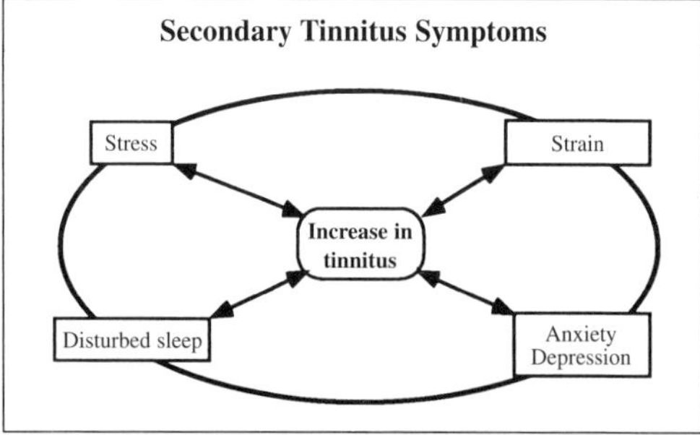

Fig. 1.4 Vicious circle of tinnitus, with supporting factors that lead to formation of secondary symptoms (from: Lenarz, 1990).

acoustic trauma which affects high frequencies, while roaring sounds point to hearing loss at lower frequency ranges (e.g. Ménière's disease).

Tinnitus may be unilateral, as in sudden deafness, or bilateral, as in chronic exposure to loud noise. Tinnitus is localized to the affected ear, as different forms of tinnitus usually do not have the same frequency and loudness characteristics on both sides and therefore can be differentiated. If these parameters are nearly identical bilaterally, the perception is that of roaring located between both ears. Noises in the head (cerebral tinnitus), in contrast, are always reported to be deep within the head. This argues against a peripheral cause of tinnitus in the middle or inner ear; rather, it indicates a cause in the central nervous system.

1.4 Etiology and pathophysiology

While objective ear noises are caused by an acoustic signal from pathological or muscular processes (Table 1.1), the pathophysiological mechanism of subjective ear noises remains unclear. Certain conclusions may be drawn from the type of hearing loss being experienced, from the medical history and other diagnostic data in a specific case. Theoretically, measurement of the electrophysiological processes in the region of the inner ear, the auditory nerve and the auditory path is possible through invasive procedures with electrodes introduced into these structures. However, the risk of further injury and the associated surgical procedures under anesthesia preclude this to a large extent. It is possible only through neurosurgical or otosurgical interventions required for other indications (Møller, 1984).

Contemporary brain research has clarified important details concerning the process of hearing (Zenner, 1986). Unfortunately, no valid animal experimental model of tinnitus exists yet. Specific injuries which lead to tinnitus in man can be produced in the auditory system. In animals, the invasive procedures noted above are possible, and the changes occurring with the injuries can be measured, but the correlation with human tinnitus is questionable because the animal cannot describe the subjective perceptions that result. This highlights the basic dilemma of tinnitus research. Research can depend on animal studies only to a limited extent because of the absence of subjective experiences, while objective findings on patients are difficult because invasive procedures must be limited. It is not surprising that for this reason and because of the complex and therefore incompletely understood physiology of hearing that only hypothetical pathophysiological models exist at this time to integrate basic research with clinical studies and experience.

Despite being hypothetical, pathophysiological models provide useful service in the development of points of departure for research, therapeutic measures, and clinical treatment (counseling, cognitive therapy), because they can serve as an explanation of the complicated process of hearing and its disturbances. Thus they can provide the patient with some understanding of the course of the disease (Feldmann, 1988). This chapter will proceed with a brief explanation of the basic research results of the anatomy and physiology of hearing, followed by a hypothesis relating to the pathogenesis of tinnitus with regard to its significance for diagnosis and treatment.

1.4.1 Anatomy and physiology of the auditory system

The auditory system includes:

—the outer ear, with the auricle (ear lobe) and the external auditory canal,
—the middle ear, with the eardrum (tympanic membrane), auditory ossicles (stapes, incus, malleus) and Eustachian tube,
—the internal ear (Fig. 1),
—the central auditory system, with auditory nerve, auditory path in the brain stem and diencephalon, and the auditory cortex in the region of the temporal lobe.

Numerous connections exist in the region of the central auditory system to other sensory organs, to the autonomic nervous system, to the motor system and to the limbic system. In addition to an *afferent auditory system*, which leads the converted acoustic information from the inner ear centrally (Fig. 1.2), the *efferent auditory system*, which runs to the inner ear and the auditory nerve, provides control for adapting hearing to the existing auditory situation (i.e. to differentiate between eavesdropping and hearing under noisy conditions).

While the external ear is responsible primarily for locating the source of sound and thus for directional hearing, the middle ear assumes the function of sound uptake via the eardrum. A transformation of the mechanically transferred sound waves follows at the base of the stapes, which is directly connected with the liquid-filled inner ear. Due to the mechanical leverage of the auditory ossicles, the sound stimulus is amplified by a factor of 10, i.e. 20dB. The tensor typani muscle of the malleus, and the stapedius muscle of the stapes (see Fig. 15.1) decrease excessive vibration and undesirable ringing via a reflex arch in the brain stem. The Eustachian tube provides the needed balance in pressure between the exterior and the middle ear by opening when swallowing (Fig. 1.1).

The *inner ear* is the actual organ of hearing, as it changes the acoustic signals into electric potentials which the central auditory system requires. This is accomplished by the hair cells, the sensory cells of hearing. The hair cells are situated on the basilar mem-

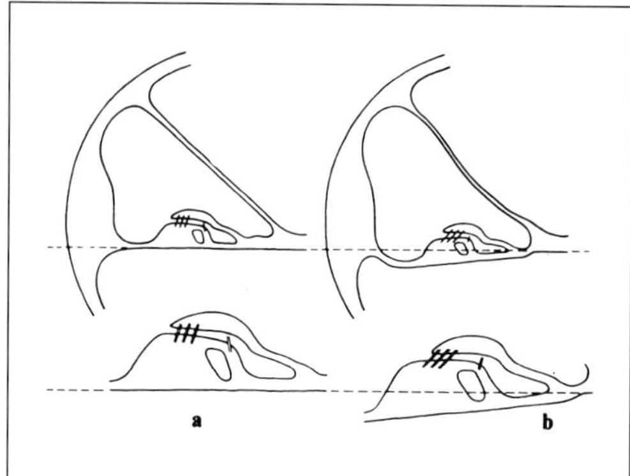

Fig. 1.5 Function of the organ of Corti: a = at rest; b = basilar membrane displaced. Displacement of the tectorial membrane leads to shearing forces acting on the hair cells (from Boenninghaus, 1990).

brane and are covered by the tectorial membrane at their upper ends, where the hair-like stereocilia are located (Fig. 1.5). The entire cochlea is filled with liquid. Connections to the middle ear are through an oval window in which the base of the stapes is free to swing, and a round window which is covered by an eleastic membrane and serves to balance pressure caused by the movement of the stapes. The afferent auditory nerve fibers run from the lower end of the inner hair cells in the direction of the brain stem. About

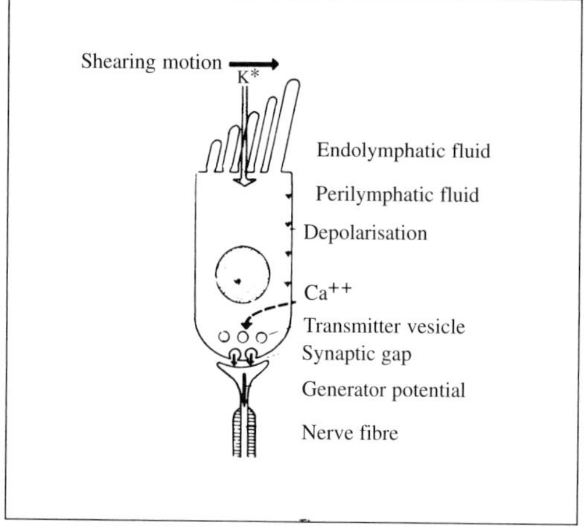

Fig. 1.7 Mode of function of the hair cells: The shearing motion of the hair cells, with deflection of the stereocilia, leads to opening of the ion channels with inflow of potassium-ions. The resulting receptor potential releases transmitters into the synaptic gap at the lower end of the cell, which build up a potential in the afferent auditory nerve fibres.

90% of the afferent fibers arise from the inner hair cells; only 10% from the external ones. The efferent auditory nerve fibers arise from the region of the olivary nucleus of the medulla oblongata and end predominantly at the external hair cells (Spöndlin, 1985).

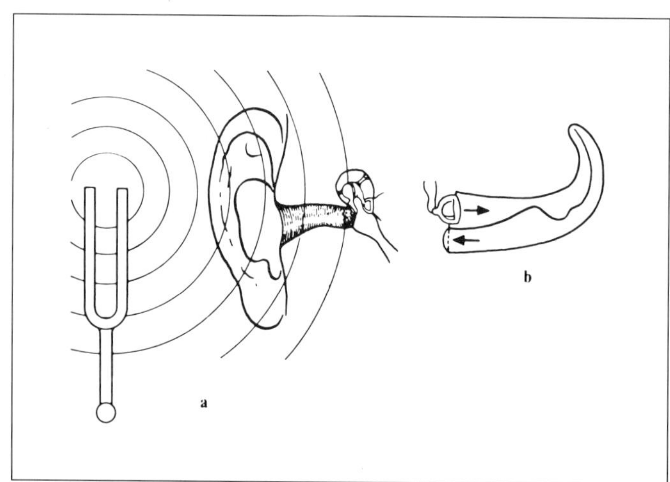

Fig. 1.6 Mode of function of the inner ear: vibrations of the eardrum elicited by sound waves are transferred to the liquid filled passages of the cochlea (scala vestibuli, scala tympani, cochlear duct via the ossicles. The waves thus elicited displace the basilar membrane. At higher frequencies, the maximum lies closer to the stapes, at lower frequencies closer to the tip of the cochlea.

The sound waves, traveling via the eardrum and the ossicles to the inner ear, set the basilar membrane in motion. Maximum displacement occurs at different points, depending on the frequency of the stimulus. Due to this frequency-location transformation, high frequencies are directed predominantly toward the base of the cochlea and lower frequencies toward the tip of the cochlea (Fig. 1.6). The displacement leads to a shearing movement against the tectorial membrane, which bends the stereocilia of the hair cells.

Inflow of potassium ions from the surrounding fluid leads to a build-up of a receptor potential, which then leads to a release of a transmitter substance (probably glutamate) for transfer of information to the auditory nerve fibers, where an electric potential develops (Fig. 1.7). This is conducted to the central auditory path where it is converted to conscious hearing in the auditory cortex of the temporal lobe.

While the internal hair cells bring about actual hearing, the external hair cells have an amplifying effect through active

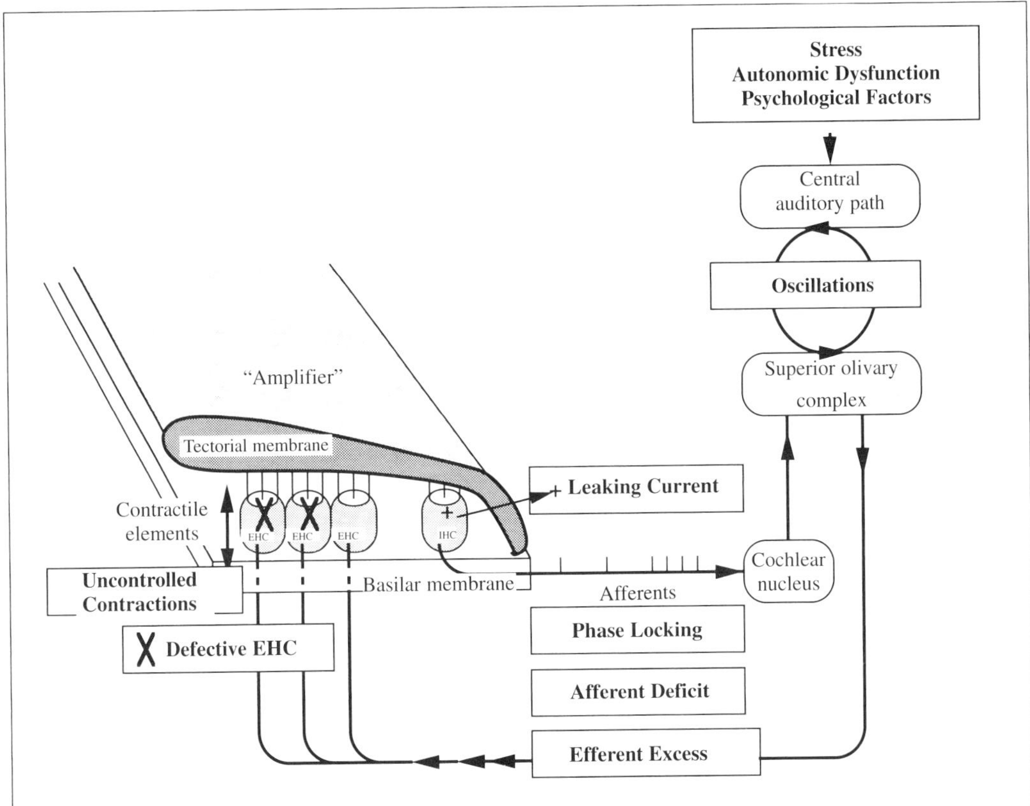

Fig. 1.8 Schematic representation of the cochlea and its central regulation. EHC = external hair cells; IHC = internal hair cells; 1 = single potentials of the auditory nerves. Pathophysiological processes are assumed in cochlear tinnitus.
When EHC are injured, loss of active amplification occurs and thus an afferent deficit, that should be balanced by efferent overstimulation. The increased activity of the EHC stimulates the IHC and thus elicits tinnitus, i.e., constantly open ion channels of the IHC lead to current leaks with permanent release of transmitters (from Lenarz, 1992).

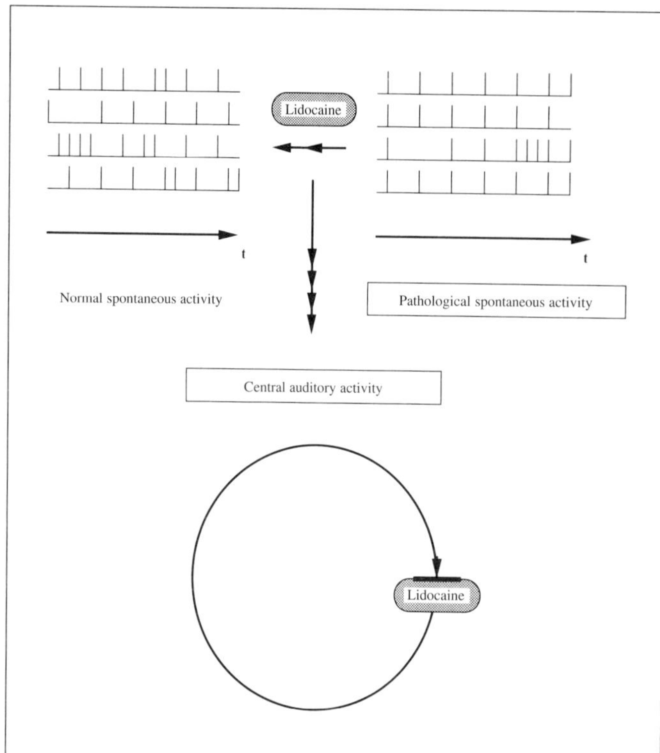

Fig. 1.9 Model of neural tinnitus. Represented are afferent nerve fibers at rest in the form of single action potentials (| |) and in injured condition with loss of coincidendal electrical activity over time. The abnormal rhythm of one or more acoustic nerve fibers (phase locking) without acoustic stimulus is misinterpreted as auditory information by the central auditory path. The abnormal neural activity manifests itself centrally in the form of self-produced circular stimuli. Lidocaine normalizes both forms of pathological activity (from Lenarz, 1989).

contraction. When the sound stimulus is weak, they can actively amplify the passive movement of the basilar membrane; when the stimulus is very strong, they can decrease it (Fig. 1.8). This increases sensitivity significantly in the first instance, and avoids injury from overstimulation in the second. Thus, displacements of the size of the diameter of a hydrogen atom can be recognized (Zenner, 1986). The function of the external hair cells is modified by the efferent auditory path system and adapted to the existing hearing conditions. This also explains effects caused by the autonomic nervous system, other sensory systems and the limbic system.

The electric potentials of the auditory nerve fibers and the neurons in the central auditory path codify the acoustic stimulus sequentially. For this reason, even at rest, i.e., in the absence of an acoustic stimulus, the constantly present spontaneous discharges are modified. This is a stochastic process. Under the influence of a sound stimulus on the hair cells and by release of the transmitter, the latter is transformed into electric potentials at regular periodic intervals (Fig. 1.9).

1.4.2 Pathophysiological objective ear sounds

Objective ear noise is caused by sound-producing events in the petrosal bone or its surroundings. In the region of the middle ear, the cause is spasm or spontaneous single contractions of the tensor tympani or stapedius muscles. Myoclonus of the palatal (otopharyngeal) musculature leads to sudden clicking movements of the Eustacian tube. Causes of extrapyramidal-motor disturbance include encephalitis or drug abuse. Streaming sounds arise from blood vessel malformations, glomus tumors, arteriosclerotic alterations of the carotid or vertebral arteries, heart valve malformations and anaemia, and have a predominantly hissing character. Ear sounds, synchronous with breathing, occur when the Eustachian tube gapes, thus transferring the sounds of breathing directly into the middle ear.

1.4.3 Pathophysiology of subjective ear sounds

Usually damage to the hair cells exists; this, together with the tinnitus, causes hearing loss. As the external hair cells, because of their active contractions, consume more oxygen than the internal hair cells, they are much more sensitive to damage such as noise, ototoxic drugs, effects of age and trauma. The damaged external hair cells lose their function and may show uncontrolled contractions that stimulate the internal hair cells (Fig. 1.8). Such stimulation elicits nerve potentials that are conducted to the brain and are interpreted there as sounds. Injury to the internal hair cells also leads to hearing loss. The ion channels, otherwise open only when the stereocilia are deformed, probably remain open permanently. The resulting leaks release transmitters constantly and thus elicit potentials continuously. In turn, these are guided to the auditory canal and are interpreted there as noise (Feldmann, 1988).

In addition to such damage to the hair cells, the auditory nerve fibers may be damaged themselves, e.g., by tumors (acoustic neurinoma), inflammation (neuritis), and multiple sclerosis. The pathophysiological result is identical, in that stochastic spontaneous activity is changed to interval/time-oriented activity. Each such coordinated sequence of potentials is interpreted in the central auditory path as a situation differing from the base-line electric potential and therefore as an acoustic signal (Fig. 1.9) (Evans & Norerwe, 1982; Moller, 1984; Salvi & Ahroon, 1983).

In the central auditory path, hair cell and auditory nerve damage leads to oscillating electrical stimuli. This repetitive, self-inducing electrical activity is distributed over broad regions of the auditory system and forms a self-contained vicious circle (Fig. 1.9). This also explains why ear noises continue to exist even after destruction of the inner ear or dissection of the 8th nerve (Lenarz, 1990).

1.5 Diagnosis

The goal of the diagnostic process in tinnitus cannot be verification of the supposed mechanism in the particular case, or to indicate the appropriate causal therapy, because of the lack of knowledge of the etiology of the condition. Rather the purpose is to establish a differential diagnosis of possible causes and the tinnitus-exacerbating factors that may serve as a starting point for therapy. This requires individually oriented diagnosis (Table 1.3), from the point of view of the otolaryngologist.

1.5.1 Tinnitus History

The specific tinnitus history is directed at establishing the character of the tinnitus, its course over time, and its relation to loss of hearing. Of importance are factors that increase or diminish the symptoms, particularly masking effects from environmental sounds. From the description of the course of the tinnitus, of the degree of stress, and the effects of tinnitus on lifestyle (*i.e. whether compensated or decompensated tinnitus exists*) important guidelines can be obtained concerning the need for therapeutic efforts. In the case of a decompensated tinnitus the tinnitus has a decisive effect on the quality of life and is

Table 1.3 Step by step diagnosis of tinnitus aurium

I	Specific tinnitus history with determination of the following: Character, duration and loudness of the tinnitus Relationship to hearing disturbance Degree of stress Effect on lifestyle (concentration, performance, sleep) Possible or likely causes Supporting factors, masking by ambient noise
II	Otorhinolaryngological examination Inspection Nasopharyngoscopy of the palatal musculature Periauricular ausculation of the vessels of the neck and ear
III	Audiometric and electrophysiological diagnosis Tone audiometry BERA Additional tests not described here (e.g. impedance audiometry)
IV	Determination of tinnitus parameters Tinnitus matching (frequency, intensity) Tinnitus masking (matching, minimal masking level, residual inhibition) Subjective loudness scaling (visual analog scale)
V	Supplemental diagnostic measures (CAT scan, NMR, angiography) Neurological status including Doppler sonography of the arteries of the neck Medical status (heart/circulation, metabolism, kidney function, hemato-rheology) Neck/cervical spine diagnosis (X-rays, palpation, orthopedics) Orthodontic status (myoarthropathy of the temporomandibular joint) Psychosomatic and psychiatric exploration Allergy screening

perceived as unbearable. A part of the patient's history can be documented on a questionnaire.

1.5.2 Otorhinolaryngological examination

The purpose of the otorhinolaryngological examination is to determine the possible presence of any existing disease within the hearing system. This leads to a differential diagnosis of objective and subjective ear noises. The diagnostic procedure includes microscopy of the eardrum, test of function of the Eustacian tube, endoscopy of the nasopharynx and ausculation of the vessels of the neck and the ear region. This may establish the existence of perforations of the eardrum, changes in the ossicles and in the auditory path, and may indicate that operative measures in the form of a tympanoplasty are necessary. If objective ear sounds are found, further appropriate diagnostic measures are performed. Vascular ear sounds are diagnosed by means of ausculation, Doppler sonography and angiography of the vessels, or tympanometry, which, in the case of a glomus tumor shows fluctuations synchronous with the pulse. Myoclonus can be verified endoscopically or electromyographically. Signs of middle ear muscle disturbances can be verified only by tympanotomy, i.e., opening a fold of the eardrum to expose the middle ear cavity. If such muscle contractions are then visible, the muscles inserted at the ossicles are dissected.

1.5.3 Hearing tests

As tinnitus is usually caused by an injury of the hearing system and coincides with a disturbance of hearing, the greatest significance of audiometric diagnosis lies in the establishment and differentiation of hearing loss.

Two fundamental types of impaired hearing are differentiated.

In *conduction hearing loss*, a disturbance exists in sound transfer to the inner ear, for example, an eardrum perforation, or defects of the ossicles. The function of the inner ear remains undisturbed.

In *sound perception hearing loss*, sound transmission to the inner ear is intact but transformation into electrical impulses in the inner ear, conduction along the auditory nerve or conversion in the central auditory path is disturbed.

Both forms can be verified with a sound-threshold audiogram (Fig. 1.10). Sinus tones of various frequencies at (half) octave intervals between 125 and 10,000 Hz are emitted for each ear separately through earphones with increasing intensity until the subject hears the sound. Then the sound intensity is decreased until the subject perceives the sound no longer. In addition, a bone conduction test is performed for both ears using the same method. In this test, one takes advantage of the fact that the head of an oscillating body, e.g., a tuning fork, when placed against the cranial bone, causes the latter to oscillate. These oscillations are perceived directly by the inner ear, bypassing the middle ear.

Audiometers are calibrated so that the sound thresholds for air conduction and bone conduction are superimposed for normal hearing. If sound conduction hearing loss exists, the air conduction hearing threshold is weaker, as the sound is not transported optimally to the inner ear. Greater sound intensities are required to reach sound perception. In sound perception hearing loss with reduced inner ear efficiency, sound transport is undisturbed, the thresholds for both air and bone conduction are superimposed, but both are higher than in the normal ear because greater sound intensity is required to elicit a response.

As the disturbance in sound perception hearing loss may be located in the inner ear, the auditory nerve or in the central auditory path, further differentiation into cochlear, retrocochlear and central hearing loss is required. An important procedure here is the measurement of early acoustically evoked potentials by Brainstem Electronic Response Audiometry (BERA). Retrocochlear and central injuries become evident early through latency delay and loss of potentials. These provide indications for use of x-ray techniques, e.g., computer-assisted tomography and nuclear-spin tomography. The otorhinolaryngologist's role is important because he may be able to identify serious disease, e.g., *acoustic neurinoma*, early, and initiate the required surgical therapy. One can assume "idiopathic" tinnitus and begin additional diagnostic tests and treatment only after such "symptomatic" forms of ear noises have been excluded.

1.5.4 Measurement of the parameters of tinnitus

Tinnitus analysis must differentiate between comparative measurements of tinnitus intensity and subjective loudness scales. The results of both methods correlate (Fig. 1.11). Thus, one frequently observes that the masking level in the region of the principal tinnitus frequency is only a few decibels above the hearing threshold in this region, while the

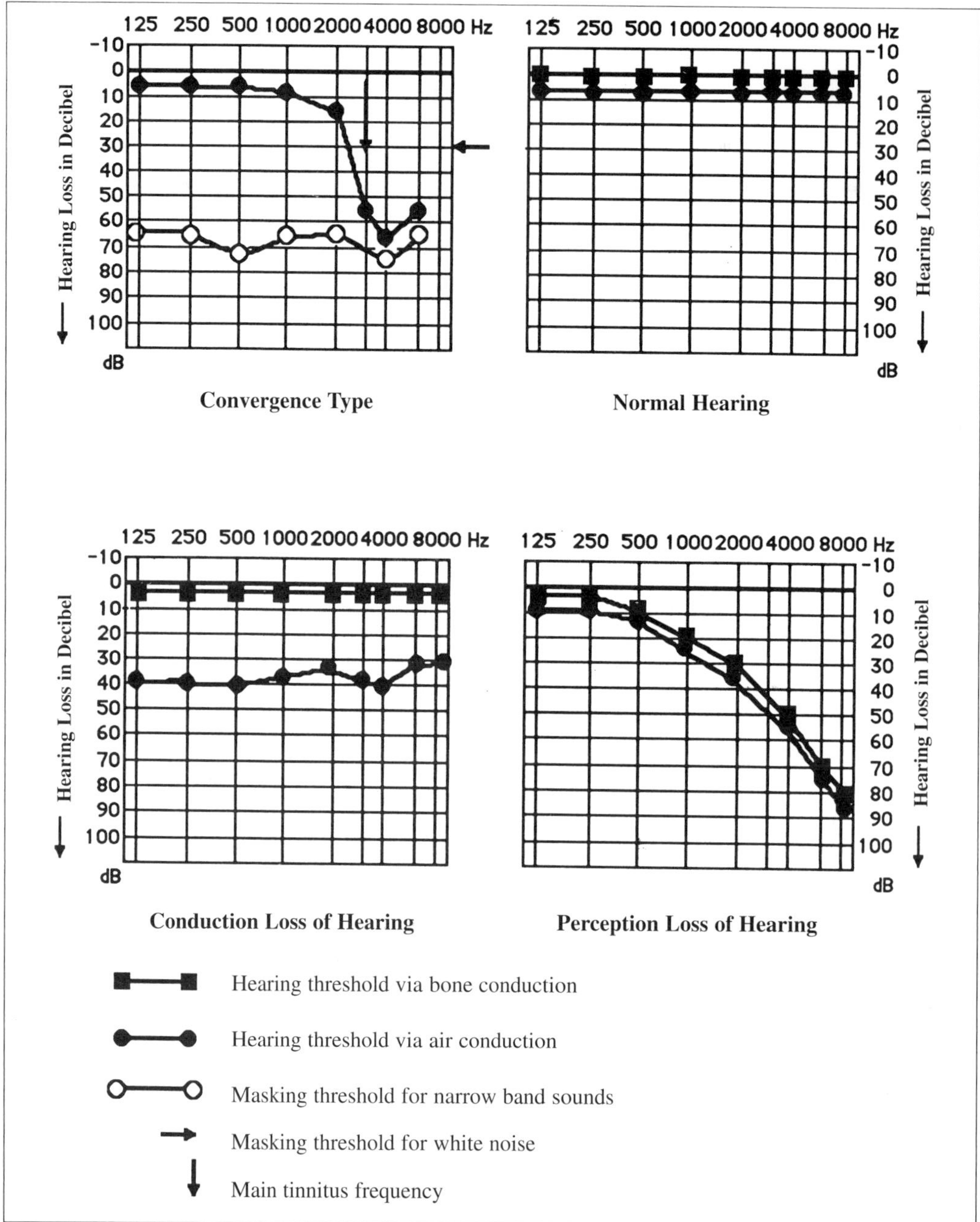

Fig. 1.10 Tone audiogram depicting an ear with normal hearing (upper right), an ear with conduction loss of hearing (lower left), and an ear with sound perception loss of hearing (lower right). Results of tinnitus matching (determination of frequency and intensity of tinnitus) and the masking curve are shown as an example of an inner ear hearing loss with a whistling tinnitus following acoustic trauma (upper left). The bone conduction threshold, which is identical to the air conduction threshold, is not shown here.

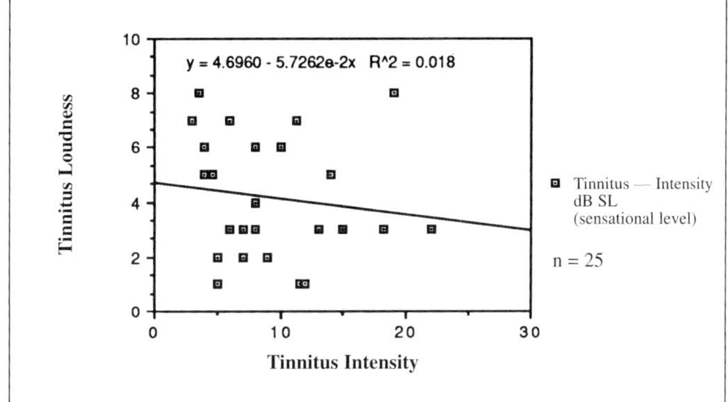

Fig. 1.11 Relationship between psychometrically measured subjective tinnitus loudness and psychoacoustically measured tinnitus intensity among 25 patients. The correlation coefficient is -0.134, therefore no correlation.

subjective loudness of the tinnitus is described as unbearably strong. This shows to what extent tinnitus is subject to subjective experience. Loudness of tinnitus is best documented on visual analog scales to record the course and effects of therapy. Visual analog scales (see Chapters 7 and 10) or rating scales with standard acoustic situations of increasing loudness (rustle of leaves, normal speech, street noise, jet-engines) are useful for psychometric measurements as they are better suited for determining the degree of subjective stress than psychoacoustic comparative measurements (see tinnitus loudness/tinnitus loudness scales in the glossary).

Comparative psychoacoustic scales provide better information than analog scales about the relation between subjectively experienced loudness and an underlying hearing loss. They also form the basis of the masking characteristics of the tinnitus and thus for masking therapy. These tests can all be performed with a normal audiometer. *Tinnitus matching* includes the determination of the principal frequency and intensity of the tinnitus by means of comparative sinus tones, narrow band sound and white noise. *Tinnitus masking* relates to possible masking characteristics of the individual tinnitus and serves as the essential prerequisite for the fitting of a tinnitus masker. By offering sinus tones or narrow band noise of adjacent frequencies to the same ear or, less frequently, to the contralateral ear, tinnitus sounds can often be masked with sounds just above the sound threshold, i.e., tinnitus is no longer perceived in the presence of an external acoustic signal. When the external acoustic signal is removed, the tinnitus returns. This "maskability" differentiates the tinnitus fundamentally from an external acoustic signal. In addition to the minimal masking sound intensity of white noise, the frequency-dependent masking sound intensity of sinus tones and narrow band noise are determined in the audiogram, as described by Feldmann (1971) (Fig. 1.10). Often the audiogram curve of the hearing threshold and the tinnitus masking converge at the principal tinnitus-frequency, which is also often located at the point of maximum hearing loss.

The convergence character is related to the changed perception of loudness in patients with inner ear hearing loss. These patients have a distinct sensitivity to noise, which may be explained by the fact that low intensity sounds are not registered at all initially. With increasing intensity, they become audible when they exceed the hearing threshold, become disproportionately loud as the sound intensity increases, and are perceived as unpleasantly loud or even painful at lower sound intensities (unlike persons with normal hearing). This limitation of hearing dynamics is defined as *recruitment* and is caused by loss of function of external hair cells which no longer amplify weak sound stimuli and cannot decrease loud ones (*see section 1.4* and addendum). The degree of convergence permits conclusions about the importance of recruitment and its significance for the subjective loudness of tinnitus. Thus it is understandable that in the region of maximum hearing loss, only comparatively low intensity sounds are necessary to mask tinnitus. The more one proceeds away from the maximum hearing loss toward normal hearing, the greater becomes the masking intensity. The relation of the masking level at maximum hearing loss and that at normal hearing correlates well with the subjectively experienced tinnitus. However, this holds true only for tonal ear sounds, and much less for those of a roaring character.

Residual inhibition is particularly important for the success of masking therapy (see section 6). After exposure to a masking tone or noise for the duration of one minute, the time until recurrence of the original intensity of the tinnitus is registered. The longer the interval the better are the chances for a masking therapy.

1.5.5 Additional diagnostic procedures

The tinnitus-exacerbating factors described above must be supplemented and verified by special examinations and tests according to the needs of the individual and the standards of otolaryngology and audiology. It is not intended to subject the patient to all possible tests. Rather, it is the task of the otolaryngologist to obtain specific consultations from other specialties so as to gain a comprehensive picture, particularly in chronic forms of tinnitus. Radiological diagnostic techniques, a thorough differential diagnosis of cardiac and circulatory as well as metabolic diseases, an orthopedic examination as well as an examination according to the diagnostic criteria of manual therapy of the cervical spine for degenerative diseases and functional blockage (*Biesinger*, 1989) and an orthodontic examination to exclude temporomandibular joint myoarthropathy, have to be considered. It is of no use to the patient to claim that the cervical spine or the dental status is the main cause in the absence of qualified diagnostic procedures to verify and substantiate the claim. Only in this way can therapeutic approaches to alleviate what is usually only an exacerbating – but not causal – factor (see Fig. 7.7 and Chapters 15 and 16). Psychosomatic or psychiatric examinations may be required (see Chapter 4) which lead to valuable insights for behavioral therapy or psychotherapy.

1.6 Treatment of tinnitus from the otolharyngological point of view

1.6.1 General therapeutic guidelines (Table 1.4)

Classification is required between compensated tinnitus, which is accepted by a patient whose quality of life is not significantly restricted, and decompensated tinnitus, in which secondary disease sequelae such as sleeping disorders or psychoneurotic alterations have special significance.

As the pathophysiology of most forms of tinnitus remains unknown, no causal or rational treatment is available. Therefore, treatment must be limited to symptomatic measures, particularly in chronic tinnitus, except in the much less frequent instances of objective ear sounds. As tinnitus is an otological symptom which may signal serious diseases such as acoustic neurinoma, careful diagnosis is indicated in all instances. Emphasis is given to explaining the possible causes and nature of tinnitus to the patient

Table 1.4 Therapeutic principles in tinnitus

1 Determination and elimination of possible causes
2 Counseling
3 Attempts at therapy with rational treatment methods
  a) Medication: calcium antagonists, rheologic agents
     anti-arrhythmic agents, anticonvulsive agents
     glutamate
     psychopharmaceuticals
  b) masker/hearing aid
  c) electrostimulation: iontophoresis
     transtympanic
     cochlea implant
4 Psychotherapy
  a) relaxation therapy (autogenic training, biofeedback, etc.)
  b) cognitive therapy (What significance does tinnitus have in my life?)
  c) behavioral therapy (How do I deal with my tinnitus?)
5 Self-help groups, self-help books

(counseling). In this way, the frequency expressed fears of brain tumor or a cerebrovascular accident can be reduced and the prerequisites for cognitive therapy (Hallum, 1987) can be established. The patient can cope with the symptom and, in most instances, learns to live with his tinnitus, i.e., to integrate the tinnitus into his life and to eliminate the secondary symptoms (Goebel et al., 1991). The purpose of such counseling is to alter decompensated tinnitus into compensated tinnitus. The patient should be instructed in preventive measures, e.g., avoidance of exposure to excessive noise, avoidance of stressful situations, and in the significance of a regular, balanced lifestyle. In general, only cases of chronic decompensated tinnitus require additional treatment. Acute tinnitus and objective ear sounds provide exceptions to this general rule.

1.6.2 Treatment of objective ear sounds

The therapeutic principle is the elimination of the cause of the sound source within the body. Frequently, objective ear sounds can be approached through surgical treatment of the underlying cause. This is particularly true of diseases of the blood vessels. Thus, partially blocked vessels must be cleared and malformed vessels must be eliminated as far as possible. For spasms of the internal muscles of the middle ear, the tendons are dissected at their insertion of the ossicles after tympanotomy. In palatal myoclonus, treatment with the anticonvulsant carbamazepine or the anti-parkinson drug biperidene may be successful. Because of the complex etiology, such attempts should always be made in cooperation with a neurologist.

1.6.3 Treatment of subjective ear sounds

The best treatment of tinnitus would be the elimination of the underlying functional disturbance in the hearing system, with normalization, for example, of hair cell function. This also would eliminate loss of hearing. This goal frequently can be reached in acute tinnitus. A good example for this type of treatment is the treatment of circulatory disturbances, as is the case with sensorineural hearing loss in sudden deafness. In this situation, it may be assumed that the functional disturbance of the hair cells is not yet morphologically established and is thus reversible. In all other instances, the lack of knowledge of specific pathophysiological mechanisms does not allow causal treatment directed specifically at the faulty electrical activity of the hair cells, the auditory nerve, or the central hearing path. Only a few of the numerous therapeutic suggestions fulfil the requirements of rational clinical therapy tested in clinical studies for clinical efficacy. For this reason, the entire programme is characterized by trial and error and by polypharmacy. Three main focuses have been developed: drug therapy, electrostimulation and masking therapy.

1.6.3.1 Drug therapy (Table 1.5)

Every acute development of tinnitus can be understood as the equivalent of sudden deafness. If one assumes a disturbance in circulation, treatment to improving circulation is appropriate (Boenninghaus, 1988). Experience shows that complete elimination of tinnitus can be achieved in approximately 50% of patients. With increasing duration of the tinnitus, chances for success diminish, as the initially reversible functional disturbance becomes morphologically fixed, which can be recognized by the absence of hair cell function.

Table 1.5 Pharmacotherapy of tinnitus

1. Acute tinnitus (duration less than 3 months) rheological therapy with plasma expanders and vasodilators e.g. poly (0-2-ethyl) starch (mean molecular size 200,000) 10% 500ml + 400 mg naftidrofuryl-hydrogenoxalate as infusion daily for 10 days.

2. Chronic tinnitus (duration more than 3 months) substances as listed according to clinical experience, frequency of employment as well as severity of side-effects.

2.1 Vasodilators p.o.
e.g. 3 × 100 mg naftidrofuryl hydrogenoxalate daily
3 × 16 mg betahistine (n-methyl-2-12-pyridyl) ethylamine) daily

2.2 Calciumantagonists
e.g. 2-3 × 5 mg flunarizine (1-Cinnamyl-4-(4,41-difluorbenzhydryl) piperazine) daily
4 × 30 mg nimodipine daily

2.3 Antiarrythmic agents (after positive xylocaine test – 100 mg i.v.)
e.g. 3-4 × 400 mg tocainide-HCL daily

2.4 Anticonvulsive agents
e.g. 3 × 400 mg carbamazepine daily

2.5 Infusion therapy with glutamine-acid-diethyl-ester and glutamate (only chemically pure substances exist, which influence transmitter metabolism and should only be used by specialized clinics).

2.6 Antidepressants, neuroleptics (major tranquilizers)
e.g. amitriptyline
doxepine
sulpiride

Fundamentally different conditions exist in chronic tinnitus (*duration greater than 3 months*), for which a curable circulatory disturbance may no longer be assumed. Vasodilators/anticoagulants are no longer promising, nor sensible. Risk factors for the development of arteriosclerosis (high blood pressure, diabetis mellitus, hyperlipidemia, hyperuricemia) should, however, be treated in all instances. Nicotine and alcohol abuse should be eliminated.

Assuming irreversible damage of the inner ear or, less frequently, to the auditory nerve treatment must be directed at the suppression of pathological electrical discharges within the auditory system (Goodey 1987, 1988). Here, drugs can affect the stimulation of neuronal structures. As certain processes within the hair cells are calcium dependent, calcium antagonists such as flunarizine or nimodipine may be effective. For the auditory nerve and the central auditory path, anti-arrhythmic agents (Lenarz 1987, 1989) of the lidocaine type, tocainamide (3 × 400 mg p.o.) or anticonvulsants such as carbamazepine are effective in that they normalize increased spontaneous activity and interrupt circular stimuli (Fig. 1.9) (Lenarz, 1987). Glutamate, a transmitter-like substance, acts in the region of the sensorineural synapse between hair cell and afferent auditory nerve fiber. Infusion therapy has led to limited success, but remains in the experimental stage (Ehrenberger & Brix, 1983). Antidepressants such as amitryptiline may provide relief through modulation of the efferent auditory system. Non-specific effects, such as general improvement in mood or a sedating effect, should be noted with these substances.

The success rate of drug therapy, defined as a reduction of at least 25% in loudness vs. placebo, is about 15-20%. Notable in this context is the relatively high rate of side effects of some substances; for that reason, strict indications should be followed and close cooperation with a neurologist or cardiologist is required.

1.6.3.2 Electrostimulation

The excitation threshold can be altered by an externally applied current. Anodic current (+ polarization) in direct current leads to hyperpolarization and thus to reduced excitability of the afferent auditory nerve fibres; cathodic current (– polarization) has the opposite effect (Aran & Cazals, 1981). Electrostimulation attempts to take advantage of this effect. For experimental purposes the electrode is pierced through the eardrum and placed directly on the bone in the inner ear. In routine practice, stimulation proceeds transcutaneously via a surface electrode placed behind the ear or in the external meatus via a conductive liquid instilled into the meatus (iontophoresis). Direct or alternating currents can be used for excitation, with frequencies varying between 50 Hz and several kHz. Reduction in tinnitus loudness, usually temporary, can be achieved in approximately 10% of patients without permanent effects even after repeated exposure. Potential side effects in the form of additional injury to the inner ear should be considered, particularly with a high current and continuous stimulatin (von Wedel et al. 1989, Zeuner et al. 1989). In conclusion, electrostimulation has a minor role at present.

1.6.3.3 Hearing-aid

When hearing loss is not amenable to surgery which is most successful in the case of sound conduction hearing loss, and if treatment aimed at improving circulation fails (as in chronic inner ear hearing loss), fitting a hearing aid is the final option. A hearing aid should be prescribed as soon as possible, even in the case of unilateral injury, as amplification of external sounds tends to mask tinnitus more successfully (v. Wedel, 1987). More than 30% of patients benefit from such devices, even over long observation periods (v. Wedel et al., 1989). Fitting must be done by an acoustic technician. This treatment is especially successful in patients with a tinnitus that can be masked (see section 1.5.4).

A tinnitus masking device can be fitted experimentally when hearing loss is not present. These devices, which resemble a hearing aid, are battery operated and take advantage of a masking effect by emitting an artificially produced noise into the auditory canal. They do not amplify external sound, as is the case with a normal hearing aid. These measures are indicated in decompensated, maskable tinnitus. Tonal forms of tinnitus of high frequency with accompanying inner ear hearing loss are best suited to masking measures, as the masking tone interferes least in such cases with hearing ability. The tinnitus becomes bearable in approximately 15% of these patients. Because of the similarity between hearing aids and masking devices and the monotony of the emitted sound, its acceptance is limited. Improvement in compliance can be anticipated from devices with variable masking sounds as they are more adaptable to the individual patient. Best results are obtained with a combination of masking and behavioral therapy (= retraining therapy). An attempt to use a "Walkman" (cassette tape recorder) is sensible, as such a device permits individual adjustment to music perceived as pleasant or specifically altered music.

1.6.3.4 Other forms of therapy

Destructive surgical procedures such as labyrinthectomy or neurectomy of the auditory nerve usually lead only to temporary diminuation of tinnitus as they are not able to affect the circulatory stimuli and the oscillations in the region of the central auditory path. Furthermore, new sites of injury arise in the region of the auditory nerve leading to a deterioration of the tinnitus. Non-ablative procedures such as saccotomia that are aimed only at improving hearing can lead to a permanent reduction of tinnitus. In deaf patients, implantation of a cochlear implant, i.e., an electronic stimulatory device which replaces the non-functioning inner ear, can lead to tinnitus suppression. The opposite effect is also possible, but rare.

In the case of demonstrated functional disturbances, orthopedic, manipulation and massage therapy of the cervical spine (see Chapter 16), and orthodontic therapy for myofunctional disturbance of the temporomandibular joint may be significant, and should be attempted. These measures belong in the hands of qualified experts. Neural therapy and acupuncture may also be sensible.

1.7 Limitations of medical treatment and alternative treatment

Very frequently, the otolaryngologist selected by the patient simply must admit defeat when faced with the problem of tinnitus. Despite all the diagnostic and therapeutic measures, the situation has not improved for the patient. Rather, it has deteriorated as a result of the increased attention to the tinnitus and associated conditions. What can the physician do in this situation? How can he cope with a situation that demonstrates his helplessness and may be experienced as evidence of his incompetence and therefore perhaps as a personal insult?

He may discharge the patient conscious of the fact that no true physical condition exists and that therefore there is no need for further treatment. With the advice that the patient should learn to live with his tinnitus, the case is closed. Or he can refer the patient to a tinnitus expert. The author of this chapter is considered a tinnitus expert by his colleagues and is occasionally taken advantage of for this reason. The expert accepts the time-consuming patient who usually asks many questions, and knows how to manage such patients who do not fit into the accepted medical scheme of things. The truth is that the author has dealt intensively with the medical aspects of tinnitus, but because of his specialized training in otology and audiology, he cannot cover all aspects of tinnitus as a psychosomatic disease. He relies on other experts from case to case, e.g., a psychotherapist or a psychiatrist. This step is not taken lightly; it must be determined in each instance which patients actually require this additional help, due to the patients' anxiety in response to being classified as psychiatric cases.

This fragmented description must suffice to describe how easily patient careers can be initiated or encouraged by insufficient guidance. It also demonstrates how easily a patient can feel lost, and left alone. In his despair, because his tinnitus persists, the patient turns to anyone who promises help; persons whose competence and intentions he is unable to judge. The patient falls prey to detrimental polypharmacy and inefficient guidance.

Behavioral therapy and psychotherapy may be used to reduce the secondary symptoms of tinnitus and thus to guide the overdominating symptoms to a bearable level that permits the patient to live with "his" tinnitus. This is described extensively in the main part of this book. Numerous other therapeutic measures are not mentioned in this chapter, as there has been no evidence of their effectiveness in clinically controlled studies, or they are beyond the limits set by otorhinolaryngology. This chapter however does not make any implications on the effectiveness of these therapeutic measures in any particular case.

1.8 References

Aran, J. M., Y. Cazals (1891): Electrical suppression of tinnitus. In: *Evered D., G. Lawrenson* (Ed.): Tinnitus. Ciba Foundation 85, Pitman London S.217-231.

Biesinger, E. (1989): Funktionelle Störungen der Halswirbelsäule in ihrer Bedeutung für die Hals-Nasen-Ohrenheilkunde. In: *H. Ganz, W. Schätzle* (Ed.): HNO-Praxis Heute Bd 9. Springer, Berlin, S. 129-147.

Boenninghaus, H.-G. (1988): Der idiopathische Hörsturz. Dt. Ärztebl. 85: 2215-2217.

Boenninghaus, H.-G. (1990): Hals-Hasen-Ohren-Heilkund für Medizinstudenten. Springer, Berlin – Heidelberg – New York, 8. Auflage).

Coles, R. R. A. (1984): Epidemiology of tinnitus: prevalence. *J. Laryng* Otol Suppl. 9:7.

Ehrenberger, K., R. Brix (1983): Glutamic acid and glutamic acid diethylester in tinnitus treatment. Acta Otolaryngol. 95: 599-605.

Evans, E. F., T. A. Borerwe (1982): Ototoxic effects of salicylates on the responses of single cochlear nerve fibers and on cochlear potentials. Brit J. Audiol 16: 101-108.

Feldmann, H. (1971): Homolateral and contralateral masking of tinnitus by noise-bands and by pure tones. Audiology 10: 138-144.

Feldmann, H. (1988): Pathophysiology of tinnitus. In: *M. Kitahara* (Ed.): Tinnitus. Pathophysiology and management. Igaku-Shoin, Tokyo – New York S. 7-35.

Goebel, G., W. Keeser, M. Fichter, W. Rief (1901): Neue Aspekte des komplexen chronischen Tinnitus. Die verlorene Stille: Auswirkungen und psychotherapeutische Möglichkeiten beim komplexen chronischen Tinnitus. Psychother, med. Psychol. 41: 123-133.

Goodey, R. J. (1987): Drug therapy in tinnitus. In: *J. W. Hazell* (Ed.): Tinnitus. Churchill Livingstone, Edinburgh S. 176-194.

Goodey, R. J. (1988): Drugs in the treatment of tinnitus. In: *M. Kitahara* (Ed.): Tinnitus. Pathophysiology and management. Igaku-Shoin, Tokyo – New York, S.64-73.

Hallam, R. S. (1987): Psychological approaches to the evaluation and management of tinnitus distress. In: *J. W. Hazell* (Ed.): Tinnitus. Churchill Livingstone, Edinburgh, S. 131-143.

Lenarz, T. (1987): Medikamentöse Beeinflussung der Hörbahn. Klinische und tierexperimentelle Untersuchung mit besonderer Berücksichtigung der Tinnitus-Therapie. Habil.-Schrift. Heidelberg.

Lenarz, T. (1989): Medikamentöse Tinnitus-Therapie. Thieme, Stuttgart.

Lenarz, T. (1990): Tinnitus: Pathophysiologie, Diagnostik und Therapie. In: *H. Ganz, W. Schätzle* (Ed.): HNO Praxis Heute, Bd. 10. Springer, Berlin - Heidelberg - New York S.1-20.

Lenarz, T. (1992): Medikamentöse Therapie. In: *H. Feldmann* (Ed.): Tinnitus. Thieme, Stuttgart - New York, S. 101-111.

Møller, A. R. (1984) Pathophysiology of tinnitus. Ann. Otol. Rhinol. Laryngol. 93: 39-44.

Salvi, R.J., W. A. Ahroon (1983): Tinnitus and Neural Activity. J. Speech Hear Res. 26: 629-632.

Spoendlin, H. (1985): Anatomy of cochlear innervation. Am. J. Otolaryngol 6: 453.

von Wedel, H. (1987): A longitudinal study in tinnitus-therapy with tinnitus-maskers and hearing aids. In: *H. Feldmann* (Ed.): Proceedings IIIrd Int. Tinnitus Seminar. Harsch, Karlsruhe, 257-260.

von Wedel, H., U. Strahlmann, P. Zorowka (1989): Effektivität verschiedener nicht medikamentöser Therapiemaßnahmen bei Tinnitus. Eine Langzeitstudie Laryngo-Rhino-Otol 68: 259.

Zenner, H. P. (1986): Aktive Bewegungen von Haarzellen. Ein neuer Mechanismus beim Hörvorgang. HNO 34: 133-138.

Zeuner, H. A., T. Lenarz, H. E. Trost (1989): Wirkungsweise und Stellenwert der Lidocain-Iontophorese bei Tinnitus aurium. Audiol. Akustik 3: 84-95.

Addendum

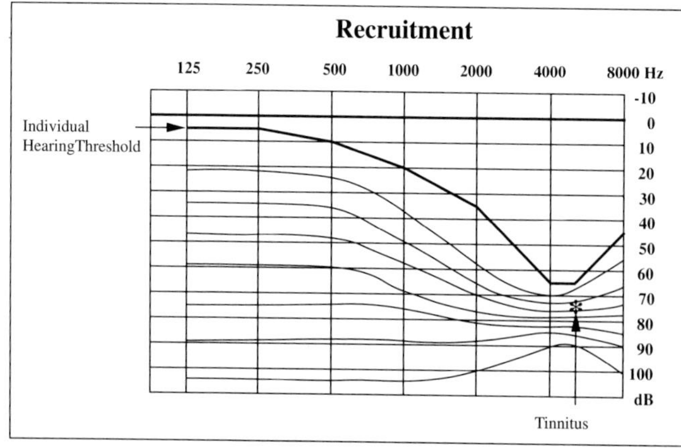

Depiction of loudness perception in the case of inner ear damage, e.g., following acoustic trauma. In the region of the damage, the perceived loudness curves converge (SISI test). This is described as positive recruitment, corresponding to increased noise sensitivity in this region.
In the tone audiogram: reduction of the hearing threshold of 65 dB at 4000 to 6000 Hz; tinnitus intensity 75 dB HL and 10 dB SL at approximately 6000 Hz.

Chapter 2

The incidence of tinnitus and its effects

Berit Scott and Per Lindberg

2.1 Summary

Tinnitus is a widespread phenomenon present in all age groups, and is a considerable impairment for 1–5% of affected patients. In the first part of this chapter, data from available epidemiological studies will be presented. In addition, various psychological methods of examination are delineated which describe characteristic features of personality and the quantitative classification of tinnitus in varying degrees of severity.

In the second part of the chapter, the results of our research will be presented, using a questionnaire available in all public institutions responsible for those suffering from impaired hearing in Sweden. The goal of this study was to determine factors which are important for dealing with the problem of tinnitus. In the process, it seems that the two most important prognostic parameters are the loudness of the tinnitus, and the ability to gain control. The findings, however, are only descriptive and further research in this area is urgently needed.

2.2 Introduction

The word tinnitus is of Latin origin and means buzzing, humming or ringing in the ears. Most, if not all, of those who suffer from tinnitus, find this general description accurate; to be exact, however, the number of different sound sensations is at least as large as the number of people who claim to suffer from such noises in the ear. Some describe tinnitus as a barely disturbing, slight buzzing in the ears. Others, on the other hand, are so disturbed by their tinnitus that, for example, they cannot sleep, concentrate or tolerate stress. In a soundproof room, almost everyone can hear humming sounds or tones of various types. According to Heller & Bergmann (1953), 94% of those tested in such a room hear sounds. Tinnitus therefore can be a normal physiological phenomenon under certain conditions. Nevertheless, this type of tinnitus, which is easily suppressed by surrounding sounds and to which one can become accustomed without effort, is completely different from the severe "terrorizing" tinnitus.

2.3 Prevalence of Tinnitus

2.3.1 In adults

The fact that almost every person is acquainted with tinnitus makes it difficult to verify the prevalence of the occurrence of this phenomenon. Earlier studies of prevalence did not differentiate between a burdening, insistent tinnitus and "normal" tinnitus, nor did they examine the differences between people with normal hearing and those with hearing impairment (McFaden, 1982). In earlier studies, more value was placed on a clear definition, in order to avoid the inaccuracy of the term "tinnitus".

One of the most thorough and often quoted studies concerning prevalence was the National Study of Hearing in England (Institute of Hearing Research, 1981; Coles 1984 a, b). This study, which dealt with different aspects of hearing, and also with the disorders associated with tinnitus, was based on a questionnaire which had been sent to 6804 randomly selected individuals in Cardiff, Glasgow, Nottingham and Southampton. "Serious" tinnitus was distinguished from "common" tinnitus by a duration of tinnitus of more or less than 5 minutes. The authors found that the total prevalence in adults (i.e. older than 17 years) was 17% for tinnitus of longer duration and 35% for tinnitus of shorter duration. A clear impairment of the quality of life due to tinnitus was cited by 1% of those questioned.

If one extrapolates the numbers of this study to other west European countries, up to 750,000 people in Germany (including the new provinces after reunification) and up to 60,000 in Sweden would be affected.

Sleeping disturbances of varying degree are also familiar consequences of tinnitus as approximately 8% of those questioned complained about them (Coles, 1984a). This corresponds to 4 million people who suffer from some form of tinnitus-related sleeping disturbance in Great Britain, and approximately 6 million in Germany. In 1987, Smith & Coles reported that approximately 7% of the adult population of Great Britain seek medical attention because of intolerable tinnitus.

In Sweden, Axelsson & Ringdahl (1987) also ran a survey among 3,600 people between the ages of 20 and 80. Although the questionnaire differed from the one used in the British study, it resulted in similar numbers for the prevalence of long lasting (14%) or disabling (2.4%) tinnitus.

These figures indicate that a large number of people are indirectly or directly affected by tinnitus, and the importance of attending to this problem especially in respect to that one per cent which is severely disabled.

2.3.2 In children

The first study concerning the prevalence of tinnitus in children was done by Nodar (1972). He observed the occurrence of tinnitus in school children between the ages of 17 and 18.

During the entire 3 year study, tinnitus occurred among approximately 15% of the participants; in this evaluation, however, tinnitus of short duration, even in healthy individuals, was not distinguished from longer lasting tinnitus. In every year of the 3 year study, approximately 2000 young people participated in the study and tinnitus was more frequent in those between the ages of 13 and 15 years.

Graham (1987) examined children and adolescents, between the ages of 12 and 18 from the London area, who suffered from decreased hearing or deafness (i.e. students from schools for the deaf). An initial part of the study concerning 74 hearing impaired subjects, showed that 64% suffered from tinnitus, but only 2.7% suffered from long lasting tinnitus. Approximately 40% of those examined described the tinnitus as disturbing. In the second part of the study with 158 participants, 49% indicated that they suffered from tinnitus. The lower percentage in the second questionnaire is due to the participation of completely deaf students. The prevalence of tinnitus was twice as high in the hearing impaired participants as in the deaf participants. This finding may initially be surprising; but Kemp (1981; cited by Graham, 1987) already stated that it may be difficult for a deaf child to distinguish between actual tinnitus and the perception of environmental sounds.

2.4 Tinnitus and demographic data

In a series of studies, it was shown that tinnitus very often occurs in association with hearing impairment, after exposure to noise and in old age; people who have been exposed to long-term noise suffer from tinnitus twice as often as others (Coles 1984 a,b; Reed, 1960).

In old age, a significant increase of tinnitus associated with disease is observed. However, no evidence has been found that tinnitus becomes more of a health problem with increasing age (Lindberg et al., 1984; Scott et al., 1990). In patients with decreased hearing, it appears that those who are most frequently affected by tinnitus are those who suffer from presbycusis or who experienced noise that caused trauma. Some authors claimed that left-sided tinnitus occurs more frequently than right-sided tinnitus, and women more often experienced tinnitus as disturbing than men (Institute of Hearing Research, 1981). Others, however (Harris et al., 1980; Axelsson & Ringdahl, 1989) reported a slightly higher number of men among those affected. A significant difference in gender for the prevelance of tinnitus was found, however, only in the group of men between ages 40-59 in the Axelsson & Ringdahl study. All in all, the results of the different studies correspond.

2.5 Tinnitus, personality structure and psychiatric aspects

A number of authors believe, because of their results, that people who suffer from tinnitus already have certain (premorbid) personality characteristics or develop them. An attempt was made to establish these characteristics of personality using different psychological tests (test designs): Minnesota Multiphasic Personality Inventory (MMPI) (House, 1981; Reich & Johnson, 1984), Eysenck Personality Questionnaire (EPQ), Beck Depression Inventory (BDI) (Wood et al., 1983), Crown-Crisp Experiential Index (CCEI) (Stephens & Hallam, 1985) and Hopkins Symptom Checklist (SCL-90) (Horrop-Griffiths et al., 1987).

The design of the MMPI was suitable to provide evidence regarding a depressive disposition of tinnitus patients. The evaluation of the EPQ and the MMPI resulted in a more frequent occurrence of neurotic behavior among those affected. The CCEI demonstrated depressive symptoms as a striking characteristic and that dizziness in conjunction with tinnitus could lead to phobic anxiety and more frequent somatic complaints than in the normal population. Using DSM-III criteria, Harrop-Griffiths et al. (1987) found that tinnitus patients suffered more frequently from somatic complaints than others.

Other authors, on the other hand, found opposite results after evaluation of the aforementioned tests. For example, Gerber et al. (1985) found no correlation between tinnitus and MMPI scales. Kearny et al. (1987) examined patients with headaches, with tinnitus, as well as a control group of healthy participants, using following tests: Emotional Control Scale (ECS), Taylor Manifest Anxiety Scale (MAS), Stress Cognitions Inventory (SCI), Unpleasant Events Schedule (UES) as well as the EPQ and the BDI. They found that patients who suffered primarily from headaches were best identified with the MAS, the EPQ, and the SCI; tinnitus patients, on the other hand, were not conspicuously different from the control group in these tests.

In conclusion, most studies could not prove beyond doubt that tinnitus was the result of a certain premorbid (psychopathological) personality structure.

2.6 Tinnitus and accompanying handicaps

A number of studies examined the degree of handicap as a result of tinnitus.

Thus, Coles (1984a) attempted to establish to what extent tinnitus limited the quality of life or the possibility of a "normal" lifestyle. Approximately 0.5% of the tinnitus patients questioned stated that tinnitus severely affected their daily lives.

Another approach was used by Tyler & Baker (1983). A tinnitus self-help group determined the 15 most troublesome problems related to tinnitus in the degree of severity. 72 of the 97 questionnaires were returned and evaluated.

The main problem of the patients appeared to be "falling asleep" (n=35,3.6). The third most frequent handicap cited by the questioned patients was difficulty in understanding speech (n=27,3.3). In fourth place was the problem tinnitus posed after waking up in the morning (n=12,3.25). Ranked according to average weight, emotional problems i.e. "concentration and confusion problems" were ranked fifth (n=24,3.08). Depression, despair, or frustration (=26,2.7) and the feeling that the tinnitus created an annoyance or irritation and an inability to relax (n=25,2.6) were also mentioned often. Headache, giddiness and avoidance of quiet surroundings were also considered as important problems. The evaluation resulted in a significant correlation between the length of time patients had suffered from tinnitus and the weighting of the resulting problems. Patients who had already suffered longer claimed to have had fewer problems. Even with an age adjustment of data, this finding was valid and agreed with our personal examinations of patients with hearing impairment (Lindberg et al., 1984; Scott et al., 1990).

Another ranking system consisting of only three grades of severity, was first described by Klockhoff & Lindblom (1967), and is another approach to the degree of handicap due to tinnitus:

Grade I: Tinnitus is audible only in silence.

Grade II: Tinnitus is audible at a low external noise level, but is masked by normal environmental noise. Beyond that, it makes falling asleep difficult, but, as a rule, does not disturb sleep.

Grade III: Tinnitus is audible at all levels of external sound. Falling asleep and sleep are disturbed, and result in a constantly increasing series of problems, which affect the entire lifestyle of the patient.

Lindberg et al. (1984) asked 1091 persons who had visited a public clinic for impaired hearing for an assessment of their tinnitus complaints. After evaluation, using the Klockhoff & Lindblom scale, the following results were reached: 35% of those questioned suffered from Grade I, 51% from Grade II and finally 14% from Grade III tinnitus. Patients with tinnitus problems were very interested in all possibilities for a specific treatment. This correlated with the degree of handicap by tinnitus (Grade I: 74%; Grade II: 85%; Grade III: 91%).

2.6.1 Incidence of tinnitus and degree of handicap in a population with impaired hearing

In 1990, Scott, Lindberg, Lyttkens and Melin studied patients of public clinics for hearing impairment. The results of the study will be described briefly and special attention will be given to the process of adaptation to tinnitus. In addition to questions concerning demographic data, the questionnaire was mainly concerned with specific tinnitus characteristics and psychological and somatic factors which were possible important predictors of discomfort from, tolerance of, and adaptation to tinnitus.

2.6.1.1 The questionnaire

In order to comprehend the duration of disturbances due to tinnitus, we also used the questionnaire of a previous British study (Institute of Hearing Research, 1981, Coles 1984a, b): "Did you ever have buzzing, humming or other sounds in the ear or head, which lasted longer than five minutes ('tinnitus')?"

All 69 medical centers for hearing impairment in Sweden were asked to participate in the study. The centers were requested to use the questionnaire for the duration of one week with a normal workload. The questionnaire had 2, 3 and 5 response categories and were concerned with subjective hearing impairment, tinnitus characteristics and psychosomatic factors. Fifty-two centers eventually participated in the study; those centers that did not participate did not differ geographically or in size. A total of 3372 patients were asked to complete the questionnaire. Nine percent refused to answer the questions, 53% of the answers received came from men and 47% from women: the average age was 62.3± 16.2 years. Age or gender-specific differences between those who answered the questions and those who did not were not noted.

2.6.1.2 Descriptive Results

Hearing impairment was experienced by 93%.

Sixty percent needed a hearing aid because of their handicap, 49% claimed to suffer from tinnitus, of whom two thirds again stated that tinnitus had had a gradual onset. Almost half (47%) had experienced tinnitus for more than 5 years and no specific laterality of the tinnitus was found. The rate of interest in receiving treatment was high (73%). When asked about the tolerance of their tinnitus, 2% of those questioned found it absolutely intolerable, while a total of

18% rated their tinnitus as very disturbing.

There was a strong correlation between the side affected by hearing impairment and by tinnitus.

In answer to the question whether the impaired hearing or the tinnitus was a greater handicap, the younger participants (aged 18–30) stated tinnitus as the major handicap more often than the older participants (over 65 years of age).

In approximately half of those questioned, increased tolerance of tinnitus developed, and only 7.5% reported a decreased tolerance.

2.6.1.3 Measurement

In order to establish to what extent tinnitus characteristics may predict adaption to tinnitus, the questions in the questionnaire were posed as follows. An adaption variable was determined by combining the question concerning tolerance of tinnitus over time with the question concerning change of the degree of discomfort/annoyance over time. Approximately 14% of the participants had to be omitted from the analysis because of inconsistent answers (such as better tolerance and a simultaneous increase of personal discomfort).

Definition of the degree of adaptation:

Category I: Poorer tolerance of tinnitus and increased general discomfort from tinnitus.

Category II: Unchanged tolerance to tinnitus and unchanged general discomfort from tinnitus.

Category III: Increased tolerance to tinnitus and decreased discomfort from tinnitus.

Those who had tinnitus as well as a hearing impairment suffered significantly more from psychosomatic disturbances than those who only complained about impaired hearing.

As Table 2.1 shows, it seems that dizziness, depression and decreased concentration are the main problems of those who have both tinnitus and hearing impairment. This has also been reported by other researchers (Harrop-Griffiths et al., 1987).

Further evaluation of the raw data, with the aid of regression analysis, showed that successful adaptation correlated mainly with an improvement in the following symptoms: depression, sleep disturbances, decreased concentration and dizziness. Those who suffered only a little or not at all from the aforementioned symptoms, statistically showed a better adaptation to tinnitus (declared variance, 8%). These symptoms served as predictors for the annoyance variable or change of discomfort over time, and together they comprised 3% of the variance.

Discrimination analysis was also conducted.

Category III tinnitus showed the following characteristics/variables compared to category I tinnitus:

1. Lower sound intensity ($p > 0.001$).
2. Less variation of sound intensity ($p > 0.001$).
3. A higher feeling of control ($p > 0.001$).
4. More intermittent perception ($p > 0.001$).
5. Better masking due to environmental sounds ($p > 0.001$).
6. Shorter duration of tinnitus ($p > 001$).

Here, the most important characteristics were the volume and the feeling of being able to control tinnitus (a multiple regression analysis of data supported this result). These two characteristics explained the variance of 22%. The other variables did not increase the variance. The omission of the question concerning the volume of the tinnitus from the regression analysis, led to a different result.

Table 2.1 Comparison of questions concerning primarily psychological or somatic disturbances between participants with or without tinnitus (*t*-test): $***P < 0.001$.

	Tinnitus mean (standard deviation)	**No tinnitus mean (standard deviation)**	***t***
anxiety	2.49 (1.04)	2.21 (0.97)	7.12***
disturbances in sleep	2.99 (1.19)	2.93 (1.16)	n.s.
disturbances of equilibrium	2.21 (1.18)	1.89 (1.13)	7.10***
depression	2.48 (1.02)	2.14 (0.94)	9.04***
dizziness	2.46 (1.12)	2.01 (1.05)	10.86***
gastrointestinal disorders	2.21 (1.09)	2.08 (1.07)	n.s.
headaches	2.49 (1.04)	2.20 (0.93)	7.75***
insomnia	2.62 (1.28)	2.30 (1.24)	6.78***
difficulties in concentration	2.36 (1.03)	2.05 (0.97)	8.14***

* Falling asleep again after awakening

The most important predictor variable represented in all dependent variables was the degree of control, i.e. the active influence on above-mentioned symptoms.

The second most important variable was the ability to mask ear noises by external noises. Frequent variation of volume was the third most important variable and appeared to be associated with a high degree of discomfort and a decreased tolerance. According to the theory of habituation (Horvath, 1980), the constant changes in sound intensity prevent tolerance of tinnitus, due to their unpredictability and degree of interference. Our recent results support this hypothesis (Scott et al., 1990).

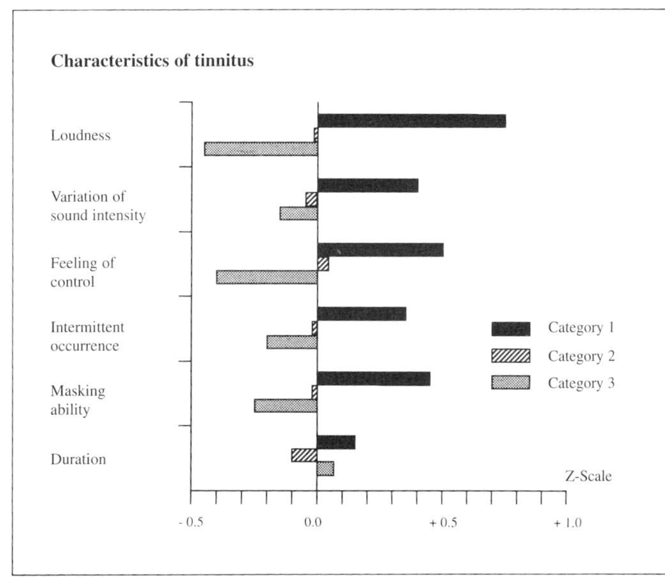

Fig. 2.1 Mean (Z-value) of the three tinnitus adaptation categories for six characteristics of tinnitus. For the definition of each category see section 2.6.1.3.

Table 2.2 Regression analysis: features of tinnitus as predictors for three independent variables (changes in tolerance, changes in discomfort, and adaptation). All predictors significantly contribute in forecasting the dependent variables, at least at the 1% level. ( ) = rank of the predictor variable.

	Predictor variables		
	Change in tolerance ß	**Changes in discomfort ß**	**Adaptation ß**
Ability to control	0.31 (1)	-0.19 (1)	-0.27 (1)
Ability to mask using external noises	0.15 (2)		-0.11 (2)
Duration of disorder: (< 6 months to > 5 years)	-0.09 (3)		
Variations in sound intensity	0.08 (4)	-0.10 (2)	-0.08 (3)
Tonal quality of tinnitus		0.09 (3)	
R^2	0.18	0.07	0.13

2.7 Conclusion

The results of our research highlighted how important it is for the patient to gain control over his unfortunate situation or — better yet — to keep control. In order to do this, the affected person must, as a rule, resort to his inner resources, which enable him to ignore the disturbing aspects and to tolerate the disorder. As noted above, environmental noises often help the patient to mask the tinnitus. Treatment with masking elements (maskers) is therefore designed to mask ear noises (masking therapy) for a better adaptation to tinnitus. The usefulness of this method was already documented in 1985 in a multicenter study by Hazell et al. In this study, we came upon patients who always had their maskers within reach without resorting to them, but had also found a way to control their tinnitus. We assumed that a patient who does not use his masker has developed a problem-oriented coping behavior. Actively perceiving environmental sounds can lead to distraction from "problem sounds" and, therefore, to better adaptation. A patient who is accustomed to his disturbing tinnitus, uses, according to the situation, his emotional control, as well as external control or maskability to control the disorder. For this reason, every treatment of tinnitus should teach patients different approaches of handling the disorder. Other symptoms, such as sleep disturbances, decreased concentration and dizziness must also be included in such coping strategies.

Psychosomatic complaints were significantly more frequent among patients, who suffered from tinnitus in addition to a hearing impairment. An interpretation of this finding is difficult, considering other results (Kearny et al., 1987).

One can argue whether a study on a selected population (in this case, patients who seek help at a center for hearing impairment) is representative. But the choice of this population group is correct, if one considers the assumption that tinnitus primarily occurs in those with hearing impairment. It is feasible that the results of this study also apply to people with normal hearing.

This type of research has certainly

not come to a conclusion. To find empirical support in intervention studies concerning the importance of such factors as lack of control or insomnia as complications of a potentially successful treatment of tinnitus, is one possibility to obtain more reliable data and reproducible results.

2.8 References

Axelsson, A. & Ringdahl, A. (1987). The occurrence and severity of tinnitus – a prevalence study. In: *H. Feldmann* (Ed.): Proceedings III International tinnitus Seminar Münster. Karlsruhe: Harsch Verlag.

Axelsson, A. & Ringdahl, A. (1989). Tinnitus – a study of its prevalence and characteristics. British Journal of Audiology 23: 53-62.

Coles, R.R.A. (1984a). Epidemiology of tinnitus: (1) Prevalence. Journal of Laryngology and Otology 98 (Suppl. 9): 7-15.

Coles, R.R.A. (1984b). Epidemiology of tinnitus: (1) Demographic and clinical feature. Journal of Laryngology and Otology 98 (Suppl. 9): 195-202.

Gerber, K.E., Nehemkis, A.M., Charter, R.A. & Jones, H.C. (1985). Is tinnitus a psychological disorder? Journal of Psychiatry in Medicine 15: 81-87.

Graham, J.M. (1987). Tinnitus in hearing-impaired children. In: *J. Hazell* (Ed.): Tinnitus. London: Churchill Livingstone.

Harris, S., Broms, P. & Reimer, A. (1980). 60-åringars hörsel och hjälpmedelsbehov. Läkarsällskapets Riksstämma. Acta Societatis Medicorum Suecanae 89: 404.

Harrop-Griffiths, J., Katon, W., Doibie, R., Sakai, C. & Russo, J. (1987). Chronic tinnitus: association with psychiatric diagnosis. Journal of Psychosomatic Research 31: 613-621.

Hazell, J.W.P., Wood, S.M., Cooper, H.R., Stephens, S.D.G., Corcoran, A.L., Coles, R.R.A., Baskill, J.L. & Sheldrake, J.B. (1985). A clinical study of tinnitus maskers. British Journal of Audiology 19: 65-146.

Heller, M. & Bergman, M. (1953). Tinnitus aurium in normally hearing persons. Annals of Otology Rhinology Laryngology 60: 73-83.

Horvath, T. (1980). Arousal and anxiety. In: *G.D. Burrows & B. Davies* (Eds.): Handbook of Studies in Anxiety. Holland: Elsevier, Biomedical Press.

House, P.R. (1981). Personality of the tinnitus patient. In: *D. Evered & G. Lawrenson* (Eds.): Ciba Foundation Symposium 85: Tinnitus. London: Pitman Medical.

Institute of Hearing Research. (1981). Epidemiology of tinnitus. In: *D. Evered & Lawerenson* (Eds.) Ciba Foundation Symposium 85: Tinnitus. London: Pitman Medical. 16-25.

Kearny, B.G., Wilson, P.H. & Haralambous, G. (1987). Stress appraisal and personality characteristics of headache patients: Comparisons with tinnitus and normal control groups. Behaviour Change 4: 25-32.

Klockhoff, I. & Lindblom, U. (1967). Menière's disease and hydrochlorothiazide (Dichlotrideʀ) – A critical analysis of symptoms and therapeutic effects. Acta Otolaryngolica (Stockholm) 63: 347-365.

Lindberg, P., Lyttkens, L., Melin, L. & Scott, B. (1984). Tinnitus-Incidence and handicap. Scandinavian Audiology 13: 287-291.

MacFadden, D. (1982). Tinnitus: Facts, Theories and Treatments. Washington DC: National Academy Press.

Nodar, R.H. (1972). Tinnitus aurium in schoolchildren: A survey. Journal of Auditory Research 12: 133-135.

Reed, G.F. (1960). An audiometric study of two hundred cases of subjective tinnitus. Archives of Otolaryngology 71: 94-104.

Reich, G.E. & Johnson, R.M. (1984). Personality characteristics of tinnitus patients. Journal of Laryngology and Otology 98 (Suppl. 9): 228-232.

Scott, B., Lindberg, P., Lyttkens, L. & Melin, L. (1990). Predictors of tinnitus discomfort, adaptation and subjective loudness. British Journal of Audiology 24: 51-62.

Smith, P. & Coles, R.R.A. (1987). Epidemiology of tinnitus: An update. In: *H. Feldmann* (Ed.): Proceedings III International Tinnitus Seminar Münster. Karlsruhe: Harsch Verlag.

Stephens, S.D.G. & Hallam, R.S. (1985). The Crown-Crisp Experiential Index in patients complaining of tinnitus. British Journal of Audiology 19: 151-158.

Stephens, S.D.G. (1987). Historical aspects of tinnitus. In: *J. Hazell* (Ed.): Tinnitus. London: Churchill Livingstone.

Tylor, R.S. & Baker, L.J. (1983). Difficulties experienced by tinnitus sufferers. Journal of Speech and Hearing Disorders 48: 150-154.

Wood, K.A., Webb, W.L., Orchik, D.J. & Shea, J.J. (1983). Intractable tinnitus: Psychiatric aspects of treatment. Psychosomatics 24: 4.

Chapter 3

Psychiatric problems due to tinnitus: results of a survey of patients with chronic tinnitus

Reinhard Gefken and Heike Kurth

3.1 Summary

Results of a survey of 165 tinnitus patients are presented. They deal in particular with the psychological effects of chronic tinnitus and the coping strategies of patients.

The statements of those surveyed make it clear that a coping strategy based on distraction definitely achieves short-term relief and relaxation, but for a permanent and long-term decrease in impairment, cognitive restructuring processes and changes which include the entire personality are necessary. Patients have to learn to live to a greater extent according to their own needs, a process which effects a change of life-style, attitudes and self-perception.

The results are presented in a coping model. Furthermore the theory that the tendency to functionalize tinnitus corresponds significantly with increased impairment is confirmed.

3.2 Introduction

What is the significance of tinnitus for the individual? How do patients experience impairment from tinnitus? How do they cope with it?

We asked ourselves these questions when we developed a questionnaire to investigate psychological impairments from chronic tinnitus. The goal was to investigate various attitudes, feelings, and types of behaviour and methods which have an influence on the patient's psychic condition (Gefken and Kurth, 1990).

The following chapter is derived from results of the survey which we conducted in 1990 among approximately 30 tinnitus self-help groups and individuals in Germany. Our results refer to 165 analyzed questionnaires (reverse quota 33%). Our information is statistically the most comprehensive psychologically oriented study of this subject in Germany. The great number of similar publications in English speaking countries confirms the enormous deficit in this country in respect of scientific research into the psychological aspects of chronic tinnitus.

3.3 Study design

3.3.1 Questionnaire

The first part of the questionnaire contains 30 open questions about case history data, together with questions about tinnitus-related experiences.

The second part consists of nine scales: Four scales are taken from the Deusinger Frankfurt self-concept scale (FSCS) (1986); they are concerned with the following self-concepts:

FSIA — irritability due to other people
FSSW — general assessment of self-esteem
FSST — relationship in respect to persons and groups
FSEG — sensitivity and mood

Four scales are based on observations which we made in various interviews and at the Hamburg self-help group meetings. These scales describe various attitudes towards tinnitus. The following functional classifications are possible.

- tinnitus as an admonisher
- tinnitus as a scapegoat
- tinnitus as a cover-up/concealing function which deters the patient from constructively working on his own psychological problems
- tinnitus as a way of obtaining care and attention

The ninth scale (subjective impairment) forms the main point of reference of the questionnaire. It serves as an assessment of the subjective impairment of every patient independent of the frequency and volume of the tinnitus because the reaction to these two qualities is very individual (Scott et al., 1985; Goebel, 1989).

3.3.2 Description of the random sample

The results of our investigation are based on the statements of 165 persons who, at the time of the survey, suffered from tinnitus of varying degrees. The tinnitus had already persisted for more than 3 months for all of the participants and accordingly was assessed as chronic (Lenarz, 1989).

One hundred and twelve patients had belonged or still belonged to a self-help group (68%).

The participants were between 23 and 83 years old with a mean age of 53.4 years (Table 3.1).

Table 3.1 Age in relation to tinnitus (n = 165)

Age	At the first occurrence n (%)	At the beginning of impairment n (%)	At the time of examination n (%)
1-10	1 (0.6)	—	—
11-20	8 (4.9)	7 (4.2)	—
21-30	17 (10.3)	13 (7.9)	7 (4.2)
31-40	29 (17.6)	24 (14.6)	22 (13.3)
41-50	45 (27.3)	44 (26.7)	40 (24.2)
51-60	38 (23.0)	45 (27.3)	43 (26.1)
61-70	18 (10.9)	21 (12.7)	41 (24.9)
71-80	3 (1.8)	3 (1.8)	11 (6.7)
81-90	—	1 (0.6)	1 (0.6)
no number	6 (3.6)	7 (4.2)	—

The results largely confirm the peak period of incidence between 51 and 60 years of age, as found in other studies (Coles, 1984).

Duration of impairment was reported as 3 months to 45 years; however, half the participants reported a duration of impairment of less than 4.5 years.

Fifty-five percent of the random sample were men (n=90) and 45% women (n=75).

Fifty-four reported an accompanying hearing impairment; this was somewhat more frequent among men (34%) than women (31%).

3.4 Results

3.4.1 Psychological aspects of tinnitus

Everyone has an individual way of reacting to stress. Nevertheless, tinnitus patients' reactions to stress correspond to a great extent. Different coping phases are discernible (similar feelings, sensations and types of behavior). We will attempt to describe the sequence of these phases on the basis of our research results.

3.4.1.1 The "black hole"

The onset of tinnitus does not always correspond directly with the onset of associated impairment. The interval between first perception of tinnitus and initial impairment of a patient varied to a great extent with intervals as long as two years. This indicates that the psychological factors acting as interindividual differences in the reaction to tinnitus and the stress play a significant role. The question concerning the significance of tinnitus in the daily experience of the patient must, for this reason, be especially considered. What role does the "disease" play, what does it cause, which function does it have and why is it significant at the given moment? These questions in general are not the most important ones in the initial phase of confrontation with this new phenomenon. The first reaction of a patient is a physician's appointment. In the random sample examined here, this resulted in only minor success. Twenty percent were very disappointed by their appointment. They reported that their doctor had reacted with disinterest, helplessness, inexperience, and lack of information and understanding. Ten percent reported having experienced sympathy and encouragement. The remaining 70% made no comments.

3.4.1.2 Previous treatment attempts

The statements about previous treatments were relatively discouraging. Most of those questioned had experienced various therapies which showed no or minor results.

The methods concerning the psychological problems of the patients were more positively judged. Self analysis and analysis of the problems due to tinnitus, and actively learning to live with tinnitus, produced the greatest improvements. 41% of those patients who had prior experiences with self-help groups, client-centered therapy, behavior therapy or meditation judged these as helpful. What is of importance is that the patient with chronic tinnitus finds his own individual way of coping with himself and his present condition and does not continue searching for newer medication and somatically oriented therapy.

The same is true of psychopharmaceuticals. At the time of our study, 22% of the participants took such drugs and, according to our results, patients who suffered more severely from tinnitus used mood-influencing medication and sleeping pills more often.

Only a few subjects used tinnitus maskers and hearing aids. Only one person (among a total of four who tried them) was satisfied with the effect of a masker.

All in all, the impression emerged that in this phase of confrontation with a disturbing impairment, no help is to be expected from any quarter. Even the attempt to find information about the phenomenon "tinnitus" fails. In contrast to the large quantity of scientific publications, very little information exists for the patient (Ganz, 1986), a situation which has begun to improve (Tonnies, 1991; "Tinnitus Forum" of the German Tinnitus League*).

* Tinnitus Forum: quarterly journal of the German Tinnitus League, G-42353 Wuppertal (circulation 12000).

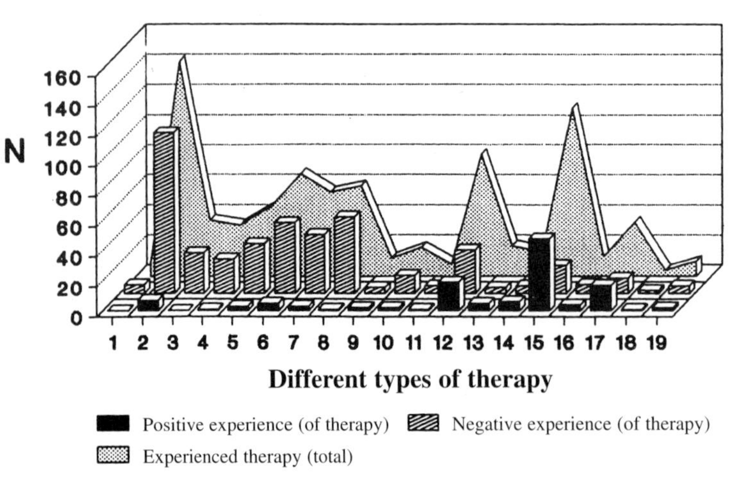

Fig. 3.1 Prior therapy

1 Surgery
2 Medication with vasodilators/anticoagulants
3 Oxygen therapy
4 Orthopedic methods
5 Non-allopathic methods
6 Massage
7 Physical therapy
8 Acupuncture
9 Biofeedback
10 Yoga
11 Tomatis-sound therapy
12 Autogenic training
13 Meditation
14 Encounter group
15 Self-help group
16 Behavioral therapy
17 Client centered psychotherapy
18 Gestalt therapy
19 Psychoanalysis

3.4.1.3 Social aspects of impairment

It is not surprising that many patients who are confronted with this situation despair. They do not always find the support that they desire from family or spouse. Thirty-five percent of those asked indicated they lacked help. In contrast, 35% were satisfied with the help received, while 16% were dissatisfied with it. The remaining 14% did not receive any support from their family or spouse, but neither lacked or expected it. Those subjects who had found ways to cope, suffered the least from their tinnitus, while those who received help but found it inadequate were most seriously impaired by their tinnitus. Presumably their high expectation level was a handicap in developing coping strategies. In this respect, self-responsibility is another important aspect of coping with tinnitus.

3.4.1.4 Emotional effects

The most frequent negative feelings toward tinnitus were helplessness, followed by anxiety, anger, resignation and depression. This was noted mainly by persons who felt severely impaired by tinnitus in their quality of life (Table 3.2). Subjects felt helpless and no longer able to actively search for new coping strategies (Table 2).

Feeling calm and collected as well as accepting the tinnitus were most often cited as positive coping strategies. The goal of treatment should therefore be to succeed in an active acceptance of tinnitus and to overcome feelings of anxiety and helplessness.

Facing the facts, e.g. confronting the tinnitus and realizing the inevitability of a life with tinnitus often leads to an acute life crisis. For this reason there is a need, in addition to thorough diagnosis and exclusion of possible somatic causes, for an active

Table 3.2 Correlation of various feelings pertaining to tinnitus in relation to subjective impairment (t-test for independent random samples: $n = 155$; N1 = naming; N2 = no naming)

	Correlation subjective impairment	**N1**	**N2**
helplessness	−.34**	84	71
anxiety	−.33**	59	96
anger	−.27**	41	114
resignation	−.22*	13	142
feeling of confinement	−.14	2	153
pessimism	−.09	4	151
despair	−.05	8	147
depression	−.03	9	146
optimism	.004	3	152
sadness	.03	11	144
abandonment	.04	15	140
endurance	.05	11	144
defiance	.07	3	152
indifference	.10	4	151
acceptance	.20	26	129
composure	.38**	27	128

$n = 155$ significance (one sided) * $p < .01$ ** $p < .001$

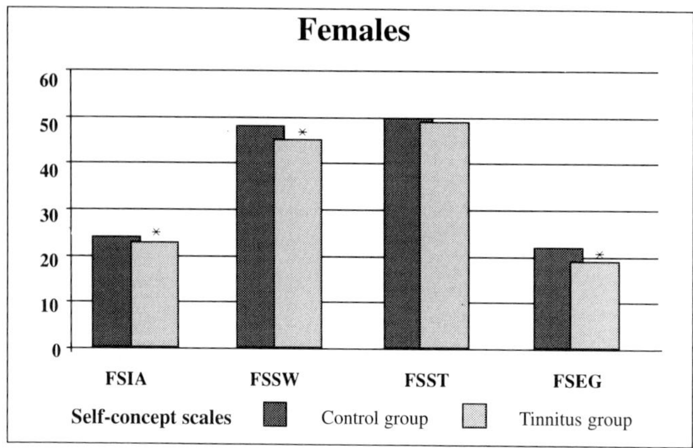

Fig. 3.2 Mean comparisons (*t*-test) of the Frankfurt self-concept scale (FSCS) (Deusinger, 1986): control group and tinnitus group, female; FSIA: irritability due to other people; FSSW: general assessment of self-esteem; FSST: relationship in respect to persons and groups; FSEG: sensitivity and mood.

* significant

development of coping strategies and psychotherapy, when necessary.

3.4.1.5 Change in self-concepts

Our subjects differed in almost all aspects from the norm in their tendency for a more negative self concept.

Female respondents rated themselves as more irritable, had less self-esteem and were more sensitive. Their values corresponded more closely to those of the norm only in the scale of stability toward partners and family (Fig. 3.2).

Similarly, male participants in our random sample also assessed their feelings of self-esteem as lower and perceived themselves as more sensitive than their normal male counterparts. In contrast to the women examined by us, they were not more irritable; instead they felt they were less able to assert their individual needs and opinions.

In dealing with tinnitus, it is of crucial significance for the patient to recognize that tinnitus has nothing to do with their self-esteem. Physicians and therapists make an important contribution by helping patients to reestablish a more positive feeling of self-

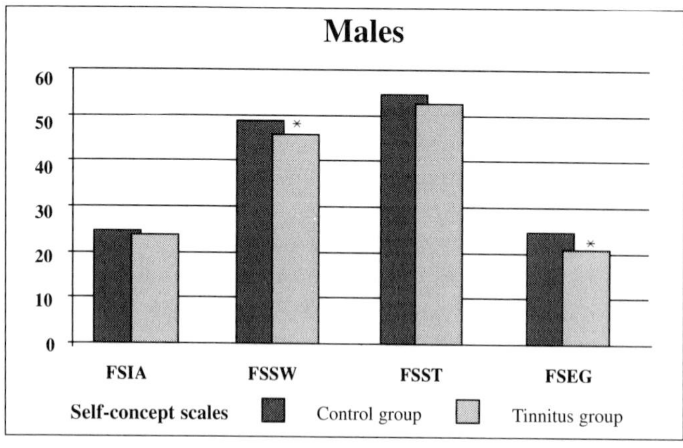

Fig. 3.3 Mean comparisons (*t*-test) of the Frankfurt self-concept scale (FSCS) (Deusinger, 1986): control group and tinnitus group, male: FSIA: irritability by others; FSSW: general assessment of self-esteem; FSST: relationship in respect to persons and groups; FSEG: sensitivity and mood.

* significant

esteem. This measure decreases fixation on tinnitus and an important step can be taken toward tinnitus management. Following an improved feeling of self-esteem, as a rule, sensitivity and mood change caused by tinnitus are altered positively.

3.5 Change of cognition

3.5.1 Diversion/Distraction

The second coping phase is characterized by patients beginning to distract

Table 3.3 Coping behavior in tinnitus of varying degrees of impairment (n = 165)

Coping behavior in varying degrees of impairment	High impairment		Average impairment		Slight impairment	
	number/group		number/group		number/group	
	n=40	%	n=77	%	n=48	%
distraction (general)	11	28	40	52	21	44
having fun	4	10	6	8	2	4
Activities:						
— travel/vacation	7	18	13	17	12	25
— work	5	13	14	18	7	15
— hobby	6	15	10	13	2	4
— music	19	48	37	48	24	50
— reading	2	5	15	20	6	13
— television	2	5	12	16	4	8
— sports	9	23	28	36	12	25
— hiking	5	13	7	9	3	6
— taking a walk	9	23	15	20	7	15
— gardening	4	10	9	12	6	13
— being outdoors	5	13	8	10	5	10
Silence:						
— absolute quiet	5	13	6	8	2	4
— resting	9	23	20	26	8	17
— sleeping	4	10	8	10	2	4
— relaxing	2	5	10	13	5	10
— excessive sleep	4	10	5	7	6	13
— decreased level of activity	5	13	1	1	—	—
Sounds:						
a) producing noises	4	10	7	9	7	15
b) avoiding noises	2	5	12	16	3	6
Work strategies:						
— working more consciously, at a slower pace	5	13	8	10	5	10
Contact behavior:						
— joining self-help group	9	23	19	25	15	31
— enjoying encouraging company	7	18	12	16	7	15
— leading interesting conversations	5	13	8	10	6	13
— withdrawing	11	28	11	14	2	4

themselves, at least temporarily, in order to avoid the constantly present tinnitus (Table 3.3).

The most common method consisted of listening to music, which also partially masked the tinnitus. Many patients pursued those hobbies more often which had been previously neglected, in order to distract themselves.

These efforts seemd to be characterized by the fact that this was not done as a way of positively coping with the problem of tinnitus and its integration into individual life, but rather as a superficial measure which was ultimately inadequate in decreasing the long-term impairment from tinnitus (flight mechanism).

3.5.2 Functionalization

A reframing in the direction of actively coping with the tinnitus is impeded by the tendency to functionalize the tinnitus. We assume that a symptom can also be maintained by fulfilling a function or a purpose.

Functionalization was found to be associated with a high to very high subjective impairment (Table 3.4).

We cannot speak of causal triggers of tinnitus in this context because it is not clear if significant impairment promotes functionalization behavior, or is caused by it. If medical treatment is not successful in chronic tinnitus, analysis is the only method that remains. Under these conditions, the question of causes is irrelevant because in this case it must be of therapeutic interest to interrupt the existing vicious circle.

Patients whose tinnitus had the function of obtaining more attention or care or avoiding existing problems were also more fixated on their tinnitus.

Our study confirms that functionalization also strongly decreases with diminishing impairment. Therefore focusing on tinnitus must be stopped early, so that patients do not resign themselves to psychic dependence.

Behavior was different when tinnitus was attributed to an admonishing function. In this case it appeared that this attribution frequently became an additional stress factor. The consciously perceived admonishment was probably not clearly defined enough for the patient to be able to recognize which changes in his life would lead to improvements. The "raised finger" was constantly heard, and admonishing did not lead to any positive changes in most patients. In this case, patients should be instructed to give this admonishment a positive meaning which, in time, leads to a positive change of the situation and the degree of impairment. If the patients recognize the changes the tinnitus points out and they become aware that they can influence these changes themselves, they achieve a large step in the direction of decreased impairment.

The path leading from passive impairment to active confrontation with the new life situation in most cases promotes a

Table 3.4 Correlation of functionalization with subjective impairment

	subjective	**impairment**
function as scapegoat	.91**	$n = 165$
function as cover-up	.68**	$n = 163$
function to achieve increased care	.52**	$n = 165$
function as admonishment	.22**	$n = 164$

* $p < 0.01$ * $p < 0.001$

change in cognitions relating to this condition.

3.5.3 Changes in attitudes

To investigate the extent to which a direct correlation exists between negative attitudes toward tinnitus and increased fixation and impairment due to tinnitus, we classified the answers of our random sample into four categories of attitude (Fig. 3.4).

Category 1 consists of the most negative attitudes: tinnitus was associated with feelings of hate and the impression of being confronted with an overwhelming enemy. These patients felt dominated by the tinnitus and were by far the most impaired.

Category 2 consists of attitudes that suggest an initial acceptance of tinnitus:

"I tolerate it well sometimes and poorly other times."
"I try to adjust my life to it."
"I must try to live with it", etc.

There was significantly less impairment than in Category 1. This positive tendency clearly improved in the next two categories. The less antagonistic the attitude toward tinnitus was, the better it was for the patient's well being.

Least impairment was found in the category which accepted tinnitus as a friend and as an integral part or perceived it as a teacher and a helpful admonisher (category 4).

The attitudes shown here appeared to reflect the result of an intensive confrontation with the tinnitus, which possibly also contributed to integrating tinnitus.

The patients should, for this reason, be encouraged to give up an antagonistic attitude toward tinnitus. Instead, a constructive analysis of tinnitus and, finally, the acceptance of its unavoidability is beneficial.

3.5.4 Lifestyle

Certain cognitive changes in individual attitudes towards one's own life and lifestyle appear to be very important in dealing with tinnitus. Only these changes can achieve a permanent decrease in impairment.

It can be ascertained from the answers of a random sample that attitudes which aimed strongly at developing a different attitude to self correlated significantly with less impairment from tinnitus.

The following changes in attitude appeared to be fundamental:

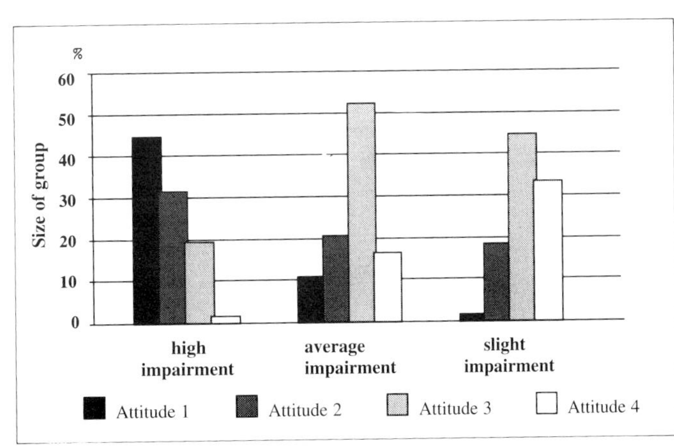

Fig. 3.4 Level of impairment depending on the attitude towards tinnitus (n = 146).
Attitude 1: very antagonistic attitude towards tinnitus
Attitude 2: negative, passive attitude towards tinnitus
Attitude 3: initial phase of acceptance
Attitude 4: positive, accepting attitude

— to take more care of oneself
— to concentrate more on oneself
— to increase regard for one's own feelings
— to work on oneself

Accordingly, a need exists to change the lifestyle in the direction of extensive reduction of stress and calmer daily activities.

Furthermore, it requires confrontation with the current lifestyle and the consequences resulting from it, in order to realize that a more conscious perception of individual needs and feelings is necessary for an improvement.

Patients must become more aware of their feelings and their individual stress factors. This means being more heedful of themselves in order to contribute to improved tinnitus management.

If it is possible to implement these new goals, defocusing the attention initially paid to the tinnitus can result. As a rule, this leads to a decrease of tinnitus impairment.

3.6 Coping

Our results indicate that the most important factor of tinnitus management is to change the specific perception of tinnitus continuously. The goal should be to reduce a fixed perception of tinnitus as much as possible and to displace it as the principal centre of attention and awareness. This requires a change in lifestyle as well as attitudes and the conscious perception of the patient in many ways. Finally, the following tinnitus promoting factors should be reduced:

— a negative body perception triggered by constant excessive demands and the resulting stress
— problems and conflicts that are constantly avoided, therefore not resolved
— functionalization of tinnitus leading to reinforcement

Only when patients are able to achieve consistent and careful self–awareness can they find and develop the necessary energy for constructive confrontation with tinnitus. Only then will it be possible to defeat the predominance of tinnitus and assume individual responsibility for all areas of life.

Patients must become aware that they can change something actively and considerably influence the extent of impairment. Furthermore, they must be convinced to give up their exclusively passive and expectant hope for future successes of somatic medicine in order to take control of their lives.

Finally, we have summarized extracts from our study and have presented them as a model for coping (Fig. 3.5).

3.7 Consequences

The unsatisfactory situation of the tinnitus patient requires the following future efforts:

1. A psychological consultation should be part of the diagnostic programme of out-patient facilities specializing in tinnitus. This can be helpful to the patient by means of goal-oriented interventions (counseling) or, if need be, referral to out-patient psychotherapy facilities (see Chapter 9).
2. Promotion of self-help groups.

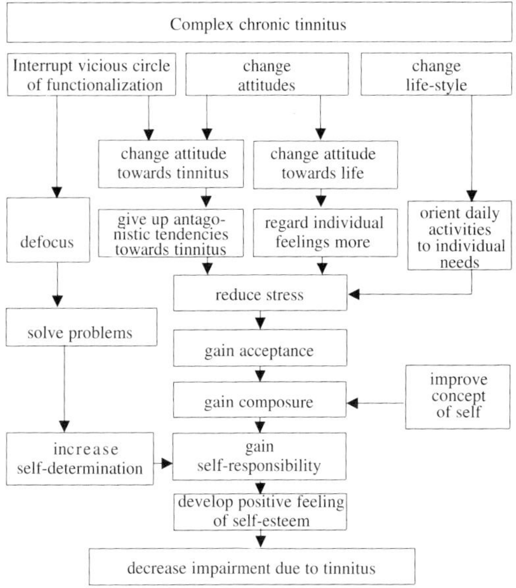

Fig. 3.5 Coping model for chronic tinnitus with high degree of impairment (Gefken and Kurth, 1990).

3. Improvement of out-patient and in-patient psychosomatic treatment options for patients with complex chronic tinnitus. This also includes the continuous training of physicians and medical personnel including hearing aid consultants (psychosomatic study groups, Balint groups, tinnitus conferences, etc.).
4. Scientific research should be intensified in the somatic and psychological fields and be promoted by research projects.
5. Increase in public relations work (by means of the German Tinnitus League, health insurance companies, etc.).

To improve the situation of tinnitus patients, collaboration is of great importance. The results of new research must be made available to the general public, so that a maximum understanding of tinnitus and concomitant possibilities of improvement is achieved for all.

3.8 References

Deusinger, I. M. (1986): Frankfurter Selbstkonzeptskalen (FSKN), Testmanual Hogrefe, Göttingen.

Ganz, F. J. (1986): Ohrgeräusche: Tinnitus-Sprechstunde. G. Thieme Verlag, Stuttgart, New York.

Gefken, R., H. Kurth (1990): Tinnitus aurium - Einflußfaktoren und Bewältigungsstrategien. Diplomarbeit am Psychologischen Institut der Universität Hamburg.

Goebel, G. (1989): Tinnitus. In: *Hand, I., H. U. Wittchen,* (Eds.): Verhaltenstherapie in der Medizin. Springer, Berlin - Heidelberg - New York - Tokyo - Hong Kong: S.207-228.

Coles, R. R. A. (1984): Epidemiology of tinnitus: (1) Prevalence. Journal of Laryngology and Otology. 98 (Suppl. 9): 7-15.

Lenarz, T. (1989): Ohrgeräusche, Pathophysiologie, Diagnostik und Therapie. Deutsches Ärzteblatt 23: 1246-1253.

Scott, B., P. Lindberg, L. Lyttkens, L. Melin (1985): Psychological treatment of tinnitus. An experimental group study. Scand. Audiol., 14: 4, 223-230.

Tönnies, S. (1991): Leben mit Ohrgeräuschen. Ein Selbsthilfebuch. Asanger Verlag.

Chapter 4

Co-morbidity of psychological disorders in patients with complex chronic tinnitus

Wolfgang Hiller and Gerhard Goebel

4.1 Summary

The prevalence and types of psychological disorders according to the DSM-III-R classification system were determined in a clinical study of 26 patients with complex chronic tinnitus. All patients were examined at the beginning of psychotherapeutic treatment in a comprehensive diagnostic interview with the aid of the Munich Diagnostic checklists (MDCL). At least one pre-existing or current psychiatric diagnosis (lifetime) was made in 96% of the patients. Found most frequently were affective disorders (85%), followed by anxiety disorders (31%) and substance-related disorders (23%). Chronological interdependence between tinnitus and psychological disorders is illustrated through individual profiles of the course of the disease. Therapeutic implications are also discussed with the aid of a conditional model describing the combination of tinnitus and psychiatric symptoms.

4.2 Introduction

Chronic and uninterrupted tinnitus is more than a mere physical symptom for many of those affected. Helplessness toward the uninterrupted nature of the ear noises — their often considerable loudness and tone, which is often perceived as dissonant — leaves its mark on the emotional state and thinking to a considerable and dramatic extent (Jakes et al., 1985, Goebel et al., 1991). Psychiatric problems can thus be experienced by patients as more strenuous and worse than the tinnitus or a concomitant decrease of hearing ability. According to Duckro et al. (1984), complex tinnitus (or tinnitus that is not compensated) exists when the tinnitus is experienced in combination with a serious psychiatric problem.

The type and range of psychiatric complaints in tinnitus patients have been investigated and documented thoroughly in a series of studies with questionaires or self evaluations (compare with House, 1981; Typer & Baker, 1983; Reich & Johnson, 1984; Jakes et al., 1985; Stephens & Hallam, 1985; Hallam, 1987; Goebel, 1989; Goebel et al., 41991). Furthermore, the question arises whether the extent of the psychiatric disorder associated with tinnitus is so serious that it attains psychiatric relevance.

Initial investigations, in which psychiatric conspicuousness of tinnitus patients was described with the aid of well-defined psychiatric diagnoses, come from Harrop Griffiths et al. (1987) and Simpson et al, (1988). Both studies rely on the new DSM-III (Diagnostic and Statistical Manual of Mental Disorders) system of diagnoses, which is considerably better than the traditional psychiatric classification. The DSM-III was issued in 1980 by the American Psychiatric Association (APA) and is still available in revised form (DSM-III-R, APA, 1987; German: Wittchen et al., 1989). DSM-III or DSM-IIIR define psychiatric disorders by extensive, precisely described diagnostic criteria (symptoms, duration and characteristics of the disease) and thereby enable considerably more dependable and reproducible diagnoses than in the past (Semler et al., 1987; Hiller et al., 1990a).

In addition to the psychiatric examination of tinnitus patients, structured and standardized interviews were incorporated in the studies of Harrop-Griffiths et al, (1987) and Simpson et al, (1988). Both studies showed a high prevalence of psychiatric disorders. According to Simpson et al., 63% of tinnitus patients (and even 80% according to Harrop-Griffiths et al.) had satisfied the criteria of a psychiatric disorder according to DSM-III at least once in their lives.

Both studies agree that tinnitus is most frequently associated with depressive disorders. In 62% of cases (Harrop-Griffiths et al.) or 33% (Simpson et al.), the diagnosis was a so-called major depression, which is a massively pronounced depressive syndrome lasting at least 2 weeks. Simpson et al. determined that 21% of patients additionally had distinctive dysthymic disorders characterized by chronic or residual depressive despondency. In addition, random tinnitus surveys point to 48% alcohol dependence and abuse (Harrop-Griffiths et al.) and to 29% anxiety (Simpson et al.).

4.2.1 Primary versus secondary psychiatric disturbance

The sequential relationships between tinnitus and psychiatric disturbances have not been analyzed in detail. Harrop-Griffiths et al. (1984, p. 615f.) state that 70% of those patients who suffered from a major depression reported that both tinnitus and depression had begun within the same year, whereas the remaining 30% reported the onset of depression at a later date. A more precise investigation of the sequential interdependencies, especially in the area of the non-depressive psychiatric disorders, was not undertaken.

In patients with multiple psychiatric disorders, and perhaps additional somatic disorders, it appears that the sequence of occurrence has prognostic and therapeutic significance (compare with Winokur et al., 1988). Therefore, primary and secondary psychiatric disorders are differentiated. If the beginning of the tinnitus is taken as the critical point in time, a primary psychiatric disorder exists if the symptoms relevant to the psychiatric disorder have already existed before the onset of tinnitus. A secondary psychiatric disorder exists if the psychiatric symptoms develop following the onset of tinnitus.

4.2.2 Co-morbidity of psychiatric disorders

At this time the composition and pattern of the psychiatric disorders that occur in addition to tinnitus are also unclear. New systems of diagnoses, such as the DSM-III (and to a greater extent DSM-IIIR), favour the so-called principle of co-morbidity (or multiple diagnoses), whereby several psychiatric disorders can be diagnosed for a single patient. According to this concept, clinically relevant anxiety and depression, for example, are not summarized in a single primary psychiatric diagnosis; rather they are denoted as two separate diagnoses (anxiety and depressive disorders).

4.2.3 Examination goals

In order to obtain a more accurate impression of co-morbidity and the relationship between tinnitus and psychiatric disorders during the course of the whole medical history of the individual patient, we examined tinnitus patients according to primary and secondary psychiatric disorders as well as differences in the sequence of onset. The random survey of our study comes from a specialized psychosomatic and behavioral-therapy clinic. It is possible that another pattern of psychiatric disorders exists in patients who seek treatment for tinnitus in a psychosomatic clinic than in patients of a university clinic (where the studies of Harrop-Griffiths et al. at a tinnitus clinic and those of Simpson et al. at an ENT clinic were carried out). The psychiatric assessment of our patients was based on DSM-III-R (APA, 1987; Wittchen et al., 1989).

4.3 Methods

4.3.1 Random survey

A random sample of 26 patients with chronic and clinically relevant tinnitus was examined. They were admitted consecutively to the special ward for tinnitus and pain treatment at the Roseneck Clinic (Prien am Chiemsee) for psychotherapeutic treatment. Patients included 17 men (65%) and 9 women (35%), average age of 45.1 years (mean variation $s = 9.3$ years). Age varied between 28 and 63 years. At the time of admission, the patients had an (uninterrupted or recurring) duration of tinnitus of between 1 and 28 years (average duration 6.5 years; $s = 6.4$). In 20 patients (77%) an organic etiology of tinnitus (sudden deafness, noise trauma, other impairment from noise, acute infection) was present. In 21 patients (81%), slight to profound decrease in hearing in the ear affected by tinnitus or bilaterally was diagnosed. Twenty-one of the patients were married, 3 were single and 2 were divorced.

4.3.2 Diagnostic questionnaire: MDCL

All patients were interviewed comprehensively at the beginning of their treatment. At this time attention was given to the type, degree and previous course of the tinnitus and the entire spectrum of the most important and frequent psychiatric disorders was examined. Past as well as present disorders (in the sense of so-called 'lifetime' diagnoses) were taken into consideration. The Munich Diagnostic Checklist served as a questionnaire and introduction (MDCL; Hiller et al 1990 b; compare with tables in the appendix). This is a set of 30 checklists that can be used systematically to check diagnostic hypotheses and diagnoses according to DSM-III-R. The MDCL was developed especially for the demands of routine clinical diagnosis and diagnoses comparable in reliability to those made from structured and standardized interviews are possible (Hiller et al., 1990 a).

4.3.3 Disease profile

In addition, an individual so-called disease profile was constructed for every patient, which graphically clarified sequential relationships between tinnitus and psychiatric disorders as well as between different psychiatric disorders. The disease profiles were based extensively on the self-evaluations of the patients. During the initial examination, they were requested to date the beginning and end of the individual disorders as accurately as possible and to specify the course of the disorder on a subjective scale of intensity between 0% and 100%. The differentiation between primary and secondary psychiatric disorders resulted from the evaluation of the disease profile.

4.4 Results

4.4.1 Prevalence of psychiatric disorders

According to DSM-III-R a total of 25 of the 26 tinnitus patients examined (96%) fulfilled the criteria of at least one lifetime psychiatric disorder. In approximately half the patients in whom psychiatric symptoms occurred, the psychiatric symptoms were extensively described by a single diagnosis (13/25 = 52%). In the framework of the co-morbidity concept, 20% had two diagnoses (5/25) and in each of 12% of the patients, three or four diagnoses were made (3/35 each). The criteria for a total of six diagnoses were fulfilled in one patient. Panic disorders and agoraphobia have been treated as separate diagnoses in these figures (the combination diagnoses of panic disorder with agoraphobia cited in DSM-III-R was made in two cases).

Figure 4.1 shows the prevalence of psychiatric disorders (lifetime), of the random survey using bar graphs. An affective disorder was diagnosed most frequently at 85%. All patients of this group fulfilled the diagnostic

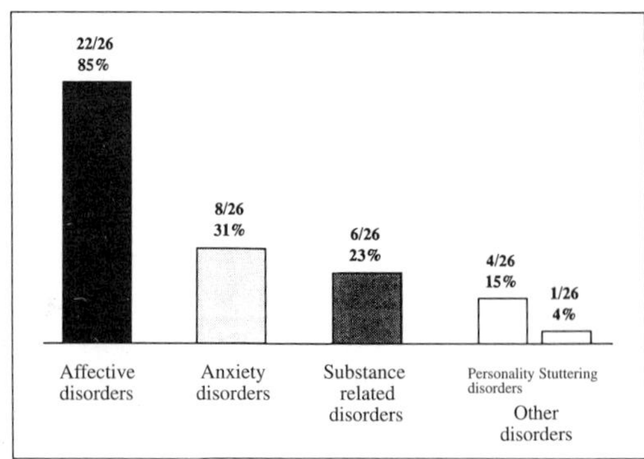

Fig. 4.1 Prevalence of psychiatric disturbances in patients with complex chronic tinnitus.

criteria of a disorder with depressive symptoms according to DSM-III-R. The numbers for anxiety and disorders due to the use of psychotropic substances were significantly smaller (31% and 23%, respectively). Personality disorders were seldom (15%). Chronic and clinically relevant stuttering was diagnosed in one patient (4%).

4.4.2 Affective disorders

Figure 4.2 gives an overall picture of the individual psychiatric diagnoses made in the random survey. A massively distinct depressive syndrome with the diagnosis of major depression was present in most cases in the affective disturbance group (65%), while dysthymia (mental depression), characterized by less serious depressive symptoms, was diagnosed significantly less frequently (15%). Three of the patients with major depression also satisfied the criteria for dysthymia because chronic distinctive symptoms had been present, which were often weaker or fluctuated initially, with additional episodes of major depression at a later point. If these patients were included in the group with dysthymia (instead of major depression), the average prevalence for dysthymia increased from 15% to 27% (7/26). In one of the three patients with the double diagnosis of dysthymia and major depression, an intensification of the depressive disorder (in the sense of a major depression) resulted after the onset of tinnitus, with a less serious depression (in the sense of a dysthymia) having existed previously. According to conventional nosology (Degkwitz et al., 1980) all patients with major depression and/or dysthymia would have been diagnosed as neurotic depression or a longer lasting depressive reaction, but in no case as endogenous depression.

All in all, the categories of diagnoses for affective disorders (Figure 4.2) show that serious and/or chronic depression in the patients examined were prevalent and short-term depressive reactions (4%) in the sense of an adaptive disorder were the exception.

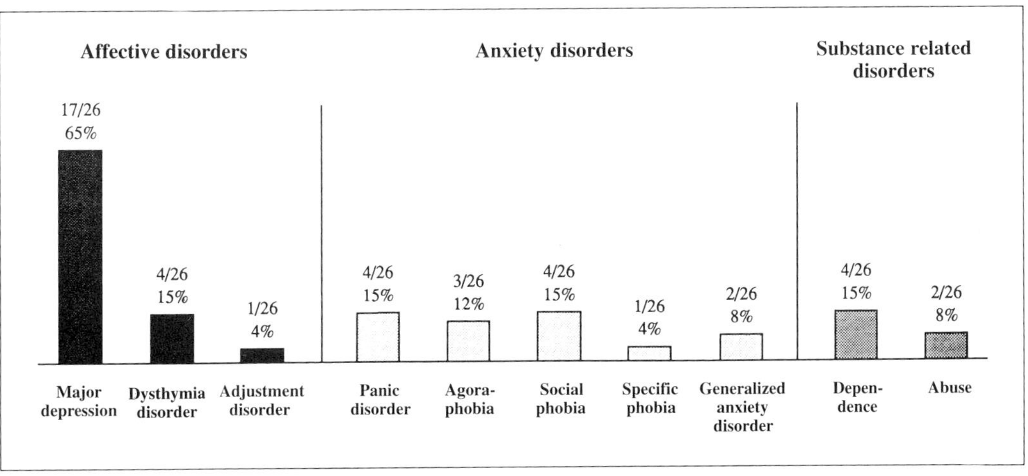

Fig. 4.2 Comorbidity of psychological disorders in patients with complex chronic tinnitus.

4.4.3 Anxiety

All forms of anxiety classified in DSM-III-R were diagnosed less frequently than depression. As Figure 4.2 shows, panic disorder was the most frequent (with 15% each time). In comparison, simple phobias were most seldom diagnosed (4%). The diagnosis of agoraphobia was made in 12% and generalized anxiety in 8% of tinnitus patients. In the case of anxiety, the number of diagnoses (14) exceeds the number of patients (8) (as a comparison of Figures 4.1 and 4.2 demonstrates) because the concept of co-morbidity allows multiple diagnoses. Only four of the eight patients had a single diagnosis in respect to possible anxiety disorders, whereas in the case of two patients, the criteria for two diagnoses and in two other patients, the criteria for three diagnoses were fulfilled.

4.4.4 Substance-related disorders

A similar frequency was found for the use of psychotropic substances as for anxiety and for slight distinctive depressive disorders. The diagnosis of alcohol dependence was made in two patients and (along with simultaneous chronic neuralgia of the trigeminal nerve) in one case each for benzodiazepine or carbamazepine. The abuse of psychotropic substances and alcohol was noted in one patient and of alcohol plus captagone in a second patient.

4.4.5 Personality disorders

Among the diagnosed disorders in personality (compare with Figure 4.1), anxiety and insecurity characteristics were predominant. One patient fulfilled the criteria for two personality disturbances (insecurity and dependence). In two patients, we diagnosed a personality disorder of insecurity, and in another patient a compulsive personality disorder.

4.4.6 Pain syndromes

In the analysis of symptoms and preliminary clinical findings, it was also apparent that 58% of the tinnitus patients examined complained of a clinically relevant chronic pain syndrome in the form of headache and back pain with insufficient organic etiology to explain the severity of experienced pain. One patient suffered from a chronic pain syndrome due to ankylolising spondylitis (Bechterev's disease).

4.4.7 Number of psychiatric diagnoses

In the 26 patients with complex chronic tinnitus, a total of 47 psychiatric diagnoses was made. This corresponded to an average of 1.81 diagnoses. If chronic pain is also accepted as psychiatric (in the sense of the aforementioned DSM–III–R category of pain syndrome), then there are an average of 2.38 diagnoses per patient, of a total of 62 diagnoses, in addition to the tinnitus (which was frequently accompanied by other physical disorders such as disturbances in hearing and dizziness).

4.4.8 Sequential relationships

Sequential relationships between tinnitus on the one hand and psychiatric disorders on the other hand are portrayed graphically in Figure 4.3. Here the percentage of the examined random survey group with psychiatric disorders arising before or after the beginning of tinnitus is shown. For all the psychiatric disorders and also for the subgroup of affective, anxiety and substance-related disorders, we determined nearly identical proportions for the differentiation of primary vs. secondary (between 45% and 55%) occurrence. According to this finding, psychiatric disorders occur nearly as often as preceding and thereby eventually predisposing conditions, as well as consequential complications. As Figure 4.3 shows, a tendency towards more serious depressive disorders in the sense of major depression occurs more often following onset of tinnitus (59%), whereas dysthymic disorders (with or without major depression), with their more often chronic course pre-existed more frequently (71%). Differentiation of preceding and subsequent disorders was omitted for the other diagnoses because of the small number of cases.

4.4.9 Course of disease

4.4.9.1 Example 1

Interdependencies between tinnitus and psychiatric disorders can be clarified with the aid of our diagrams. Figure 4.4 shows the course of tinnitus and psychiatrically relevant syndromes in a 34-year-old patient. The duration (in this case from 1985 until 1990) is marked on the abscissa and the degree of severity of the existing symptoms on the ordinate (between 0% and 100%).

The course portrayed in Figure 4.4 can be viewed as a typical example for a secondary psychiatric disorder. A major depression developed after the initial occurrence of tinnitus (beginning in 1988). As the diagram shows, tinnitus abruptly began immediately after sudden deafness and was perceived from the beginning as unbearable (rated by the patient as extremely loud = 100%). The depressive syndrome which developed in this situation was the result of decreased interest and happiness and characterized by lack of drive, severe self-doubt, pessimism and transient suicidal tendencies. The patient experienced this psychological condition for the first time in his life, because he had only identified brief changes in mood with slight passing despondency (clearly under the critical threshold for making a psychiatric diagnosis previously). The depressive syndrome decreased gradually, as did the tinnitus, over several months. A chronic pain syndrome (cervical syndrome) already existed before the beginning of the tinnitus. It was, however, perceived as serious and unbearable only after the onset of tinnitus.

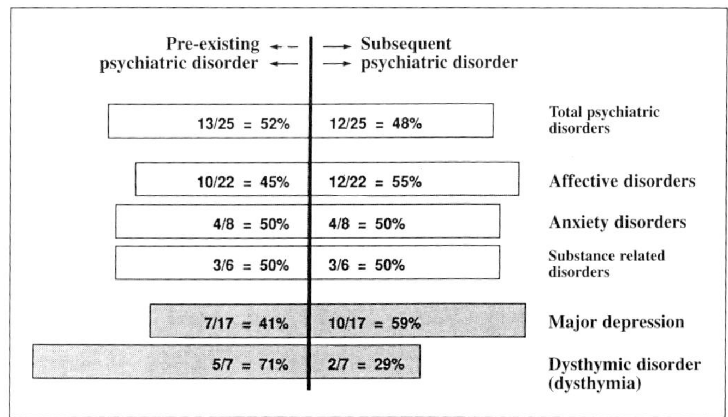

Fig. 4.3 Differentiation of pre-existing and subsequent psychiatric disorders in patients with complex chronic tinnitus.

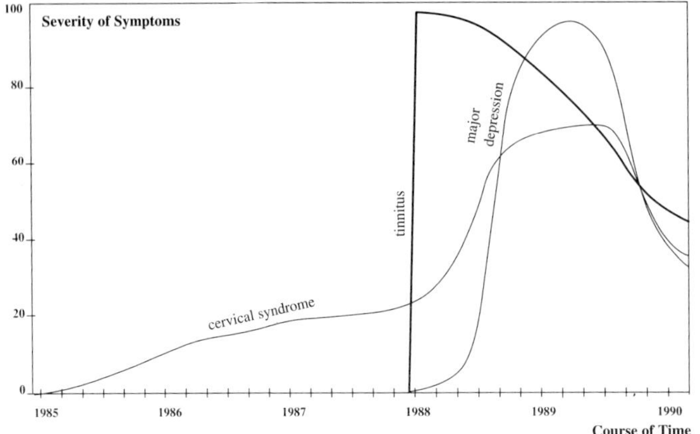

Fig. 4.4 Course of disease for tinnitus and psychiatric disorders in a 34-year-old patient. Central tinnitus (BERA) in the high frequency range, bilateral, maskable in the vicinity of the hearing threshold; first occurrence during an influenza infection and psychological stress.

4.4.9.2 Example 2

Finally, Figure 4.5 demonstrates the symptoms of a 28-year-old patient, in whom the psychiatric disorder preceded the beginning of tinnitus. The tinnitus occurred initially in 1989 following an acute infection and lasted (except for a period of complete remission of approximately three weeks) until the beginning of hospitalization. This patient had already suffered from pronounced anxiety since childhood. In the beginning, the symptoms were characterized by fear of thunder (under the diagnostic threshold), and later by social phobia, panic attacks, and subsequent agoraphobic fears (accompanied by a personality disorder with traits of self-doubt and anxiety). In addition, it resulted in development of depression since childhood (dysthymia with later episodes of a major depression). It is of interest that the tinnitus began at a point in time when the symptoms of anxiety were already fading (resulting from intensive out-patient psychotherapy); the depression, however, still existed.

4.5 Discussion

In this study, the revised edition of the psychiatric classification system DSM-III of 1987 (DSM-III-R) was incorporated for the first time to examine the type and extent of

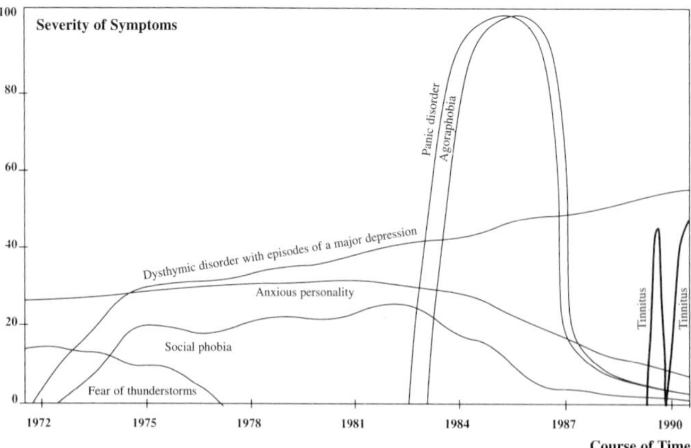

Fig. 4.5 Course of disease for tinnitus and psychiatric disorders in a 28-year-old patient. Bilateral cochlear tinnitus in high frequency range, indication of cervicogenic involvement; maskable in the vicinity of the hearing threshold (bilateral BERA, hearing threshold 20 dB).

psychiatric disorders in patients with complex, chronic tinnitus. In a random survey of patients who sought in-patient psychotherapeutic treatment because of tormenting ear noises and associated psychiatric disorders, we found almost without exception (96%) serious and psychologically relevant disorders of experience and behaviour. This corresponds with results from other studies which were carried out in clinics specializing in tinnitus and ENT diseases and in which just as many well-defined and criterion-based psychiatric diagnoses were used (Harrop-Griffiths et al., 1987; Simpson et al., 1988).

In the co-morbidity profile which we established, tinnitus was by far most frequently associated with pronounced affective disorders (85%). Serious depression developed in approximately half of the examined patients only after the beginning of tinnitus. In pre-existing and often chronic depressive disorders with tinnitus as an additional 'stressor', a dramatic increase of the depressive symptoms was observed. Anxiety and dependency/abuse of psychotropic substances were diagnosed significantly less frequently (31% and 23%) than affective disorders.

Depressive disorders in the form of a major depression were predominantly diagnosed in our tinnitus patients. This corresponds with the results of Harrop-Griffiths et al. (1987) and Simpson et al. (1988). Goebel et al. (1991; p. 117) came to contrary results as the diagnosis of dysthymia was made more frequently than major depression (75% vs. 11%). This study deals, however, with clinical routine diagnoses, which were given without an instrument and often without a systematic evaluation of individual diagnostic criteria. According to our observations, many clinical physicians and psychologists tend to classify long-term depression as dysthymia while, on the other hand, major depression is dealt with as being equivalent to endogenous depression. This corresponds neither with diagnostic criteria, nor with the basic concept of the category of major depression (APA, 1987). In a comparative study, it was shown that even long-lasting depression (in the sense of the earlier diagnosis of neurotic depression) is frequently so serious that the criteria of a major depression are satisfied (Hiller et al., 1988).

Our findings demonstrate that psychiatric disorders are the presumably most severe side-effect (or complication) in chronic tinnitus. The symptoms characterized in the present study clearly can be isolated from the normal fluctuation of psychological findings, because psychiatric diagnoses are justified only in clinically serious cases and, as a rule, imply consultation or treatment. DSM-III-R presupposes an objectively minimal degree of severity of the given characteristic psychiatric symptoms for all disorders that were taken into consideration in our study (for example, at least five depressive symptoms over at least 2 weeks for the diagnosis of a major depression).

Prevalence rates for psychiatric disorders in tinnitus, however, may not be interpreted independently from the selection and composition of the random sample we examined. It may be assumed for the patients in our study, that the motivation for psychotherapeutic treatment (admission to the clinic as selection criterion) was increased by the severity of the psychiatric symptoms. In patients with pre-existing (primary) psychiatric disorders, the tinnitus was the decisive factor for psychotherapeutic treatment which had already been necessary at an earlier date because of the primary disorder. If, on the other hand, tinnitus patients were examined who were not selected from the general population or were patients from ENT or a general practice, psychiatric disorders may have occurred significantly less frequently than in our clinical population (also compare Hallam, 1987).

Unexplained to great extent until now are the mechanisms of the presumably complex combined effects of tinnitus and psychiatric symptoms. Because tinnitus does not inevitably lead to serious psychiatric disorders (McKenna, publishing date in the near future), other etiologically relevant conditions must be taken into consideration. The acceptance of an individual variable such as psychological vulnerability could be helpful. Figure 4.6 depicts a model according to which such a psychological vulnerability in the sense of a reactivity or disposition can occur in varying degree (shaded area) in persons whose symptoms are not noticeable (compensated).

If a critical threshold of stress is crossed, decompensation or the development of a psychiatric disorder results (unshaded area), (Figure 4.6). Tinnitus can be seen as a stress factor that can trigger a psychiatric disorder only with considerable pre-existing vulnerability. In psychologically stable persons (i.e. persons with slight psychological vulnerability) the tinnitus disorder can be overcome without decompensation. Figure 4.6 contrasts two cases with tinnitus of the same degree, but with varying levels of vulnerability. The decompensation threshold is crossed only in one case by the combined effects of vulnerability and tinnitus disorder. According to this model, the existence of a psychiatric disorder must always be viewed as a function of tinnitus and a pre-existing psychological vulnerability.

4.6 Final conclusions

Different therapeutic goals and procedures can be deduced from the outlined concept. Adaptation to tinnitus, a presumably chronic physical symptom, should be encouraged primarily (acceptance and coping). In this way, a decrease in the acute psychological stress and a remission of the psychological disorder may be expected (compare with the declining line in Figure 4.6). What also appears to be decisive is the reduction of psychological vulnerability (e.g. stress reduction and coping strategies), in order to increase the 'psychic padding' of the patient so as to allow him to be more stable when faced with future burdens (including exacerbation of tinnitus). The psychiatric diagnoses determined in our random sample suggest that developing goal-oriented, antidepressive patterns of thinking and behaviour, as well as strategies to overcome anxiety, are important and should be available to the patient.

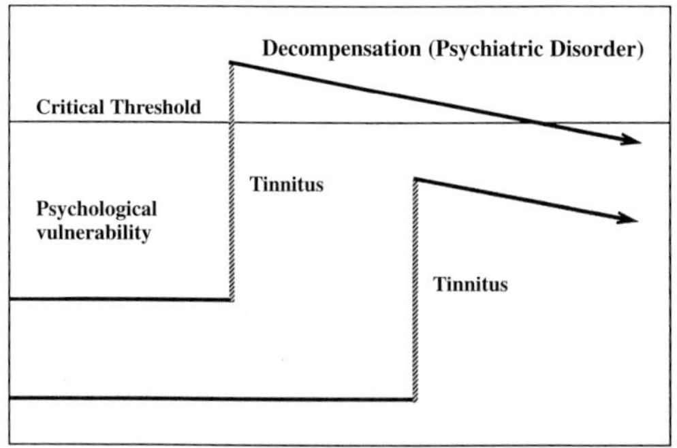

Fig. 4.6 Model of the combined effects of tinnitus and psychological vulnerability on psychiatric disorders.

4.7 References

American Psychiatric Association, APA (1980): Diagnostic and Statistical Manual of Mental Disorders, 3rd edition (DSM-III). APA, Washington DC.

American Psychiatric Association, APA (1987): Diagnostic and Statistical Manual of Mental Disorders, revised 3rd edition (DSM-III-R). APA, Washington DC.

Degkwitz, R., H. Helmchen, G. Kockott, W. Mombour (1980): Diagnoseschlüssel und Glossar psychiatrischer Krankheiten. Deutsche Ausgabe der Internationalen Klassifikation der Krankheiten der WHO, ICD, 9. Revision. Springer, Berlin.

Duckro, P.N., C.A. Pollard, H.D. Bray, L. Scheiter (1984): Comprehensive behavioral management of complex tinnitus: a case illustration. Biofeedback and Self-Regulation, 9, 459-469.

Goebel, G. (1989): Tinnitus. In: *Hand, I., H.-U. Wittchen* (Eds): Verhaltenstherapie in der Medizin. Springer, Berlin, 207-228.

Goebel, G., W. Keeser, M. Fichter, E. Rief (1991): Neue Aspekte des komplexen chronischen Tinnitus. Teil I: Überprüfung eines multimodalen verhaltensmedizinischen Behandlungskonzeptes; Teil II: Die verlorene Stille: Auswirkungen und psychotherapeutische Möglichkeiten beim komplexen chronischen Tinnitus. Psychother. med. Psychol. 41: 115-133.

Hallam, R.S. (1987): Psychological approaches to the evaluation and management of tinnitus distress. In: *Hazell, J.* (Ed.): Tinnitus. Churchill Livingstone, Edinburgh.

Harrop-Griffiths, J., W. Katon, R. Dobie, C. Sakai, J. Russo (1987): Chronic tinnitus: association with psychiatric diagnoses. Journal of Psychosomatic Research, 31: 613-621.

Hiller, W., W. Mombour, R. Rummler, J. Mittelhammer (1988): Divergence and convergence of diagnoses for depression between ICD-9 and DSM-III-R. European Archives of Psychiatry and Neurological Sciences, 238: 39-46.

Hiller, W., M. von Bose, G. Dichtl, D. Agerer (1990a): Reliability of checklist-guided diagnoses for DSM-III-R affective and anxiety disorders. Journal of Affective Disorders, 20: 235-247.

Hiller, W., M. Zaudig, W. Mombour (1990b): Development of diagnostic checklists for use in routine clinical care. Archives of General Psychiatry, 47: 782-784.

House, P.R. (1981): Personality of the tinnitus patient. In: Tinnitus: CIBA Foundation Symposium 85. Pitman Books, London, 193-203.

Jakes, S.C., R.S. Hallam, C. Chambers, R. Hinchcliffe (1985): A factor analytical study of tinnitus complaint behaviour. Audiology, 24: 195-206.

McKenna, L., R.S. Hallam, R. Hinchcliffe (at press): The prevalence of psychological disturbance in neuro-otology outpatients. Clinical Otolaryngology.

Reich, G.E., R.M. Johnson (1984): Personality characteristics of tinnitus patients. Journal of Laryngology and Otology, 9: 228-232.

Semler, G., H.-U. Wittchen, K. Joschke, M. Zaudig, T. von Geiso, S. Kaiser, M. von Cranach, H. Pfister (1987): Test-retest reliability of a standardized psychiatric interview (DIS/CIDI). European Archives of Psychiatry and Neurological Sciences, 236: 214-222.

Simpson, R.B., J.M. Nedzelski, H.O. Barber, M.R. Thomas (1988): Psychiatric diagnoses in patients with psychogenic dizziness or severe tinnitus. The Journal of Otolaryngology, 17: 325-330.

Stephens, R.D.G., R.S. Hallam (1985): The Crown-Crisp Experiential Index in patients complaining of tinnitus. British Journal of Audiology, 19: 151-158.

Tyler, R.S., L.J. Baker (1983): Difficulties experienced by tinnitus sufferers. Journal of Speech and Hearing Disorders, 48: 150-164.

Wittchen, H.-U., H. Saß, M. Zaudig, K. Köhler (Eds) (1989): Diagnostisches und Statistiches Manual Psychischer Störungen, DSM-III-R. Belz, Weinheim.

Winokur, G., D.W. Black, A. Nasrallah (1988): Depression secondary to other psychiatric disorders and medical illnesses. American Journal of Psychiatry, 145: 233-237.

Appendix

International Diagnostic Checklist for DSM-IV (IDCL): psychiatric diagnosis checklist according to Diagnostic and Statistical Manual of Mental Disorders IV. The IDCL (Hiller et al, 1996) was published and copyrighted by Hogrefe & Hüber Publishers, Toronto, Canada. In general only minor differences exist between DSM-III-R criteria as mentioned in this article and updated DSM-IV criteria.

IDCL *International Diagnostic Checklist for DSM-IV*

Generalized Anxiety Disorder

Name: ______
Age: ___ Date: ______

A *Excessive anxiety and worry* (apprehensive expectation), occurring more days than not for at least *6 months*, about a number of events or activities (such as work or school performance).

No ☐ (Stop) Probably ☐ Yes ☐

Describe the anxiety and worry:

B The person finds it difficult to *control* the worry.

No ☐ (Stop) Probably ☐ Yes ☐

C **• Determine which symptoms are usually present in the period coded above**

	Probably	Yes
(1) Restlessness or feeling keyed up or on edge	☐	☐
(2) Being easily fatigued	☐	☐
(3) Difficulty concentrating or mind going blank	☐	☐
(4) Irritability	☐	☐
(5) Muscle tension	☐	☐
(6) Sleep disturbance (difficulty falling or staying asleep, or restless unsatisfying sleep)	☐	☐

Criterion C: At least 3 of the symptoms (1) to (6) with at least some symptoms present for more days than not for the above period of at least 6 months.
Note: For children, only 1 symptom is required.

No ☐ (Stop) Probably ☐ Yes ☐

D The focus of the anxiety and worry is *not* confined to features of an Axis I disorder

e.g. the anxiety and worry is not about having a Panic Attack (as in Panic Disorder), being embarrassed in public (as in Social Phobia), being contaminated (as in Obsessive-Compulsive Disorder), being away from home or close relatives (as in Separation Anxiety Disorder), gaining weight (as in Anorexia nervosa), having multiple physical complaints (as in Somatization Disorder), or having a serious illness (as in Hypochondriasis), and the anxiety and worry do not occur exclusively during Posttraumatic Stress Disorder.

not met ☐ (Stop) Probably ☐ met ☐

Generalized Anxiety Disorder *Page 2*

Specify if symptomatology is current or previous:

☐ Yes ☐ Probably	☐ Yes ☐ Probably	☐ Yes ☐ Probably
Current: Symptomatology exists currently for the first time.	**Current and previous:** Symptomatology exists currently, and it had also been present in past history.	**Previous:** Symptomatology existed in past history (specify: ______)

E The anxiety, worry, or physical symptoms cause clinically significant *distress* or *impairment* in social, occupational, or other important areas of functioning.

No ☐ (Stop) Probably ☐ Yes ☐

F <u>Rule out:</u> Direct organic causes of the disturbance and some specific other mental disorders

The disturbance *is due* to the direct physiological effects of a substance (e.g., drugs, medication) or a general medical condition (e.g., hyperthyroidism) <u>or</u> occurs *exclusively* during a Mood Disorder, a Psychotic Disorder, or a Pervasive Developmental Disorder.

Yes ☐ (Stop) Probably ☐ No ☐

If criteria A to F are met:

Generalized Anxiety Disorder | 3 | 0 | 0. | 0 | 2 |

☐ not met ☐ probably met ☐

• If a clinically relevant symptomatology is or was present, consider other possible categories (use the corresponding IDCL):

Specific Phobia (300.29) or Social Phobia (300.23)	Probably ☐	Yes ☐
Anxiety Disorder due to a General Medical Condition (293.89)	Probably ☐	Yes ☐
Substance-Induced Anxiety Disorder	Probably ☐	Yes ☐
Residual Category: Anxiety Disorder NOS (300.00)	Probably ☐	Yes ☐

IDCL *International Diagnostic Checklist for DSM-IV*

Panic Disorder

Name: ______

Age: ____ Date: ______

A1 Recurrent *unexpected Panic Attacks*

Check if the below criteria for a Panic Attack are fulfilled:

A Panic Attack is defined

- as a *discrete period* of intense fear or discomfort,
- in which *at least four* of the following symptoms develop abruptly and reach a peak within *10 minutes*

	Probably	Yes		Probably	Yes
(1) Palpitations, pounding heart, or accelerated heart rate	☐	☐	(8) Feeling dizzy, unsteady, lightheaded, or faint	☐	☐
(2) Sweating	☐	☐	(9) Derealization (feelings of unreality) or depersonalization (being detached from oneself)	☐	☐
(3) Trembling or shaking	☐	☐	(10) Fear of losing control or going crazy	☐	☐
(4) Sensations of shortness of breath or smothering	☐	☐	(11) Fear of dying	☐	☐
(5) Feeling of choking	☐	☐	(12) Paresthesias (numbness or tingling sensations)	☐	☐
(6) Chest pain or discomfort	☐	☐	(13) Chills or hot flushes	☐	☐
(7) Nausea or abdominal distress	☐	☐			

Decide if the above criterion (A1) of recurrent unexpected Panic Attacks is met: Stop ← ☐ not met ☐ Probably ☐ met

A2 Define some consequences of the Panic Attacks

At least one the Panic Attacks has been *followed* by 1 month (or more) of the following:

	No	Probably	Yes
(a) Persistent concern about having *additional attacks*	☐	☐	☐
(b) Worry about the *implications of the attack* or its consequences (e.g., losing control, having a heart attack, "going crazy")	☐	☐	☐
(c) A significant *change in behavior* related to the attacks	☐	☐	☐
At least 1 item out of (a) to (c)	☐ Stop ↵	☐	☐

Panic Disorder *Page 2*

Specify if the panic symptomatology is current or previous:

☐ Yes ☐ Probably
Current: Symptomatology exists currently for the first time.

☐ Yes ☐ Probably
Current and previous: Symptomatology exists currently, and it had also been present in past history.

☐ Yes ☐ Probably
Previous: Symptomatology existed in past history (specify: ______)

C Rule out: Direct organic causes of the Panic Attacks

The Panic Attacks *are due* to the direct physiological effects of a substance (e.g., drugs, medication) or a general medical condition (e.g., hyperthyroidism). Stop ↵ ☐ Yes ☐ Probably ☐ No

D The Panic Attacks are *better* accounted for by another mental disorder Stop ↵ ☐ Yes ☐ Probably ☐ No

such as Social Phobia (e.g., occurring on exposure to feared social situations), Specific Phobia (e.g., on exposure to a specific phobic situation), Obsessive-Compulsive Disorder (e.g., on exposure to dirt in someone with an obsession about contamination), Posttraumatic Stress Disorder (e.g., in response to stimuli associated with a severe stressor), or Separation Anxiety Disorder (e.g., in response to being away from home or close relatives).

If criteria A1, A2, C, and D are met:

Panic Disorder ☐ met ☐ probably ☐ not met

- If a clinically relevant symptomatology is or was present, consider other possible categories (use the corresponding IDCL):

	Probably	Yes
Specific Phobia (300.29)	☐	☐
Social Phobia (300.23)	☐	☐
Anxiety Disorder due to a General Medical Condition (293.89)	☐	☐
Substance-Induced Anxiety Disorder	☐	☐
Adjustment Disorder With Anxiety (309.24)	☐	☐
Residual Category: Anxiety Disorder NOS (300.00)	☐	☐

- Define the type of Panic Disorder: With or Without Agoraphobia (pages 3 and 4)

Panic Disorder: Diagnostic Assignment

According to criterion B of Panic Disorder, the exact diagnosis depends on the presence or absence of Agoraphobia. Therefore, check the criteria of Agorapobia:

(a) *Anxiety* about being in places or situations from which escape might be difficult (or embarrassing) or in which help might not be available in the event of having an unexpected or situationally predisposed Panic Attack or panic-like symptoms.

No ☐ (Stop ←) Probably ☐ Yes ☐

Note: Consider Specific Phobia if the avoidance is limited to one or only a few specific situations, or Social Phobia if the avoidance is limited to social situations.

Specify the agoraphobic situations:

Yes	Probably	
☐	☐	being outside the home alone/ being home alone
☐	☐	being in a crowd or standing in a line
☐	☐	being on a bridge
☐	☐	traveling in a bus, train, or automobile
☐	☐	other situations; specify:

(b) Define some consequences of the agoraphobic anxiety

The anxiety coded above under (a) leads to the following *consequences:*

	No	Probably	Yes
(a) The situations are *avoided* (e.g., travel is restricted)	☐	☐	☐
(b) The situations are *endured* with marked distress or with anxiety about having a Panic Attack or panic-like symptoms	☐	☐	☐
(c) The situations require the *presence of a companion*	☐	☐	☐
Criterion (b): At least 1 item out of (a) to (c)	☐ Stop ←	☐	☐

(c) The anxiety or phobic avoidance is *better* accounted for by another mental disorder

Yes ☐ (Stop ←) Probably ☐ No ☐

such as Social Phobia (e.g., avoidance limited to social situations because of fear of embarrassment), Specific Phobia (e.g., avoidance limited to a single situation like elevators), Obsessive-Compulsive Disorder (e.g., avoidance of dirt in someone with an obsession about contamination), Posttraumatic Stress Disorder (e.g., avoidance of stimuli associated with a severe stressor), or Separation Anxiety Disorder (e.g., avoidance of leaving home or relatives).

Specify if the agoraphobic anxiety is current or previous:

☐ Yes ☐ Probably
Current: Symptomatology exists currently for the first time.

☐ Yes ☐ Probably
Current and previous: Symptomatology exists currently, and it had also been present in past history.

☐ Yes ☐ Probably
Previous: Symptomatology existed in past history (specify: ____________)

If criteria (a) to (c) for Agoraphobia are not met:

Panic Disorder
Without Agoraphobia

☐ probably ☐ Yes

3	0	0.	0	1

If criteria (a) to (c) for Agoraphobia are met:

Panic Disorder
With Agoraphobia

☐ probably ☐ Yes

3	0	0.	2	1

IDCL — *International Diagnostic Checklist for DSM-IV*

Agoraphobia

Name: ____________

Age: _____ Date: ____________

Aa *Anxiety* about being in places or situations from which escape might be difficult (or embarrassing) or in which help might not be available in the event of having an unexpected or situationally predisposed Panic Attack or panic-like symptoms. — ☐ No (Stop) ☐ Probably ☐ Yes

Note: Consider Specific Phobia if the avoidance is limited to one or only a few specific situations, or Social Phobia if the avoidance is limited to social situations.

Specify the agoraphobic situations:

Yes	Probably	
☐	☐	being outside the home alone/ being home alone
☐	☐	being in a crowd or standing in a line
☐	☐	being on a bridge
☐	☐	traveling in a bus, train, or automobile
☐	☐	other situations; specify:

Ab Define some consequences of the agoraphobic anxiety

The anxiety coded above under Aa leads to the following *consequences:*

	No	Probably	Yes
(a) The situations are *avoided* (e.g., travel is restricted)	☐	☐	☐
(b) The situations are *endured* with marked distress or with anxiety about having a Panic Attack or panic-like symptoms	☐	☐	☐
(c) The situations require the *presence of a companion*	☐	☐	☐
Criterion Ab: At least 1 item out of (a) to (c)	☐ (Stop)	☐	☐

Ac The anxiety or phobic avoidance is *better* accounted for by another mental disorder — ☐ Yes (Stop) ☐ Probably ☐ No

such as Social Phobia (e.g., avoidance limited to social situations because of fear of embarrassment), Specific Phobia (e.g., avoidance limited to a single situation like elevators), Obsessive-Compulsive Disorder (e.g., avoidance of dirt in someone with an obsession about contamination), Posttraumatic Stress Disorder (e.g., avoidance of stimuli associated with a severe stressor), or Separation Anxiety Disorder (e.g., avoidance of leaving home or relatives).

Agoraphobia — *Page 2*

Specify if symptomatology is current or previous:

☐ Yes ☐ Probably	☐ Yes ☐ Probably	☐ Yes ☐ Probably
Current: Symptomatology exists currently for the first time.	**Current and previous:** Symptomatology exists currently, and it had also been present in past history.	**Previous:** Symptomatology existed in past history (specify: ________)

B Rule out: History of a Panic Disorder

Criteria have *ever* been met for Panic Disorder. — ☐ Yes (Stop) ☐ Probably ☐ No

Check the diagnostic criteria of Panic Disorder more carefully with the corresponding IDCL.

C Rule out: Direct organic causes of the disturbance

The disturbance *is due* to the direct physiological effects of a substance (e.g., drugs, medication) or a general medical condition. — ☐ Yes (Stop) ☐ Probably ☐ No

D If an associated general medical condition is present, the fear described in criteria Aa to Ac is clearly in excess of that usually associated with the condition. — ☐ not met (Stop) ☐ Probably ☐ met

Note: If no such associated general medical condition is present, consider criterion D as met.

If criteria Aa to Ac and B to D are met: **3 0 0. 2 2**

Agoraphobia

Without History of Panic Disorder

☐ not met ☐ probably ☐ met

- If a clinically relevant symptomatology is or was present, consider other possible categories (use the corresponding IDCL):

Other specific Anxiety Disorder (specify: ____________) ☐ Probably ☐ Yes

Residual Category: Anxiety Disorder NOS (300.00) ☐ Probably ☐ Yes

IDCL — *International Diagnostic Checklist for DSM-IV*

Dysthymic Disorder

Name: ____________________

Age: _____ *Date:* ____________

A *Depressed mood,* for most of the day, for more days than not, for at least 2 years, as indicated indicated either by subjective account or observation by others.
Note: In children and adolescents, mood can be irritable and duration must be at least 1 year.

No ☐ (Stop) — Probably ☐ — Yes ☐

B
- Define the pattern of depressive symptomatology
- All symptoms must be present in the same 2-year period
- Relate all symptoms to periods with depressed mood
- Consider only symptoms without direct organic causes

		No	Probably	Yes
(1)	*Poor appetite* or *overeating*	☐	☐	☐
(2)	*Insomnia* or *hypersomnia*	☐	☐	☐
(3)	*Low energy* or fatigue	☐	☐	☐
(4)	*Low self-esteem*	☐	☐	☐
(5)	*Poor concentration* or difficulties making *decisions*	☐	☐	☐
(6)	Feelings of *hopelessness*	☐	☐	☐
	At least 2 items from (1) to (6)	☐ (Stop)	☐	☐

C Interval *without* the symptoms in criteria A and B for more than 2 months at a time (during the period coded under criterion A).

Yes ☐ (Stop) — Probably ☐ — No ☐

Specify if symptomatology is current or previous:

☐ Yes ☐ Probably	☐ Yes ☐ Probably	☐ Yes ☐ Probably
Last 2 years: Symptomatology existed in the last 2 years for the first time.	**Last 2 years and previous:** Symptomatology existed in the last 2 years, and there have been similar periods in past history.	**Previous:** Symptomatology existed in past history over a period of 2 years or longer. (time frame: ________)

Dysthymic Disorder — *Page 2*

D The diagnoses of *Dysthymic Disorder* and *Major Depressive Disorder* exclude each other under certain conditions. In order to decide if criterion D of Dysthymic Disorder is met, it is necessary to determine if there has *ever* been a Major Depressive Episode (e.g., use the IDCL "Major Depressive Episode" for this purpose).

Criterion D of Dysthymic Disorder is met under the following conditions:

- *No* Major Depressive Episode has been present during *the first 2 years* of the disturbance (1 year for children and adolescents).
- If a Major Depressive Episode had been present *prior* to the symptomatology of a Dysthymic Disorder, an interval *without* significant signs and symptoms (i.e., full remission) of at least 2 months is required between the Major Depressive Episode and the development of the Dysthymic Disorder.
- Superimposed Episodes of Major Depression may occur in Dysthymic Disorder. However, no Major Depressive Episodes may have been present *during the initial 2 years* of Dysthymic Disorder (1 year for children and adolescents).

Decide if criterion D is met: not met ☐ (Stop) — Probably ☐ — met ☐

E Rule out: Manic and hypomanic symptoms

At some time, there has been a *Manic, Mixed,* or *Hypomanic Episode,* or criteria have been met for *Cyclothymic Disorder.*

Yes ☐ (Stop) — Probably ☐ — No ☐

F Rule out: Any chronic Psychotic Disorder

The disturbance occurs *exclusively* during the course of a chronic Psychotic Disorder (such as Schizophrenia or Delusional Disorder).

Yes ☐ (Stop) — Probably ☐ — No ☐

G Rule out: Direct organic causes of the depression

The symptoms *are due* to the direct effects of a substance (e.g., drugs, medication) or a general medical condition (e.g., hypothyroidism).

Yes ☐ (Stop) — Probably ☐ — No ☐

H The symptoms cause clinically significant *distress* or *impairment* in social, occupational, or other important areas of functioning.

No ☐ (Stop) — Probably ☐ — Yes ☐

Dysthymic Disorder *Page 3*

If criteria A to H are met:

Dysthymic Disorder

3 0 0. 4

☐ met ☐ probably not met ☐

- Specify Early or Late Onset and presence or absence of Atypical Features

Early onset:

Before age 21 years — Yes ☐ Probably ☐

Late onset:

Age 21 years or older — Yes ☐ Probably ☐

- If a clinically relevant symptomatology is or was present, consider the other diagnoses on the bottom of this page

Note: It is generally possible that criteria are met for both Dysthymic Disorder and Major Depressive Episode (c.f. criterion D of Dysthymic Disorder).

In this case, both diagnoses may be given: **Dysthymic Disorder with superimposed Episodes of Major Depression.**

Atypical Features	No	Probably	Yes
(A) Mood reactivity (i.e., brightens in response to positive events)	☐	☐	☐
(B1) Significant weight gain or increase in appetite	☐	☐	☐
(B2) Hypersomnia	☐	☐	☐
(B3) Leaden paralysis (i.e. heavy, leaden feelings in extremities)	☐	☐	☐
(B4) Long-standing pattern of interpersonal rejection sensitivity (not limited to episodes of mood distrubance) that results in significant social or occupational impairment	☐	☐	☐
(C) Criteria are not met for With Melancholic Features or With Catatonic Features for the same episode	☐	☐	☐
With Atypical Features: Item A plus item C plus at least 2 items from (B1) to (B4)	☐	☐	☐

Other diagnoses for disorders with depressive symptomatology:

Major Depressive Disorder (296.xx)	Probably ☐	Yes ☐
Bipolar Disorder (296.xx) or Cyclothymic Disorder (301.13)	Probably ☐	Yes ☐
Residual Category: Depressive Disorder NOS (311)	Probably ☐	Yes ☐

IDCL *International Diagnostic Checklist for DSM-IV*

Major Depressive Episode

Name: ______________________

Age: _____ Date: ______________

A

- Define the pattern of depressive symptomatology.
- Each symptom must have been present for at least two weeks and all symptoms must relate to the same 2-week period.
- Each symptom must represent a change from previous functioning.
- Do not include symptoms that are clearly due to a general medical condition, or mood-incongruent delusions or hallucinations.

		No	Probably	Yes
(1)	*Depressed mood* most of the day (nearly every day). Note: Mood can be irritable in children and adolescents.	☐	☐	☐
(2)	Markedly *diminished interest* or *pleasure* in or all, or almost all, activities most of the day (nearly every day).	☐	☐	☐
(3)	Decrease or increase in *appetite* (nearly every day), or significant weight loss when not dieting or weight gain. Note: In children, consider failure to make expected weight gains.	☐	☐	☐
(4)	*Insomnia* or *hypersomnia* (nearly every day).	☐	☐	☐
(5)	Observable *psychomotor agitation* or *retardation* (nearly every day).	☐	☐	☐
(6)	*Fatigue* or *loss of energy* (nearly every day).	☐	☐	☐
(7)	Feelings of *worthlessness* or excessive or inappropriate *guilt* (nearly every day) (not merely self-reproach or guilt about being sick).	☐	☐	☐
(8)	Diminished ability to *think* or *concentrate*, or indecisiveness (nearly every day).	☐	☐	☐
(9)	Recurrent thoughts of death or *suicide* (not just fear of dying), or a suicide attempt or a specific plan for committing suicide.	☐	☐	☐
	At least 5 items from (1) to (9), including (1) or (2)	☐ Stop ↵	☐	☐

Specify if symptomatology is current or previous:

☐ Yes ☐ Probably	☐ Yes ☐ Probably	☐ Yes ☐ Probably
Current: Symptomatology exists currently for the first time.	**Current and previous:** Symptomatology exists currently, and it had also been present in past history.	**Previous:** Symptomatology existed in past history (specify:_____________)

Major Depressive Episode *Page 2*

B

Rule out: Concurrent manic symptoms

The symptoms meet the criteria for a *Mixed Affective Episode*

Note: Mixed Episode is diagnosed if the criteria are met for both a Manic Episode and for a Major Depressive Episode (except for duration) nearly every day during at least a 1-week period.

Yes ☐ → Stop Probably ☐ No ☐

C

The symptoms cause clinically significant *distress* or *impairment* in social, occupational, or other important areas of functioning.

Stop ← No ☐ Probably ☐ Yes ☐

D

Rule out: Direct organic causes of the depression

The symptoms *are due* to the direct physiological effects of a substance (e.g., drugs, medication) or a general medical condition (e.g., hypothyroidism).

Stop ← Yes ☐ Probably ☐ No ☐

E

Rule out: Bereavement (V62.82)

The symptoms are not better accounted for by Bereavement.

Note: Bereavement is diagnosed if depressive symptoms develop after the death of a loved one, persist for no longer than 2 months and if there is no functional impairment, morbid preoccupation with worthlessness, suicidal ideation, psychotic symptoms, or psychomotor retardation.

Decide if criterion E is met: Stop ← not met ☐ Probably ☐ met ☐

If criteria A to E are met:

Major Depressive Episode

☐ met
☐ probably
☐ not met

- If a clinically relevant symptomatology is or was present, consider other possible categories (use the corresponding IDCL):
- Determine the appropriate diagnosis (page 3).

Dysthymic Disorder (300.4)	Probably ☐	Yes ☐
Adjustment Disorder With Depressed Mood (309.0)	Probably ☐	Yes ☐
Bipolar Disorder or Cyclothymic Disorder	Probably ☐	Yes ☐
Residual Category: Depressive Disorder NOS (311)	Probably ☐	Yes ☐

Major Depressive Episode *Page 3*

Major Depressive Episode: Diagnostic Assignment

General exclusion criteria for Major Depressive Disorder

		Yes	Probably	No
#1	*Rule out: Bipolar Disorders* There has ever been a Manic, Mixed, or Hypomanic Episode. Note: Do not count any manic-like, mixed-like, or hypomanic-like episodes that were substance or treatment induced, or due to the direct physiological effects of a general medical condition.	☐ ↓ Stop	☐	☐
#2	*Rule out: Schizophrenia and Other Psychotic Disorders* The Major Depressive Episodes are better accounted for by Schizoaffective Disorder or are superimposed on Schizophrenia, Schizophreniform Disorder, Delusional Disorder, or Psychotic Disorder NOS.	☐ ↓ Stop	☐	☐

Type of Major Depressive Disorder

	Probably	Yes	
Major Depressive Disorder, Single Episode Only a single (i.e., the first) Major Depressive Episode.	☐	☐	2
Major Depressive Disorder, Recurrent Presence (and history) of two or more Major Depressive Episodes, separated by an interval of at least 2 consecutive months in which criteria are not met for a Major Depressive Episode.	☐	☐	3

Diagnosis:

2	9	6.		

Fill in: **Fourth digit of diagnosis**
Type of Major Depressive Disorder

Fill in: **Fifth digit of diagnosis**
Severity of current state

mild symptomatology = 1
moderate symptomatology = 2
severe symptomatology, without psychotic features = 3
severe symptomatology, with psychotic features = 4
in partial remission = 5
in full remission = 6
unspecified = 0

Major Depressive Episode *Page 4*

Specify: Melancholic Features	No	Probably	Yes
(A1) Loss of pleasure in all, or almost all, activities	☐	☐	☐
(A2) Lack of reactivity to usually pleasurable stimuli	☐	☐	☐
(B1) Distinct quality of depressed mood i.e., different from feelings experienced after the death of a loved one	☐	☐	☐
(B2) Depression regularly worse in the morning	☐	☐	☐
(B3) Early morning awakening (at least 2 hours before usual time)	☐	☐	☐
(B4) Marked psychomotor retardation or agitation	☐	☐	☐
(B5) Significant anorexia or weight loss	☐	☐	☐
(B6) Excessive or inappropriate guilt	☐	☐	☐
With Melancholic Features: At least 1 item from (A1) and (A2) plus at least 3 items from (B1) to (B6)	☐	☐	☐

Specify: Atypical Features	No	Probably	Yes
(A) Mood reactivity (i.e., brightens in response to positive events)	☐	☐	☐
(B1) Significant weight gain or increase in appetite	☐	☐	☐
(B2) Hypersomnia	☐	☐	☐
(B2) Leaden paralysis (i.e. heavy, leaden feelings in extremities)	☐	☐	☐
(B3) Long-standing pattern of interpersonal rejection sensitivity (not limited to episodes of mood disturbance) that results in significant social or occupational impairment	☐	☐	☐
(C) Criteria are not met for With Melancholic Features or With Catatonic Features for the same episode	☐	☐	☐
With Atypical Features: Item A plus item C plus at least 2 items from (B1) to (B4)	☐	☐	☐

Specify: Longitudinal Course	No	Probably	Yes
With Full Interepisode Recovery full remission is attained between the two most recent mood episodes	☐	☐	☐

Specify: Chronic	No	Probably	Yes
Chronic full criteria for a Major Depressive Disorder have been met continuously for at least the past 2 years	☐	☐	☐

IDCL *International Diagnostic Checklist for DSM-IV*

Substance Dependence and Abuse

Name: ____________________

Age: _____ *Date:* ______________

- Define the characteristic maladaptive pattern of substance use
- Relate all symptoms to *the same* substance
- The single symptoms as listed below must have occurred at any time in *the same 12-month period*

	No	Probably	Yes
(1) *Tolerance* as defined by: (a) a need for markedly increased amounts of the substance to achieve intoxication or desired effects, or (b) markedly diminished effect with continued use of the same amount of the substance.	☐	☐	☐
(2) *Withdrawal* as defined by: (a) a characteristic withdrawal syndrome for the substance, or (b) the same (or closely related) substance is taken to relieve or avoid withdrawal symptoms.	☐	☐	☐
(3) The substance is often taken in *larger amounts* or *over a longer period* than was intended.	☐	☐	☐
(4) There is a persistent desire or unsuccessful efforts to *cut down* or *control* substance use.	☐	☐	☐
(5) A *great deal of time* is spent in activities necessary to obtain the substance (e.g., visiting multiple doctors or driving long distances), use the substance (e.g., chain-smoking), or recover from its effects.	☐	☐	☐
(6) Important social, occupational, or recreational activities are *given up* or *reduced* because of substance use.	☐	☐	☐
(7) The substance use is continued *despite knowledge* of having a persistent or recurrent physical or psychological problem that is likely to have been caused or exacerbated by the substance e.g., current cocaine use despite recognition of cocaine-induced depression.	☐	☐	☐

At least 3 symptoms from (1) to (7), leading to clinically significant impairment or distress:

Substance Dependence No ☐ Probably ☐ Yes ☐

- Check if criteria for Substance Abuse are met (page 3)
- Determine the appropriate diagnosis according to the specific substance and check the specifiers (page 2)

Substance Dependence and Abuse *Page 2*

Specify if symptomatology is current or previous:

☐ Yes ☐ Probably	☐ Yes ☐ Probably	☐ Yes ☐ Probably
Current: Symptomatology exists currently for the first time.	**Current and previous:** Symptomatology exists currently, and it had also been present in past history.	**Previous:** Symptomatology existed in past history (specify: ____________)

Diagnostic assignment of the Substance Dependence: Specify the drug of abuse or medication

Substance	Code	Yes	Probably
Amphetamine:	304.40	☐	☐
Cannabis:	304.30	☐	☐
Cocaine:	304.20	☐	☐
Hallucinogen:	304.50	☐	☐
Inhalant:	304.60	☐	☐
Nicotine:	305.10	☐	☐
Opioid:	304.00	☐	☐
Phencyclidine:	304.90	☐	☐
Sedative, Hypnotic, or Anxiolytic:	304.10	☐	☐
Polysubstance Dependence:	304.80	☐	☐
Other (or Unknown) Substance Dependence:	304.90	☐	☐

Specify other features of the Substance Dependence

Course Specifiers:	Yes	Probably
Early Full Remission (1-11 months)	☐	☐
Early Partial Remission (1-11 months)	☐	☐
Sustained Full Remission (≥ 12 months)	☐	☐
Sustained Partial Remission (≥ 12 months)	☐	☐
On Agonist Therapy	☐	☐
In a Controlled Environment	☐	☐

With Physiological Dependence:

There is evidence of tolerance or withdrawal (i.e., one of the items 1 or 2 is present)

☐ Yes ☐ Probably

Substance Dependence and Abuse *Page 3*

Substance Abuse

- Define the characteristic maladaptive pattern of substance use
- Relate all symptoms to *the same* substance
- The single symptoms as listed below must have occurred at any time in *the same 12-month period*

	No	Probably	Yes
(1) Recurrent substance use resulting in a failure to fulfill major role obligations at work, school, or home e.g., repeated absences or poor work performance related to substance use; substance-related absences, suspensions, or expulsions from school; neglect of children or household.	❑	❑	❑
(2) Recurrent substance use in situations in which it is physically hazardous e.g., driving an automobile or operating a machine when impaired by substance use.	❑	❑	❑
(3) Recurrent substance-related legal problems e.g., arrests for substance-related disorderly conduct.	❑	❑	❑
(4) Continued substance use despite having persistent or recurrent social or interpersonal problems caused or exacerbated by the effects of the substance e.g. arguments with spouse about consequences of intoxication; physical fights.	❑	❑	❑

At least 1 item from (1) to (4),
leading to clinically significant impairment or distress;
and criteria of Substance Dependence for the specific substance have never been met:

	No	Probably	Yes
Substance Abuse	❑	❑	❑

Amphetamine: 305.70 ❑ Yes ❑ Probably	Hallucinogen: 305.30 ❑ Yes ❑ Probably	Phencyclidine: 305.90 ❑ Yes ❑ Probably
Cannabis: 305.20 ❑ Yes ❑ Probably	Inhalant: 305.90 ❑ Yes ❑ Probably	Sedative, Hypnotic, or Anxiolytic: 305.40 ❑ Yes ❑ Probably
Cocaine: 305.60 ❑ Yes ❑ Probably	Opioid: 305.50 ❑ Yes ❑ Probably	Other (or Unknown) Substance Abuse: 305.90 ❑ Yes ❑ Probably

IDCL *International Diagnostic Checklist for DSM-IV*

Alcohol Dependence and Abuse

Name: ______________________

Age: ______ *Date:* ______________

- Define the characteristic maladaptive pattern of alcohol use
- The single symptoms as listed below must have occurred at any time in *the same 12-month period*

	No	Probably	Yes
(1) *Tolerance* as defined by: (a) a need for markedly increased amounts of alcohol to achieve intoxication or desired effects; or (b) markedly diminished effect with continued use of the same amount of alcohol.	☐	☐	☐
(2) *Withdrawal* as defined by: (a) a characteristic alcohol withdrawal syndrome; or (b) alcohol is taken to relieve or avoid withdrawal symptoms.	☐	☐	☐
(3) Alcohol is often taken in *larger amounts* or *over a longer period* than was intended.	☐	☐	☐
(4) There is a persistent desire or unsuccessful efforts to *cut down* or *control* alcohol use.	☐	☐	☐
(5) A *great deal of time* is spent in activities necessary to obtain alcohol, use alcohol, or recover from its effects.	☐	☐	☐
(6) Important social, occupational, or recreational activities are *given up* or *reduced* because of alcohol use.	☐	☐	☐
(7) The alcohol use is continued *despite knowledge* of having a persistent or recurrent physical or psychological problem that is likely to have been caused or exacerbated by alcohol e.g. continued drinking despite recognition that an ulcer was made worse by alcohol consumption.	☐	☐	☐

At least 3 symptoms from (1) to (7), leading to clinically significant impairment or distress:

Alcohol Dependence 303.90 — No ☐ Probably ☐ Yes ☐

- Check if criteria for Alcohol Abuse are met (lower part of page 2)
- Check specifiers of Course and Physiological Dependence (upper part of page 2)

Alcohol Dependence and Abuse *Page 2*

Specifications for Alcohol Dependence

Course Specifiers:	Yes	Probably
Early Full Remission (1-11 months)	☐	☐
Early Partial Remission (1-11 months)	☐	☐
Sustained Full Remission (≥ 12 months)	☐	☐
Sustained Partial Remission (≥ 12 months)	☐	☐
On Agonist Therapy	☐	☐
In a Controlled Environment	☐	☐

With Physiological Dependence:

There is evidence of tolerance or withdrawal (i.e., one of the items 1 or 2 is present)

☐ Yes ☐ Probably

Alcohol Abuse

- Define the characteristic maladaptive pattern of alcohol use
- The single symptoms as listed below must have occurred at any time in *the same 12-month period*

	No	Probably	Yes
(1) Recurrent alcohol use resulting in a *failure* to fulfill major role obligations at work, school, or home e.g., repeated absences or poor work performance related to alcohol use; alcohol-related absences, suspensions, or expulsions from school; neglect of children or household.	☐	☐	☐
(2) Recurrent alcohol use in situations in which it is *physically hazardous* e.g., driving an automobile or operating a machine when impaired by alcohol use.	☐	☐	☐
(3) Recurrent alcohol-related *legal problems* e.g., arrests for alcohol-related disorderly conduct.	☐	☐	☐
(4) Continued alcohol use despite having persistent or recurrent *social or interpersonal problems* caused or exacerbated by the effects of alcohol e.g. arguments with spouse about consequences of intoxication; physical fights.	☐	☐	☐

At least 1 item from (1) to (4), leading to clinically significant impairment or distress;

and criteria of Alcohol Dependence have never been met:

Alcohol Abuse 305.00 — No ☐ Probably ☐ Yes ☐

Chapter 5

A review of the effectiveness of psychological therapies in chronic tinnitus

Gerhard Goebel

5.1 Summary

Tinnitus is among the most common otologic disturbances diagnosed by an otolaryngologist. Up to the present day only a few medical treatments are effective, which is surprising given the frequency of this disturbance. If chronic tinnitus develops, the majority of those affected simply become accustomed to it. For the approximately 1-5% of those affected who suffer seriously from their tinnitus ('complex chronic tinnitus'), a variety of psychological treatment modalities have been developed and evaluated. In this chapter, the results of clinical studies are summarized and discussed in terms of their significance. Relaxation techniques and biofeedback have been evaluated controversially in numerous investigations, and apparently are effective only in combination with further tinnitus-oriented types of therapy (cognitive methods, deconditioning, imagination, stress immunization, etc.). In fact, with increased severity of the tinnitus, multi-modular behavioral therapy is indicated and its effectiveness can be verified. In this chapter, important studies are reviewed and critically discussed in relation to their design and their specific and unspecific tinnitus variables.

5.2 Introduction

Patients who are asked about their complaints during a medical examination initially describe different localizations, volumes and tonal qualities of the tinnitus, as well as different symptoms associated with their complaint. Etiologically, the tinnitus can then be associated with diseases such as sudden deafness, noise trauma, chronic noise exposure, Menière's disease, cervical spine syndrome, temporomandibular joint disorders, bruxism (grinding of the teeth), cerebral trauma, infections, rare brain tumors (e.g., acoustic neurinoma) and cerebrovascular diseases. Those affected, however, suffer most from being subjected to a permanent disturbance: the loss of stillness and composure. Regeneration and inner retreat are no longer possible for 1–5% of those affected, rendering these patients incapable of leading a normal life (Coles, 1984). A high percentage of patients feel considerably handicapped by tinnitus in elementary areas of daily life and show clinically relevant psychiatric syndromes.

Why those who suffer from chronic tinnitus experience this as extremely disturbing or life threatening is, in the end, an unanswered question. Numerous studies (Jakes et al., 1985, 1986; Hallam, 1986) have found only a minimal correlation between self-evaluated degrees of severity and audiological measurements of the intensity of tinnitus (see also Chapter 1). Additionally the type, quality or frequency of tinnitus does not correlate with the self-evaluation of the degree of its severity (Meikle et al., 1984).

Patients with intolerable tinnitus as a chief complaint are, for this reason, a riddle for the otologist. If the medical examination does not produce unfavourable results but ordinary treatment remains unsuccessful, it is of critical importance to establish methods of treatment together with the patient (who is often considerably impaired) which will enable him to learn to cope with tinnitus.

5.3 Psychological approaches to therapy

Psychological therapies derive from the idea that the etiology and the consequences of tinnitus can be influenced by psychological intervention. Given this fact one can proceed from different models of therapy.

5.3.1 Models of therapy

5.3.1.1 Psychosomatic model

Different psychological factors as a chain reaction may cause the emergence and persistence of tinnitus. This may be described using the cervical spine as an example.

Unreconciled chronic conflicts or life crises lead, by means of psycho-physiological mechanisms, to chronic muscular tension of the cervical spine, which then manifests itself as an aching neck or headaches originating from the back of the head as well as blocked vertebrae. Complex chain reactions which affect the afferent neurons and as a result central sites of the auditory path or cochlear circulation, together with further impairments (e.g. disturbances in blood viscosity) can lead to idiopathic/central tinnitus or cochlear/peripheral tinnitus with or without impairment of hearing (see Chapter 16). The therapeutic goal of psychotherapy here would be the reduction of the psychological trigger mechanisms using specific intervention techniques (e.g. conflict management) or unspecific intervention techniques (relaxation training, stress reduction). Hospitalization alone — and with this the removal from a conflict-laden environment — can set such a mechanism in motion and this possibly explains many 'spontaneous remissions' of hearing loss and idiopathic forms of tinnitus.

5.3.1.2 Somatopsychic model

Trauma or increasing impairment in the form of degenerative processes can lead to tinnitus (noise trauma, cerebral trauma, arthrosis of the cervical spine, defective jaw movement, presbycusis, etc.). The sudden confrontation with tinnitus symptoms which cannot be eliminated despite medical treatment can lead to psychological decompensation in the patient. This presents itself in most cases in the form of a depressive or phobic anxiety reaction (see Chapter 4). The goal of psychological intervention in this case would be to manage the psychological reaction to the tinnitus problem. Specific adjunctive treatment would be counselling, cognitive therapy, and stress immunization, or treatment which is not specific for tinnitus but has been effective in the treatment of depression and anxiety.

5.3.1.3 Personality variables and pre-existing psychic stress

Characteristics in personality which influence the experience of tinnitus are frequently described (see Chapters 2 and 4). The basic consideration is that tinnitus is triggered by an emotional trauma in a person with pre-existing psychological vulnerability and that it would not have occurred or at least have had the same severe effects in a more stable person.

This approach would require therapy related to depth psychology, which is not a specific therapy for tinnitus, but may enable the patient, for example, to consider his tinnitus as a symbolic expression of his emotional and psychic state.

Also effective here are the acknowledged therapeutic approaches dealing with crisis management aiming for emotional stabilization.

These models, however, are closely related to each other and interact. Because none of these models is superior, an individualized conditional analysis is imperative, leading to a preference of one or the other model.

5.4 Review of studies of psychological therapy

The treatment studies discussed do not concentrate on different etiological classifications of tinnitus. The patients treated, as a rule, are classified only according to ENT criteria, which makes a comparison difficult. Even the description of psychopathological symptoms, in most cases does not clarify whether the psychological intervention used is also effective. For this reason, a detailed presentation of the patient groups is omitted to a great extent.

5.4.1 Relaxation techniques and biofeedback

Since the 1970s, many studies have been published concerning the effectivity of relaxation in the treatment of tinnitus (Grossan, 1976; House et al., 1977; Borton et al., 1981; Elfner et al., 1981; Duckro et al., 1984; Carmen & Svihovic, 1984; Walsh, 1985; Hallam & Jakes, 1985; Walsh & Gerley, 1985; Scott et al., 1985; Haralambous et al., 1987; Kirsch et al., 1987, etc.). Grossan (1976) assumed that tinnitus is influenced by muscle tension and that a reduction in tinnitus would result from the physiological decrease in tension. Similar considerations and results also have been made in chronic pain syndrome (Sternbach, 1982). Biofeedback training could then specifically create a reduction in tinnitus.

Another argument for the use of biofeedback in tinnitus is the observation that the severity of tinnitus can be increased by stress, nervousness, exhaustion, and the tinnitus itself (Duckro et al., 1984).

If the patient using biofeedback concentrates on the relaxation instructions and the effect of physical relaxation, the result will be a simultaneous temporary reduction of tinnitus. This can then lead the patient to realize that he can control his tinnitus. Emotional neutrality and fewer phobic reactions can lead to greater tolerance of tinnitus. Relaxation as a coping technique already has a long tradition in anxiety therapy (Suinn, 1975).

The results of the initial studies of tinnitus treatment with biofeedback and relaxation (Grossan, 1976; House et al., 1977) were greeted optimistically at that time. However, it soon became apparent that an improvement of tinnitus could not be replicated in studies with strict control protocols (Ireland et al., 1985; Jakes et al., 1986; Kirsch et al., 1987; Haralambous et al., 1987; v. Wedel et al., 1989; see Table 6.1). With respect to tinnitus loudness, tinnitus discomfort and the effects of tinnitus on life-style, frequently no differences could be ascertained between the experimental and the control groups. In the study by Kirsch et al. (1985), an improvement was reported with regard to dealing with tinnitus in a controlled study, Scott et al. (1985) were able to prove a significant influence on tinnitus due to progressive muscle relaxation. In that study, additional cognitive relaxation techniques were used, in which relaxation was combined with directions for distraction techniques which could then be used as a coping strategy when required (see Chapter 9).

The need for implementation of studies with controlled conditions is shown in the results of Ireland et al. (1985) and Haralambous et al. (1987).

They observed a significant decrease in depression and tinnitus perception as effects of therapy (Beck Depression Inventory). However, this was also observed to the same extent in subjects on the waiting list, so that no specific effect of therapy was established (Table 6.2). An explanation for this effect could be, for example, the hope that the tinnitus would be treated effectively in the near future (8 weeks) among those subjects on the waiting list. Without a control group, this effect would have been attributed to the biofeedback treatment alone. Ireland et al. (1985) and Haralambous et al. (1987) demonstrated how important controlled studies are.

These studies verify that the effect of relaxation methods or biofeedback as monotherapy is not sufficient in seriously affected tinnitus patients. The efficacy of this method appears to depend on additive effects of further psychological factors which are associated with the design of the studies. The efforts on behalf of the patient, taking part in a treatment concept and the convictions of the researchers concerning the efficacy of the therapy are able to reduce depression in the patient. Jakes et al. (1986) reported a decrease in the tinnitus discomfort during the five various waiting phases among those affected; patients who had been given written information about tinnitus and possible coping strategies during the waiting phase experienced a decrease in tinnitus discomfort equal to that attained by the relaxation method used during a later phase of the study.

An explanation for the contradictory results of Grossan (1976) and House et al. (1977) on the one hand and studies showing negative results on the other may be ascribed to the possibility that the patients did not learn relaxation methods properly. In the studies of Ireland et al. (1985) and Jakes et al. (1986), the levels of relaxation were reviewed neither subjectively nor with physiological measurements. In contrast, Haralambous et al. (1987) demonstrated a significant decrease in the level of stress by means of biofeedback.

A further explanation may result from the fact that the studies involved patients with a different distribution of tinnitus etiologies, intensities, and psychological impairments. The description of the random studies delivers insufficient information for such a conclusion.

5.4.2 Accuracy of retrospective tinnitus assessment

A comparison of the studies is problematic because the individual variables were, in part, obtained through generalized reports on the effect of treatment or questionnaires about tinnitus in the form of a diary. Generalized reports at the conclusion of the treatment about the effect of therapy are not useful because they are not very reliable (Cahn & Cram, 1980; Blanchard, 1981; Lindberg, et al. 1988). We, as well as Lindberg et al. (1988), were able to observe this tendency in our catamnestic study. The patients were asked, 1 year after the conclusion of their treatment, how they had filled out their diaries at the beginning and the end of their therapy. A discrepancy arose, particularly among those who reported good treatment results. In retrospect these patients assessed the variables of the initial weeks of therapy as clearly more pessimistic, the variables at the time of discharge as clearly more optimistic as was the case at the time of treatment according to the entries in the tinnitus diary.

All in all, the assumption can be made that the reliability of retrospective reports do not agree with actual findings and that this criterion is insufficient for the evaluation of therapy.

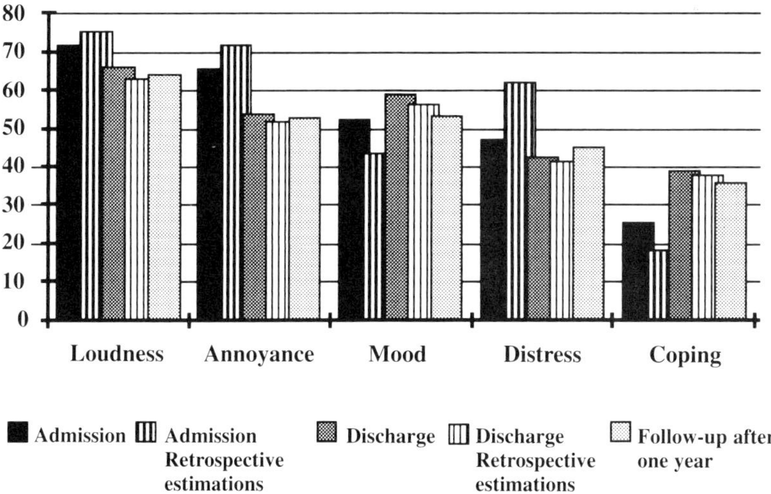

Fig. 5.1 Evaluations concerning the effect of therapy of 67 patients taking part in a multi-dimensional treatment program of complex chronic tinnitus: evaluations with daily ratings (tinnitus diary) on a visual 100 mm analog scale. The average evaluation over a 14 day period was compared to the estimates given by patients 1 year after the conclusion of therapy. In comparison with evaluations recorded during therapy, retrospective estimates were more unfavorable in respect to the beginning of therapy but in most cases more favorable in respect to the end of therapy.

5.4.3 Effects of other factors on results

Only a few studies compare groups, which makes the assessment of efficacy more difficult (Table 6.1). In clinical practice, control groups are often not control groups in the strict experimental sense; rather they are so-called waiting list control groups, established at the beginning of a study or treatment. They are, as a rule, examined with regard to specific and unspecific tinnitus variables. To maintain motivation in respect to further participation, they are informed from the beginning about the basics of the course of therapy and the purpose of therapy or they receive general information about tinnitus and its effects. Such measures alone, before the beginning of the actual therapy, can have an effect on certain parameters of tinnitus and possibly produce effects similar to a relaxation method. This effect also depends on the duration of the control phase. The waiting lists of the study by Jakes et al. (1989), Ireland et al. (1985) and Haralambous et al. (1987) were only a few weeks long. Thus, the scheduled treatment may already have had an effective psychological influence. If the waiting list lasts over a longer period of time, as was the case in our study, no significant changes in the variable tinnitus discomfort is perceivable (see Chapter 7). Ideally, the effect-variables should vary little over the entire period of the waiting list control group. Only in this case can the effects achieved by therapy be considered as reliable results.

5.4.4 Loudness and intensity of tinnitus

In a German study, deCamp & deCamp (see Chapter 10) compared the influence of relaxation (progressive muscle relaxation according to Jacobsen) in combination with EMG-biofeedback with the effect of an unspecific client-centred therapy and a waiting list (see Table 6.2). In addition to a tinnitus questionnaire and tinnitus diary (visual analog scale), psycho-acoustic measurements were also used for assessment. No effects were found in the waiting list control and the unspecific client-centred therapy groups. In comparison, the relaxation/EMG-biofeedback group had a significant decrease in the loudness and discomfort of tinnitus. The psycho-acoustic measurements also showed a significant decrease in the intensity of tinnitus.

These results of the psycho-acoustic measurements (significant decrease of the intensity of tinnitus in the tinnitus specific treatment group) contradict the results of Scott et al. (1985). Although they also found a significant decrease in the loudness of tinnitus, the intensity of tinnitus measured by audiometry at the beginning and end of treatment, showed no change. A possible explanation may be that the psycho-acoustic measurements were not made by the therapist, but rather by other individuals who were not informed about the various phases of therapy. To measure the intensity of tinnitus more accurately, a double-blind design ought to be used at least partly.

To minimize a placebo effect, deCamp & deCamp (see Chapter 10) divided the experimental groups into sub-groups who received positive or neutral instructions. As in Ireland et al. (1985), this had no influence on the results of treatment.

On the other hand, it is also conceivable that different patient groups took part in the study of deCamp & deCamp as compared to the study of Scott et al. (1985). Those whose tinnitus is influenced by muscular tension of the cervical spine and the temporomandibular joint (bruxism) can react differently to treatment from those with other tinnitus etiologies (see section 3.2). For this reason Scott et al. (1985) observed an improvement of the tinnitus comparable to a decrease of headaches and painful muscle tension as well.

Other investigators reviewed their methods of treatment with the aid of psycho-acoustic measurements without recognizing any significant influence (Kirsch et al., 1987; Ireland et al., 1985; Lindberg et al., 1989) (Tables 6.1 and 6.2).

Only Ince et al. (1984) obtained a specific decrease in tinnitus intensity by means of a specialized biofeedback technique ('matching to sample feedback procedure'). Here patients initially heard a 'tinnitus' produced by a special audiometer of the same quality and intensity as their own and were then asked to reduce the intensity of their own tinnitus according to the reduced intensity of the 'tinnitus' produced by the audiometer. When, after a 1-minute test activity, the impression arose that the intensity of tinnitus could be reduced, the external noise was reduced to 5 dB and the subjects were asked again to compare the intensity. Here almost every individual was able to achieve a significant reduction in tinnitus intensity, which was between 10 and 62 dB for 84%. Several subjects noted that their tinnitus had completely disappeared. This result was not actually compared with an untreated group, e.g. it was not determined whether the tinnitus would have taken the same course without this intervention. The results are nevertheless impressive, because they confirm the hypothesis that cognitive techniques can modulate tinnitus.

To compare psycho-acoustic measurement with a daily protocol of tinnitus volume is difficult. The recording of the tinnitus loudness (on a visual analog scale, for example) relates to the experienced tinnitus over the period of an entire day, while the psycho-acoustic measurement of the intensity of tinnitus only relates to the moment of measurement when the subject is expressly requested to consciously perceive the tinnitus intensity. In contrast, the goal of a psychologically oriented treatment often consists of ignoring the perception of tinnitus. The ability to reduce the loudness of tinnitus is consciously interrupted in the laboratory situation (e.g. during psycho-acoustic measurement) and is therefore only of little practical value for the assessment of the degree of coping with the tinnitus.

The question remains whether the varying frequencies of the recorded variables (daily recording of the loudness of tinnitus compared to the sporadic measurements of tinnitus intensity) can be compared with each other reliably.

Finally it is also important to know which method of psycho-acoustic measurement was used to identify the intensity of the tinnitus. DeCamp (1985) found a decrease in tinnitus intensity when using noise of tonal quality as compared to noise generally used for masking.

5.4.5 Controlled studies and long-term effects

Only a few studies fulfil a high standard of methodological criteria by using a sufficient amount of psychometric instruments such as daily protocols (tinnitus diary with specific variables) and psychological variables within the framework of a specific tinnitus questionnaire. Furthermore, only a few studies were made with a genuine control group. Found even less frequently are studies that report on the effect of therapy after treatment (catamnestic studies). Among these are studies by authors who have explained their research methods in this book (Goebel et al., Hallam, Lindberg, Scott, deCamp) as well as Haralambous et al. (1987), Ireland et al. (1985), Jakes et al. (1986) and Kirsch et al. (1987) (Table 6.2). Methods of therapy which could demonstrate clinically relevant results under such conditions were predominantly multimodular. Using this approach, Jakes et al. (1986) achieved an adaptation to tinnitus

Table 5.1 Summary of psychophysiological and psychotherapeutic treatment studies in complex tinnitus (without control group)

Author	*N*	Therapy	Duration	Evaluation instrument	Variables	Results	Long-term follow-up	*N*	Results
Grossam, M. 1976	51	EMG-biofeedback + relaxation training; counseling	6 sessions of 20 min. 2× per week	audiometer interview	T-loudness; T-intensity	80% noted improvement (report); 7.5% showed improvement; T-intensity; author: effect was not from biofeedback alone	no		
Goebel et al 1989	14	Integrative, multi-modular behavioral medicine, in-patient setting	7-12 weeks (average 55 days)	daily diary (visual 100mm analog scale); T-questionnaire; symptom checklist (SCL-90-R)	T-loudness; T-discomfort; T-management (coping)	no change in volume; significant decrease in discomfort (70-50); significant increase in control (13-26); normalization of affective and phobic parameters (SCL)	no		
Goebel et al 1991a	28	integrative, multi-modular behavioral medicine, in-patient setting	7-12 weeks (average 58 days)	daily diary (visual 100mm analog scale); T-questionnaire; symptom checklist (SCL-90-R); Freiburg personality inventory	T-loudness; T-discomfort; T-management (coping); general mood, general distress, evaluation of therapy	71% responder; no change in loudness; significant decrease in discomfort (65-55); significant increase in control (25-32); significant improvement in mood and distress; increase in feeling of success; normalization of feelings of insecurity	no		
House, J.W. 1981	132	EMG-biofeedback + skin temperature; biofeedback with relaxation	8 sessions weekly	interview	general change	15% complete remission; 29% major success; 33% improvement T-tolerance; 23% no effect; often decrease of pain syndromes	no		
Ince et al 1987	30	"matching to sample feedback procedure"		audiometer (matching) general self-evaluation	loudness	84% noted decrease of intensity of 10-26 db; complete remission in a few cases	no		
Marlow 1973	3	hypnotherapy		general evaluation	general	"positive effect"	no		
Brattberg 1983	32	hypnotherapy; tape cassettes for use at home	4 weeks, 15 minutes daily	general interview	T-loudness	decrease of tinnitus of 94%	8 weeks	32	significant improvement in 68% of the patients (n = 22)

Carmen & Svihovec 1983	11	EMG-biofeedback + relaxation group of 5-6 persons; 3× biofeedback each	10 sessions	11-point scale audiometer (matching)	T-loudness; general discomfort; T-intensity (audiometer)	no change with the exception of 2 patients who reported having had complete remission	18 months	11	90% noted a decrease of negative reactions to T; 63% noted decrease of T
House, J.W. 1978 House et al 1977	41	EMG-biofeedback + temperature; biofeedback with relaxation	10-12 sessions	n = daily diaries; questionnaires	T-quality anxiety, sleep, general well-being, use of medication	36% very good to good success; 40% slight success; 15% complete remission; best effect in depression and phobia	6-12 months	41	17% very good to good success; 39% slight success; 40% no change; worst results in seriously affected
Lindberg et al 1988 (see Chapter 9)	75	coping strategies; relaxation, information, cognitive therapy, desensitisation and exposure	10 × 60 minute sessions	visual 100mm analog scale; audiometer (matching)	T-loudness; T-discomfort; distress	decrease in discomfort from 6.5 to 5.4; decrease in distress from 5.4 to 4.5; no significant change in T-intensity	3 months		77% stabilization; 24% without effect; n = 1 deterioration
Lindberg et al 1989 (see Chapter 9)	27	6 × progressive relaxation and "quick relaxation" followed by exposure training vs distraction training	10 × 60 minutes 2-3 weeks	visual 100mm analog scale; T-questionnaire; tinnitus matching db HL, db SL; personal loudness units (PLU)	T-loudness; T-discomfort; T-management (coping)	decrease in volume from 7 to 5.7; decrease in discomfort from 6 to 4.5 and 6.7 to 5.2; increased control from 2.3 to 4 or 3.2 to 4.2; no difference in methods, no correlation between subjective and objective loudness	1 month	20	stabilization; decrease of other symptoms
Wedel, V., et al 1989	78	EMG-biofeedback	6 × 30 minutes	questionnaire	5 levels of change	14% small to average effect	6 months	47	13% small to average effect
Wimmer, J. 1983	10	Gestalt-therapy; bioenergetic therapy, half-structured program (relaxation, dialog with T, listening to T, awareness training)	10 sessions 2 months (4 drop-out)	questionnaire at the beginning and end of therapy (yes/no); audiometer at beginning and end of therapy	loudness, frequency, discomfort, distress, sleep, well-being, coping	no change in audiometer; improvement in coping (n = 6); decrease frequency (n = 3); loudness (n = 3); distress (n = 4); improvement of sleep (3 of 3); wish to continue and for home exercise regimen	3 months	6	general interview; decrease in disturbance (n = 6; improved well-being; irregular implementation of home work regimen

Table 5.2 Summary of psycho-physiological or psychotherapeutic studies of therapy in complex chronic tinnitus, including control groups

Author	*N*	Therapy	Duration	Evaluation instrument	Variables	Control	Results	Catamnesis	*N*	Results
deCamp 1989 (see Chapter 10)	44	1) specific relaxation + EMG-biofeedback 2) unspecific psychotherapy	8 sessions at 60 min. 6 months	visual analog scale; T-questionnaire; measurements each time before sessions (total 8×); sub-groups; each with specific instructions or non-specific instructions; 3 × audiometer (tone noises, maskability) db HL (not blind)	T-loudness; T-discomfort; T-intensity	waiting list	significant effect of specific therapy (loudness, discomfort, intensity); no effect of unspecific therapy; T-intensity: decrease compared to tone; no change in maskability	1-2 years	22	predominantly questionnaire; significant stability (value of both therapy groups together)
Goebel et al 1990	56	integrative multi-modular in-patient behavioral medicine	7-12 weeks (average 55 days)	daily diary (visual 100mm analog scale); T-questionnaire; symptom checklist (SCL-90-R) Freiburg personality inventory (FPI-R)	T-loudness; T-discomfort; T-control (coping); general distress; assessment of therapy	waiting list 6 months (stable)	68% responder; significant decrease of loudness (2%); significant decrease of discomfort (65-57); significant increase in T-coping (22-28); significant improvement distress and mood (10%); increased success of therapy (n.s.); significant improvement of mood, phobia, insecurity, introversion and emotional liability and inhibition (SCL/FPI)	1 year	30	significant stabilization of discomfort, T-coping, distress, mood, physical complaints, inhibition, stress, introversion
Goebel et al (see Chapter 7)	155	integrative multi-modular in-patient behavioral medicine	7-12 weeks (average 55 days)	daily diary (visual 100mm analog scale); T-questionnaire; symptom checklist (SCL-90-R) Freiburg personality inventory (FPI-R)	T-loudness; T-discomfort; T-control (coping); general mood; general distress; assessment of therapy; T-tolerance stimulus	waiting list 5.7 months (6-12 months $n = 79$)	70% responder; significant decrease in loudness (70-63); significant decrease of discomfort (65-52); significant increase of T-coping (27-40); significant improvement of mood/distress; normalization of depression, phobia, insecurity, introversion, etc (SCL and FPI)	12 months	63	significant stabilization of loudness, discomfort, T-coping, depression, phobia, insecurity, somatisation, emotional lability; no lasting effect on distress and mood

Jakes et al 1992 (see Chapter 8)	69	cognitive group therapy in comparison to masker, placebo masker or combination with masker	5 sessions 90 minutes per week	T-diary; T-questionnaire	discomfort, distress; T-perception; sleep disturbances	waiting list 7 weeks (n = 9)	group therapy with masker had best effect, masker initially slightly better than group, no effect of placebo masker	1-2 years (phone interview)	69	effect 46% group; effect 10% masker; effect 17% placebo masker
Haralambous et al, 1987	26	1) EMG-biofeedback 2) EMG-biofeedback with negative instructions (no specific relaxation instructions in either case)	8 × 90 min. weekly	T-diary; T-questionnaire (at beginning and end of therapy)	distress, anxiety, depression; T-perception	waiting list	no change of variables; T-perception decreased in therapy group and waiting list to the same extent	4-5 weeks	30	no change
Ireland et al 1985	30	progressive relaxation 1) relaxation + neutral instructions 2) relaxation + negative instructions (groups with 4-7 participants)	7 sessions 1 × 90 min. week, daily at home	T-diary; T-questionnaire; audiometer	T-loudness; frequency of disturbance; sleep disturbances; depression, anxiety	waiting list 8 weeks	no effect; no decrease of T-intensity, only decrease of depression, but no difference between groups	6-8 weeks	30	no change
Jakes et al 1986	24	orientation phase (info., counseling, coping strategies) followed by waiting period, followed by 1) progressive relaxation vs 2) relaxation perception training	5 × 30 min.	daily rating scale (1-7), no audiometer; T-questionnaire; depression scale (Hamilton); experimental index (Crown/Crisp)	T-loudness; discomfort, urgency distress, activity, sleep disturbances	waiting list	no change loudness; significant decrease of discomfort from 3.9 to 3.3 (17%); improvement of sleep (50%) + depression; no influence on activity, decrease of T-distress and impaired activity through T already in orientation phase; no difference between groups	1-4 months	24	stability of the achieved affects; positive attitude to T; less T-perception; relaxation = direct influence on T (n = 4); 7 non-responder = most seriously affected + hearing disorder
Kirsch et al 1987	6	6 × progressive relaxation + "key word"; 2 × EMG and 4 × temperature; biofeedback 40 min.	12 sessions	daily rating scale (point scale) visual analog scale: contentment, coping; multiple baseline cross-over design; audiogram (tone, narrow and	T-management (coping); T-distress; degree of tinnitus severity; effect of therapy; quality of sleep	waiting list 2-5 weeks	increased coping ability; no effect on T-distress or degree of severity; good general result; general effect exaggerated compared to specific variables	1-3 months	6	stability, relaxation and biofeedback; effective as a strategy

Continued on next page

Author	N	Therapy	Duration	Evaluation instrument	Variables	Control	Results	Catamnesis	N	Results
				broad band noise); global assessment, MMPI, BDI, STAI PSC			3 objectively louder, 3 quieter; no correlation with subjective estimation of loudness			
Marks et al 1985	14	1) hypnosis 2) "ego boosting" 3) suggestion of decreased T-loudness	6 sessions of 2 weeks 1 + 2, 6 + 7, 11 + 12, total over 3 months	cross-over design; daily visual analog scale (100mm); audiometer (matching)	T-intensity; T-tolerance; T-loudness; T-annoyance	baseline of 3 weeks	improvement in analog scale of n = 1; 5/14 were slightly more content, more able to relax; no correlation with tinnitus matching	none		
Scott et al 1985 Lindberg et al 1987 (see Chapter 9)	24	relaxation + deconditioning; imagination + exposition provocation	10 × 60 min. 3 weeks or daily 2 weeks	4 × daily visual analog scale; T-questionnaire n = 14; audiometer (matching; blind)	loudness, discomfort, distress, irritability; T-intensity (db HL, frequency)	waiting list 4 weeks	significant decrease of discomfort (24%); significant decrease of distress (24%); decrease of irritability (n.s.); significant decrease of loudness; no change of T-intensity	9 months	20	stability in discomfort (24%); no lasting effect on loudness, distress, irritability, T-intensity; 29% non-responder
Walsh & Gerley 1985	32	relaxation, audio cassette, temperature-biofeedback	8 sessions 60 min. week	10 point interval scale (measurements before and at the beginning and end of study); skin temperature	T-loudness; T-discomfort; skin temperature changes	waiting list 8 weeks (stable)	loudness and discomfort decreased by 65% (no precise data); significant increase in temperature by practice; significant correlation with temperature	none		
White et al 1986	22	motivation: "Your facial muscles show more emotion than you are able to verbalize"; EMG biofeedback: 10 × 1 minute + progressive relaxation 20 min. (audio cassettes for daily home work)	none	3 × daily 5-point rating scale; structured telephone interviews (blind)	intensity, annoyance, change	waiting list 6-9 months randomised (n = 22)	decrease in loudness and discomfort 60% compared to 5% of the control	6-9 months	22	(telephone interview) good (global assessment)

using the combination of relaxation training and cognitive therapy with emphasis on change in attitude toward tinnitus. Jakes et al. (1992) were able to achieve an increase in the effect of cognitive therapy by using a tinnitus-masker (see Chapter 8). Scott et al. (1985) and Lindberg et al. (1987) demonstrated that with the help of multi-modular therapy, significant changes could be achieved in the tinnitus variables of discomfort, distress, irritability, and loudness of tinnitus. Goebel et al. achieved similar results using an integrated multi-modular treatment approach (1990/1992, Chapter 7).

Individual techniques such as biofeedback, relaxation and hypnosis showed good general effects, but these were minor to negative (Haralambous et al. 1987; Ireland et al. 1985) in a differentiated examination of tinnitus consequences using a tinnitus questionnaire. Kirsch et al. (1987) concluded that the minor effect of their relaxation and biofeedback programmes was due to a multimodular effect and that the integration of additional techniques and interventions was necessary. White et al. (1986) attained positive results, but these cannot be verified by *quantitative* data and critical assessment due to ill-defined general categories such as decrease of tinnitus loudness and discomfort and global assessment of the course of the tinnitus using telephone interviews.

Finally, it is also important to determine the evaluated effect over a period of time after the conclusion of therapy. The results of treatment depend in part upon whether the patients regularly implement the coping strategies at home. This was noted by Lindberg et al. (1987), who found that 80% of their patients employed the techniques of self control several times weekly.

In addition, the development of somatic problems of disorders associated with tinnitus must be considered. On the one hand, a longterm impairment of the effects of therapy can, for example, develop due to a recurrence of sudden deafness or the chronic course of otosclerosis or arteriosclerosis. On the other hand the effect of therapy, evaluated over periods of 3 months to 2 years, showed a further decrease of tinnitus or a stabilization of the achieved effect of therapy in about 40-60%.

5.5 Summary

A review of the various studies leads to the conclusion that the development of psychological methods of therapy is leading to multidimensional treatment of complex chronic tinnitus. For some of those affected by tinnitus, in fact, it appears that relaxation methods and biofeedback training are sufficient. With increased suffering due to depression or anxiety, extensive additions to therapy such as cognitive therapy, hypnotherapy, stress immunization and deconditioning, as well as focusing on the management of tinnitus are important. When psychoanalytic methods are integrated, effective interventions of behavioral therapy are enriched. An individualized therapeutic approach, which does not cling to a standardized programme, often consisting of a single technique, is frequently beneficial for those most seriously affected.

It appears to be advantageous to treat those affected by tinnitus in group settings. Here, the following aspects come into play: 1. group phenomenon (the possibility of comparing one's own experience with that of others); 2. encouragement drawn from the possibility of observing other participants (increased motivation for psychotherapy: the experience of possible progress); 3. model learning (observation and imitation of methods that promote health; imitation of observed coping strategies).

An empiracally founded tinnitus therapy requires documentation of the different etiologies of tinnitus, the individualized application of therapeutic measures as well as careful and comprehensive long-term evaluation.

Specific instruments such as daily protocol (diary) of the loudness and discomfort from tinnitus as well as the coping ability are more dependable variables than general ratings relating to improvement and success of therapy. The individual results of therapy can be evaluated to a much greater extent in respect to their influence and effects using a specific tinnitus questionnaire (Jakes et al. 1985; Hallam et al. 1988; Wilson et al. 1991; Hiller & Goebel 1992). Retrospective studies should be avoided because of the above-mentioned reasons.

A verification of treatment results using audiometric methods for the assessment of tinnitus volume is only of minor value when measurements are sporadic in frequency. Of interest would be the systematic use of audiometer methods in tinnitus etiologies which are associated with significant fluctuations of tinnitus intensity and in which psychological interventions tend to be effective (cervical or myogenic tinnitus, tinnitus as a result of bruxism or disorders of the mandible). During the course of therapy as much audiometric data should be gathered as possible.

Psycho-acoustic measurements are of minor importance in the evaluation of tinnitus management, the purpose of therapy.

The results of the studies summarized in this chapter show that psychological strategies in the treatment of tinnitus have a positive long-term effect. Especially when medical intervention has little chance of success, behavioural-medicine presents a scientifically proven therapeutic alternative.

5.6 References

Biesinger, E. (1979): Funktionelle Störungen der Halswirbelsäule in ihrer Bedeutung für die Hals-Nasen-Ohrenheilkunde. In: *Ganz, H., W. Schätzle* (Ed.): HNO-Praxis Heute, 9. Springer, Berlin-Heidelberg.

Blanchard, E.B., F. Andrasik, D.F. Neff, S.E. Jurish, D.M. O'Keefe (1981): Social validation of the headache diary. Behavior Therapy, 12: 711-715.

Borton, T.E., W.M. Moore, S.R. Clark (1981): Electromyographic feedback treatment for tinnitus aurium. Journal of Speech and Hearing Disorders, 36: 39-45.

Brattberg, G. (1983): An alternative method of treating tinnitus: Relaxation-hypnotherapy primarily through the home use of a recorded audio cassette. International Journal of Clinical Experimental Hypnosis, 31: 90-97.

Cahn, T., J.R. Cram (1980): Changing measurement instrument at follow-up: A potential source of error. Biofeedback and Self-Regulation, 5: 265-273.

Camp, U. de (1989): Beeinflussung des Tinnitus durch psychologische Methoden. Unveröff. Diplomarbeit Psychologisches Institut der FU, Berlin.

Carmen, R., D. Svihovec (1984): Relaxation biofeedback in the treatment of tinnitus. A. J. Otolaryngology, 5, 5: 376-381.

Coles, R.R.A. (1984): Epidemiology of tinnitus. J. Laryngology Otology (Suppl.), 9: 7-15.

Coles, R.R.A., R.S. Hallam (1987): Tinnitus and its management. British Medical Bulletin, Vol. 43, 4: 983-998.

Duckro, P.N., C.A. Pollard, H.D. Bray, L. Scheiter (1984): Comprehensive behavioral management of complex tinnitus: a case illustration. Biofeedback and Self-Regulation, 9, (4): 459-469.

Gerber, K.H., A.M. Nehemkis, R.A. Charter, H.C. Jones (1985): Is tinnitus a psychological disorder? In: J. Psychiatry in Medicine, 15/1: 81-87.

Goebel, G. (1989): Tinnitus. In: *Hand, I., H.-U. Wittchen* (Eds): Verhaltenstherapie in der Medizin. Springer, Berlin - Heidelberg - New York - Tokyo - Hong Kong, 207-228.

Goebel, G., M. Lederer, W. Rief, M. Fichter (1990): Integrative multimodale verhaltensmedizinische Behandlung des komplexen chronischen Tinnitus: Behandlungsergebnisse und Langzeiteffekt. 61 Kongreß der Deutschen HNO-Gesellschaft, Würzburg, Poster.

Goebel, G., W. Keeser, M. Fichter, W. Rief (1991a): Neue Aspekte des komplexen chronischen Tinnitus. Überprüfung eines multimodalen verhaltensmedizinischen Behandlungskomzepts. Psychother. Med. Psychol., 41: 115-122.

Goebel, G., W. Keeser, M. Fichter, W. Rief (1991b): Neue Aspekte des komplexen chronischen Tinnitus. Die verlorene Stille: Auswirkungen und psychotherapeutische Möglichkeiten beim komplexen chronischen Tinnitus. Psychother. Med. Psychol., 41: 123-133.

Goebel, G., H. Hiller, K. Frühauf, M. M. Fichter (1992): Effects of in-patient multimodal behavioral treatment on complex chronic tinnitus. In: Tinnitus 91 (*J. M. Aran & R. Dauman* (eds.)). Proceedings of the Fourth International Tinnitus Seminar Bordeaux, 1991. Kuglev Publications, Amsterdam/New York: 465-470.

Grossan, M. (1976): Treatment of subjective tinnitus with biofeedback. Ear Nose Throat Journal, 55: 22-30.

Halford, J. B. S., D. Stewart. S. D. Anderson (1991): Tinnitus severity measured by a subjective scale, audiometry and clinical judgment. J. of Laryngology and Otology, 105: 89-93.

Halford, J. B. S., S. D. Anderson (1991): Anxiety and depression in tinnitus sufferers. J. of Psychosomatic Research, 35: 383-390.

Hallam, R. S., S. C. Jakes, R. Hinchcliffe (1988): Cognitive variables in tinnitus annoyance. Brit. J. Clin. Psychol. 27: 213-222.

Hallam, R. S. (1986): Psychological approaches to the evaluation and management of tinnitus distress. In: *Hazell* (Ed.): Tinnitus. Churchill Livingstone, London, 1-50.

Haralambous, G., P. H. Wilson, S. Platt-Hepworth et al. (1987): EMG-biofeedback in the treatment of tinnitus: An experimental evaluation. Behav. Research and Therapy, 25: 49-55.

Harrop-Griffiths, J., W. Katon, R. Dobie, C. Sakai, J. Russo (1987): Chronic tinnitus: Association with psychiatric diagnostics. Journal of Psychosomatic Research, 31: 613-621.

Hiller, W., G. Goebel (1992): A psychometric study of complaints in chronic tinnitus. Journal of Psychosomatic Research, (4): 337-348.

House, J. W., L. Miller, P. R. House (1977): Severe tinnitus: Treatment with biofeedback training (result in 41 cases). Transactions of the American Academy of Ophthalmology and Otolaryngology, 84: 697-703.

Ince, L. P., R. Y. Greene, A. Alba, H. H. Zaretsky (1987): A matching-to-sample feedback technique for training self-control of tinnitus. Health Psychol. 6: 173-182.

Ireland, C. E., P. H. Wilson, J. P. Tonkin, S. Platt-Hepworth (1985): An evaluation of relaxation training in the treatment of tinnitus. Behaviour Research and Therapy, 23: 423-430.

Jakes, S. C., R. S. Hallam, C. Chambers, R. Hinchcliffe (1985): A factor analytical study of tinnitus complaint behaviours. Audiology, 24: 195-206.

Jakes, S. C., R. S. Hallam, S. Rachmann, R. Hinchcliffe (1986): The effects of reassurance, relaxation training and distraction on chronic tinnitus sufferers. Behav. Res. Thera., 24: 497-507.

Jakes, S. C., L. McKenna, R. S. Hallam, R. Hinchcliffe (1992): Cognitive therapy in chronic tinnitus. Cognitive Therapy and Research, 6: 67-82.

Kirsch, C. A., E. B. Blanchard (1987): A Multiple-baseline evaluation of the treatment of subjective tinnitus with relaxation training and biofeedback. Biofeedback and Self-Regulation, 4: 295-312.

Lindberg, P., B. Scott, L. Melin. L. Lyttkens (1988): Behavioral therapy in the clinical management of tinnitus. British J. of Audiology, 22: 265-272.

Lindberg, P., B. Scott, L. Melin, L. Lyttkens (1989): The psychological treatment of tinnitus: An experimental evaluation. Behav. Res. Ther. 6: 593-603.

Lindberg, P., B. Scott, L. Melin, L. Lyttkens (1987): Long-term effects of psychological treatment of tinnitus. Scand. Audiol., 16: 167-172.

Marks, N. J., H. Karl Onisiphorou (1985): A controlled trial of hypnotherapy in tinnitus. Clin. Otolaryngol., 10: 43-46.

Marlow, F. I. (1973): Effective treatment of tinnitus through hypnotherapy. Am. J. Clin. Hypn., 15: 162-165.

Melzack, R., P. D. Wall (1965): Pain mechanisms: A new theory. Science, 150: 971-979.

Meikle, M. B., J. Vernon, R. M. Johnson (1984): The perceived severity of tinnitus: Some observations concerning a large population of tinnitus patients. Otolaryngology – Head and Neck Surgery, 92: 689-696.

Scott, B., P. Lindberg, L. Lyttkens, L. Merlin (1985): Psychological treatment of tinnitus: An experimental group study. Scand. Audiol., 14, 4: 223-230.

Sternbach, R. (1982): Psychologische Verfahren bei der Behandlung von Schmerz. In: *Keeser, W., E. Pöppel, P. Mitterhusen* (Eds): Schmerz: Fortschritte der klinischen Psychologie, 284-295. Urban & Schwarzenberg, Munich - Vienna - Baltimore.

Suinn, R.M. (1975): Anxiety management training for general anxiety. In: *Suinn, R.M., R.G. Weigal* (Eds): The innovative psychological therapies. New York, Harper & Row.

Walsh, W.M., P.P. Gerley (1985): Thermal biofeedback and the treatment of tinnitus. Laryngoscope, 95: 987-989.

Wedel, H. v., U. Strahlmann, P. Zorowka (1989): Effektivität verschiedener nicht medikamentöser Therapiemaßnahmen bei Tinnitus. Laryngo. Rhino-Otol., 68: 259-266.

Wilson, P., J. Henry, M. Mowen, G. Haralombous (1991): Tinnitus reaction questionnaire: Psychometric properties of a measure of distress associated with tinnitus. J. Speech and Hearing Research, 34: 197-201.

Wimmer, J. (1983): Hilfe zur Selbsthilfe: Ein Therapie- und-Übungsprogramm für Patienten mit subjektiven Ohrgeräuschen. Inaugural Dissertation Ludwig Maximilians University, Munich. (*Prof. H.H. Naumann.*)

White, T.P., S.R. Hoffmann, E.N. Gale (1986): Psychophysiological therapy for tinnitus. Ear and Hearing, 397-399.

Chapter 6

Dealing with motivational problems of tinnitus patients

Barbara Rabaioli-Fischer

6.1 Summary

This chapter deals with the specific problems in the management of tinnitus patients using a case report. The constant difficulties of motivation for therapy are highlighted and specific situations, when and how they occur in the course of treatment, are described.

Using practical examples of intervention, possibilities are presented of how the patient can achieve relief from his symptoms using cognitive therapeutic methods. Interventions will be mentioned concerning daily planning, information, stress management and stress reducing cognitions as well as problem-solving strategies.

6.2 Introduction

In this article the individual phases of motivational work will be outlined with the help of a practical example of a tinnitus patient.

These phases evolved from the out-patient treatment of patients with primary somatic diseases. Experience gained from the treatment of patients with Parkinson's disease (Ellgring & Rabaioli-Fischer 1988, 1990) is also included. These phases also implement the results of studies by Prohaska

& di Clemente (1983), who described the individual phases and steps in which the practical process of therapy develops.

A flow chart in the appendix to this chapter as well as at the end of each passage describes the different phases of interaction between therapist and patient.

6.3 Description of the phases

6.3.1 Initial Appointment

As psychotherapists, we frequently assume that the actual suffering from physical symptoms is a sufficient motivation for psychotherapy.

This is, however, not always the case. Patients begin therapy for completely different reasons. One reason may be that the physician who has treated them believes that they may profit from psychotherapy. Another may be that patients are frustrated by the "so-called success" of somatic treatment or that they recently came across information concerning psychotherapy. They nevertheless have no idea what psychotherapy itself is.

To attain successful results, the psychotherapist depends on the active cooperation of the patient and has to guide the patient in this direction. For most patients this entails a change of perspective from being passive, e.g. "enduring" therapy (an approach to therapy the patient is familiar with due to prior experience with somatic therapy) to being active, e.g. taking an active part in therapy. This also includes his readiness to give the therapist, as a stranger, detailed personal information concerning his problems, habits and convictions e.g. to actively create a working relationship with the therapist by confiding and relying on him.

Phase I: Initial appointment

Patient	**Therapist**
confides him/herself	listens
	leads/guides
	gives information

6.3.2 Expose problem areas

In order to maintain the achieved motivation, patients should feel that to be "active" leads to positive consequences. In practical terms, the therapist and the patient develop possibilities of improving symptoms mutually.

This is exemplified in the following case report.

Patient R suffered from sudden deafness in October 1987. Constant noise and occasional whistling sounds in the left ear together with inner ear hearing loss of the left ear resulted. Medical treatments did not alleviate these symptoms. She went to various ENT specialists for 9 months, until she was told that the noises probably would remain. She tried unsuccessfully to accept this fact as well as the impairment, but she developed anxiety at work because she could not understand the customers properly. She was often impatient because of constant stress due to the tinnitus but did not admit to being impatient, because she expected herself to remain constantly polite towards her customers. Her performance dropped and she became nervous and suffered from additional frequent stomach aches. She suddenly made errors in cost planning, which contradicted her opinion of herself as being extremely reliable. She became insecure and tense.

At home, she felt just as anxious, because she could not follow conversations well and did not have the courage to constantly ask her conversational partner to repeat what she had not been able to understand. She believed her nervousness and tenseness disturbed others and she isolated herself for this reason increasingly. In her marriage she felt increasingly dependent on her husband and clung to him which resulted in an increasing fear of becoming a burden. Even in this relationship, she was not able to be candid any more. She tried to fulfil her husband's wishes, but at the same time was forced to delegate more tasks such as shopping and appointments at public offices.

She was constantly aware of her symptoms and felt at their mercy. Frequently her whole body shivered; she felt tired constantly and was convinced that she was unattractive to others. When she sought help from her general physician, he told her for the first time, that she suffered from the complications of tinnitus and advised her to seek psychotherapeutic treatment.

The typical problems of this patient are constant stress due to tinnitus and the resulting nervousness and tenseness. Our patient is handicapped in social situations. Feelings of inferiority and insecurity crop up as soon as she is not able to lead a conversation properly and with self-confidence. These problems were also described as occurring with other disabilities by Brengelmann (1985) and especially for tinnitus by Lindberg et al. (1987).

Another typical result of tinnitus is that our patient suddenly feels dependent on her husband, because she perceives him as her last chance for help, understanding and care. Due to increasing isolation the partner takes over all the responsibility for care, support and activity. Most patients are aware of this dependence and become anxious, especially because they feel to what extent their partner is overwhelmed. This leads to a reduction in self-determination (Brengelmann 1985).

Tinnitus is also a handicap in every conversation especially when perfectionist tendencies are present, as is the case with this patient. Patient R is exhausted sooner and ought to learn how to adapt her reduced performance at work to her disorder as well as to reduce her ambitious demands on herself.

At this point, our patient and the psychotherapist set up a treatment plan mutually.

In order to maintain the motivation for cooperation our patient also needed the assurance that she had the right to suffer from these symptoms. This allowed her to be less perfectionistic at work.

Phase II: Problem area classification/relevant problem

Patient	**Therapist**
Reports	Provides structure
a) Stress from tinnitus	
* Helplessness	
* Disturbances of concentration	
* Nervousness	
* Increased fatigue	
b) Disturbances of social contact	
* At work	
* At home	
* During social events	
c) Stress from incorrect attribution	Provides information and explanations
Negative self-perception	

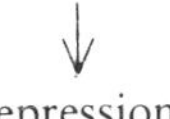

Depression

6.3.3 Practical interventions, individual support

The next step is to determine the sequence of the planned individual interventions.

Our patient says that it is the symptom itself, the disturbing tinnitus, from which she suffers most.

Because she has not learned to

think in "psychophysical relationships" it is helpful that she receives information using a descriptive model, which demonstrates the consequences of permanent stress in all possible areas of life. This knowledge stabilizes motivation for further cooperation, and relaxation exercises and distraction methods can begin (Manual I-A/B, see appendix). At this point, we comply with the principle wish, which is to find relief from the stress caused by the tinnitus syndrome.

Our patient requires support to be able to continue to practise relaxation methods at home. It is important to explain that, under stress, in this case tinnitus, relaxation techniques are much more difficult to learn than under normal circumstances. It is important to note how much patience and practice is needed before she can expect initial relief. An appropriate amount of time and a beneficial atmosphere (Manual II, see appendix), are very helpful.

Phase III: Practical interventions: individualized support

Patient	**Therapist**
Self observation	Gives feedback
practices:	explains:

relaxation exercises and cognitive distraction methods.

6.3.4 Adaptation to the disorder

Adaptation to tinnitus always means that one must make changes in daily life. Every disorder leads to a reduced stress threshold. For our patient this means that she must reduce previous demands on performance and abilities accordingly, not only in order to get along better with the tinnitus, but also to prevent deterioration (Lindberg et al. 1987).

After our patient has deduced this fact using a specific example, it is important to analyse her daily life mutually. This can be done using a weekly diary, in which she notes exactly her routine daily activities and how she spends her leisure time. Now, with the aid of specific details, which our patient has reviewed with the therapist, she examines where and when stress can be reduced (Manual III, see appendix).

This entails a change of attitude towards work and concentration. For example, our patient reduced her ambition to "function perfectly" and allowed herself to be increasingly conscious of even her negative feelings. She dared to ward off disagreeable customers and learned strategies to deal constructively with feelings and irritations in daily communication (Manual IV, see appendix).

In her leisure time, she increased the amount of enjoyable activities again, in order to "refuel". Here it is necessary to examine individually which specific activities have been enjoyable in the past (Manual V, see appendix), and are still of recreational value.

Further social isolation should be avoided at all costs and it should be conveyed to our patient that she is not inferior if she cannot always follow conversations well and has to ask her partner to repeat what he has said. Possibilities for improved socializing and improved protection of own interests are worked out in practical exercises such as role-playing.

Further therapy is only successful if our patient acquires and implements practical skills according to the self-efficacy theory described by Bandura (1977). In our case, the exercises from the Personal Effectiveness Training by Liberman et al. (1975) are particularly suitable.

This is also important because our patient regains a secure feeling of social competence and is able to relieve her marriage of additional and preventable stress.

For our patient to remain motivated, the analysis of the problems should alternate with simultaneous training of practical coping strategies. This leads to a continuous beneficial exchange between new capabilities and further analysis, and greater trust develops in personal strengths and the ability of self control (Bandura 1977, Kanfer 1989). Our patient is rewarded for her active progress and as a result no longer feels helpless in regard to her symptom.

Phase IV: Adaptation to the disorder

Patient		Therapist
	(decreased stress threshold and ability to concentrate)	
Practices self observation	Daily activities	Gathers information and gives practical advice
	Recreational activities	

6.3.5 Biographical analysis

Having learned techniques of relaxation, and cognitive distraction and after self-assertiveness training, additional factors, which promote stress and originate in the biographical development, should be analysed.

Our patient creates additional stress by means of so-called "stress inducing cognitions" and overambitiousness. Examples for such stress inducing cognitions are that our patient believes she disturbs others because of her tension or when she interrupts conversations in order to ask her conversational partner to repeat what she hasn't understood. She experiences herself as inferior, unsure of herself and feels responsible for her decreased ability to concentrate. Our patient should be told that feelings of insecurity existing prior to the disorder will reappear and increase again as a result of the disorder. This means that negative opinions of oneself, which were acquired early in childhood, are aggravated by additional stress. Our patient had learned as a child and young adult to yield to and please others in order to be loved and acknowledged, and that she must always try her best to remain acknowledged. These attitudes have, at this point in life, become a burden. Methods of cognitive restructuring are therefore incorporated.

Phase V: Biographical analysis

Patient	Therapist
Analyses stress inducing cognitions	
Analyses false attributions	
Self-incriminations instead of attributing problems to the disorder	
Collects statements:	Changes the statements:
"I have to concede to others"	provides feed-back
"I must always function."	Explains inter-dependent aspects
"I have to exert myself continuously to be loved and acknowledged."	

6.3.6 Help for self-help

As a preventive measure, it is a good idea, considering later conflicts and problems, to develop alternative problem solving strategies mutually in the sense of "help for self-help".

A specific example is better management of cost planning, an important task for our patient in her occupation. Our patient should learn to ask a colleague for help, to support her in checking cost assessments. She can also alleviate her situation by adjusting her routine in such a way as to do the cost planning when she is not being disturbed and still feels alert. In this way, she learns to function according to her own well being.

The sooner the psychological interventions are integrated into our patient's life, the sooner she will be motivated to implement them and find new personal solutions using acquired strategies of problem solving. Furthermore, it is sensible to increase the interval between individual sessions during the final phase of therapy, in order to give her time for independent learning. In this phase the activities of the therapist are often limited to accompanying support (counselling).

Phase VI: Goal: 'help for self-help'

- Improved management of the disorder
- Renewed self-acceptance
- Improved ability to recognize personal needs, feelings and thoughts
- Implementation of above mentioned capabilities

Patient	**Therapist**
Experiences —	Shows —
ability for:	high sensitivity for:
* self-regulation	* inner processes
* self-control	* motivational level
* self-competence	

6.4 Course of treatment and results

Our patient had a total of 43 sessions of individual therapy. In the beginning it was very difficult for her to learn the relaxation techniques. She overcame these initial difficulties and was able to exercise regularly.

She planned her recreational activities much more conscientiously. As she was interested in botany, she joined a botanical society. In addition, she liked gardening and began to visit meetings and social events occasionally. This made her feel more sure of herself and led to a rejuvenation of her marital relationship. She regained the ability to assert herself and had a stronger feeling of autonomy.

Her extreme ambition was reduced. She worked out a series of alternative cognitions, which she also always kept with her on a small index card and reviewed whenever she felt under pressure or, for example, made errors and felt insecure again. Her colleagues reacted very positively to her change in her work pattern and she allowed herself to be helped regularly with the bookkeeping which had a deadline.

What was still difficult for her was to ask people to repeat themselves whenever she did not understand properly. She intended to continue practising this. She experienced the tinnitus differently. She couldn't say if it had really improved, but she no longer experienced it as threatening.

The interval between therapy sessions was significantly increased after the 30th session. She came once a fortnight, later in 3-week intervals, with the aim of determining to what extent she felt able to cope with various situations. At the same time this decreased the dependence on the therapist and gave our patient an increased feeling of autonomy as well as the possibility of examining and increasing strategies of self-control.

In a telephone interview 3 months after the conclusion of treatment, she reported that she was especially happy with her new hobby and her intensified relationship to her husband, even though both pursued their own interests to a greater extent. She believed that her marriage was more fulfilling and meaningful because the exchange of individual experiences had stimulated their relationship. In respect to her requesting a conversational partner to repeat what she had not understood properly, she had informed all her acquaintances, friends and colleagues that she heard better when she assumed a certain body posture which enabled her to point her right ear in the direction of the speaker. It was still difficult for her to request this from strangers because of frequent angry reactions.

6.5 Prognosis

In general the treatment of the tinnitus patient is concerned with the analysis of psycho-physical interrelationships. Applicable models concerning the mediation of information should be available in order to convey plausibly where and when tinnitus patients can achieve behavioural changes. This demands a high level of sensitivity for the wishes and needs of the patient from the therapist. Many patients are not aware of their personal needs because they have never been asked about them. Due to the disorder they become aware that they have often neglected themselves and their wishes in the past. In addition, the perception that the patients have of themselves, of their shortcomings and inabilities, should be changed and be brought to a realistic level. Practically speaking, this means that they must develop an understanding of the fact that they cannot perform unimpaired any longer and for that reason should not attribute failure to personal incapabilities.

On the other hand, they should experience that they are able to achieve again and should develop increasing capabilities in regulation, goal-setting and self assessment as well as self-reinforcement (Kanfer 1989).

The main concern of tinnitus therapy as well as its motivational aspects is therefore to help patients develop coping strategies. In addition, they should develop a feeling of self-competence by means of the acquired methods and thus be able to reduce the degree of dependence and insecurity (Bandura 1977, Scott et al. 1990). Unbearable physical and psychological stress situations leading to depression develop only when the patient experiences the disorder as being unmanageable.

Exaggerated expectations concerning personal capabilities as well as coping skills in combination with the estimation that the tinnitus is not manageable lead into a dead end (cul de sac), in which a patient develops additional symptoms and loses his self-confidence. We can therefore deduce that constant motivation with the aim of improved self-observation and an active approach toward coping strategies is the foundation of an effective therapy.

6.6 References

Bandura, A. (1977): Self-efficacy: Toward a unifying theory of behavioral change. Psychological Review, 84, 191-215.

Brengelmann, J. C. (1985): Psychologische Aufgaben bei der Integration der Behnderten. In: Berufsverband Deutscher Psychologen (Ed.): Psychologische Hilfen für Behinderte, Band 1 Weissenhof, Weinsberg, 27-36.

Ellgring, H., B. Rabaioli-Fischer (1988): Training of coping strategies for Parkinson patients. Poster for the Behaviour Therapy World Congress in Edinburgh, Sept. 5th-10th. 1988.

Ellgring, H., B. Rabaioli-Fischer (1990): Psychological interventions for Parkinson patients. First International Congress of Behavioral Medicine, Uppsala, Sweden, June 27th to 30th, 1990.

Kanfer, F.H. (1989): Basiskonzepte in der Verhaltenstherapie: Veränderung während der letzten 30 Jahre. In: *I. Hand, H.-U. Wittchen* (Ed.). Verhaltenstherapie in der Medizin. Berlin: Springer, S. 1-16.

Liberman, R., W. King, W. de Risi, McCann (1975): Personal effectiveness. Research Press, Champaign, Ill.

Lindberg, P., B. Scott, L.A. Melin, L. Lyttkens (1987): Long-term effects of psychological treatment of tinnitus. Scandinavian Audiology 16, 167-172.

Prohaska, J., C. di Clemente (1983): Toward a comprehensive model of change. In: *Miller, W., N. Heather* (1985): Treating addictive behaviors, Plenum Press, New York, 3-27.

Scott, B., P. Lindberg, L. Lyttkens, L. Melin (1990): Predictors of tinnitus discomfort, adaptation and subjective loudness. British Journal of Audiology, 14, 51-62.

Seligmann, M. (1986): Erlernte Hilflosigkeit. Urban & Schwarzenberg, München.

Appendix

Manual I —
Information diagram

A Vicious circle of self cognitions and physical state of health

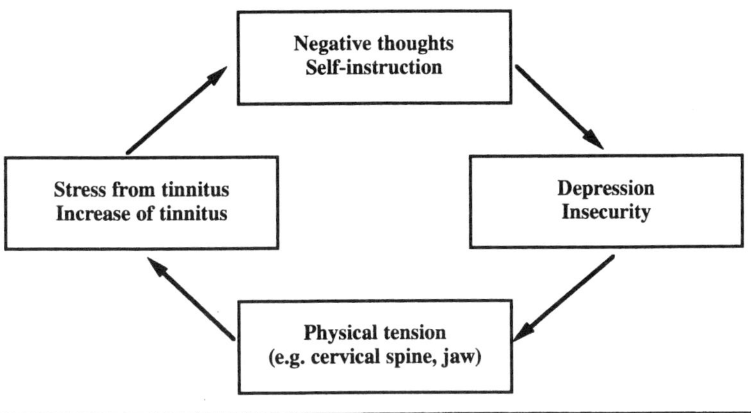

B Change in the vicious circle by cognitive restructuring and the use of relaxation methods

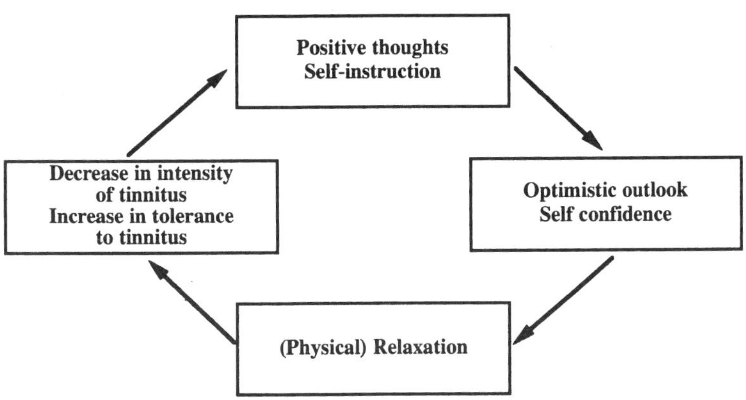

Manual II —
Daily report about the course of relaxation exercises

Saturday: approx 2.30pm — A good feeling due to relaxed atmosphere — thoughts wander — problems with relaxing the stomach

Sunday: approx 6.30pm — Easy relaxation due to composed condition. Nearly feel like slipping away — thoughts wander

Monday: approx 3.30pm — Very tense — restlessness and slight anxiety, stress from all sides — went to the toilet — relaxation had a strong relaxing effect

Wednesday: approx 7.15pm — At home — nervous — headaches (migraine) — relaxation did not work completely — nevertheless soothing — maybe stomach is too congested — slight improvement of headache — tuning out not quite successful

Thursday: approx 7.30pm — At home — a day full of stress — relaxation exercises OK — problems with the audio-cassette — in spite of quiet breathing not under control — felt calmer

Friday: approx 6.30pm — At home — nervous — relaxation relaxation exercises pretty good — even though distracting noise from the personal computer printer and music from the radio were present felt under control — felt calm and collected

Manual III — Examples of a daily protocol of events, feelings and thoughts that serve as a basis for cognitive therapy

Saturday morning (3.15am)

Important: Woke up, nausea, cramps in the legs and stomach — my period is due — a tearing headache

Conscious of: Anxious again, don't know for what reason, want to fall asleep again, listen to a record, so I can hear a voice at least

My thoughts: Once again my sleep is completely disrupted, everything is getting on my nerves — I want to feel well again

Saturday (1.30pm)

Important: Just finished breakfast, want to write a letter to S

Conscious of: Am ashamed of the fact that I didn't phone M. It was actually a fine day, I enjoy my whitewashed window frames

My thoughts: I really don't feel like going on a bike ride, want to go to bed again and read. Have to force myself again!

Saturday (5.15pm)

Important: Went cycling — am exhausted

Conscious of: Total fatigue, waver between complete lack of incentive and really wanting to experience something

My thoughts: What an embarrassment — wanted to accompany M & C to the theatre for weeks and I still can't decide

Saturday (10.00pm)

Important: Shape up!

Conscious of: Boredom. As soon as I don't have anything to do, my physical symptoms develop. I don't want to be alone

My thoughts: Should I read or write a letter to my cousin?

Sunday (2.42pm)

Important: Paid S a visit on my bicycle

Conscious of: The ride was a bit strenuous. What a joy, spring is here at last

My thoughts: Want to accomplish going out on my own tonight

Examples for learning goals including degree of difficulty

Manual IV

"Learning-Unlearning" List

Name ______________________

Behavioral training for social competence;
Formulation of specific therapy goals

	1.	2.	3.	4.	5.
Dates of evaluation	10/1	10/14			
I would like to learn	Evaluation according to an assessment scale from 1-6				
1. to tell my colleagues that they should help me with bookkeeping more	5				
2. to visit administration officials by myself again	3				
3. ask husband/friends to speak louder	6				
4. use leisure time more actively		3			

	1.	2.	3.	4.	5.
Dates of Evaluation	10/7	10/24	10/28		
I would like to unlearn	Evaluation according to an assessment scale from 1-6				
1. to withdraw whenever I don't understand others	4				
2. to be passive when I should say "no"		5			
3. to have to do everything correctly at work		3			
4. to always think about what opinion others have of me			2		

Manual V — List of Reinforcers (L-R)

Excerpt from a list of possible reinforcers with the aim of helping a patient to develop ideas concerning new and pleasant activities

List of Reinforcers

Name:______________________ Age: ______

____

Introduction

On the following pages you will find a number of experiences, hobbies, situations and activities which you and your fellow participants experience either as pleasant or unpleasant.

Please concentrate on ***every*** given activity and decide, without pondering; according to your present ***inclinations*** how much you would enjoy this activity. If the chosen activities are not possible, then try to say how much you ***would*** like to perform these activities under other circumstances.

Because the list in this questionnaire is not complete or the specific activity is not always defined exactly, it is possible that something is missing that you would enjoy. If this is the case, then please write down the missing items on the foreseen gaps which appear at various intervals.

Your ratings should be identified by a cross on the line for the appropriate category.

An example describes how you should fill out the questionnaire and which ratings are possible.

	dis-like	like nor dislike	like a little	like	like very much
cultivating roses	–	–	–	x	–
eating fish	–	–	–	–	x

Please be careful not to omit any activity and not to checkmark falsely.

Another piece of advice: There are no correct or incorrect answers in this questionnaire. This is also not a personality test, rather you should checkmark how much you enjoy or would like to enjoy the activities listed.

Please begin!

	dis-like	like nor dislike	like a little	like	like very much
eating					
ice cream	–	–	–	–	–
sweets	–	–	–	–	–
fruit	–	–	–	–	–
cake	–	–	–	–	–
pastry	–	–	–	–	–
certain dishes	–	–	–	–	–
specialties	–	–	–	–	–
....	–	–	–	–	–
drinking					
mineral water	–	–	–	–	–
milk	–	–	–	–	–
tea	–	–	–	–	–
coffee	–	–	–	–	–
fruit juice	–	–	–	–	–
lemonade	–	–	–	–	–
beer	–	–	–	–	–
wine	–	–	–	–	–
other alcoholic	–	–	–	–	–
beverages	–	–	–	–	–
....	–	–	–	–	–
solving					
crossword puzzles	–	–	–	–	–
mathematical problems	–	–	–	–	–
quizzes	–	–	–	–	–
figuring out how something works	–	–	–	–	–
puzzles	–	–	–	–	–
....	–	–	–	–	–
listening to					
symphonic music	–	–			–
chamber music	–	–	–	–	–
jazz	–	–	–	–	–
pop	–	–	–	–	–
....	–	–	–	–	–
visiting					
sporting events	–	–	–	–	–
soccer games	–	–	–	–	–
handball games	–	–	–	–	–
track & field meets	–	–	–	–	–
swim meets	–	–	–	–	–
basketball games	–	–	–	–	–
hockey games	–	–	–	–	–
tennis tournaments	–	–	–	–	–
water-sport activities	–	–	–	–	–
ice hockey games	–	–	–	–	–
boxing matches	–	–	–	–	–
wrestling matches	–	–	–	–	–
car races	–	–	–	–	–
bicycle races	–	–	–	–	–
riding tournaments	–	–	–	–	–
gymnastic meets	–	–	–	–	–
....	–	–	–	–	–
historical buildings	–		–		
museums	–	–	–	–	–
art exhibits	–	–	–	–	–
zoos	–	–	–	–	–
botanical gardens	–	–	–	–	–
....	–	–	–	–	–
dining	–	–	–	–	–
seeing panoramas of landscapes	–	–	–	–	–
....	–	–	–	–	–

Chapter 7

Integrative behavioral medicine in-patient treatment concept for complex chronic tinnitus Evaluation of therapy and long-term effects

Gerhard Goebel, Wolfgang Hiller, Winfried Rief and Manfred Fichter

7.1 Summary

Complex tinnitus describes a disorder in which the patient hears disturbing, irritating noises or tones without identifiable external sound sources, which can be described only by the patients themselves. Although tinnitus is one of the most common otologic disorders, only a few effective medical treatments exist. For this reason various psychological therapies have been developed recently to reduce symptom induced stress, to acquire relevant strategies to deal with the symptoms and possibly minimize those psychological factors which increase the amount of suffering, and finally to employ the symptom itself as a way of coping so as to be able to live as normal as possible again. In this chapter the development of an integrated multi-modular behavioral medicine concept of therapy will be presented. The results of 155 consecutively treated patients are compared with those of a control group. A significant and clinically relevant effect concerning specific tinnitus variables (loudness, discomfort, control of tinnitus) and psychological variables (depression, anxiety, introversion, etc) is evident. A 1 year follow-up study shows stability of the improvement achieved.

7.2 Introduction

In 1981 the following definition of tinnitus was established at the International Tinnitus Congress in London:

"Tinnitus is defined as the sensation of a tone which is not caused by a simultaneous mechanical-acoustic or electrical signal."

Special value was placed on the term "sensation" by the participants and it was recommended that external or objective noises should be omitted from the definition of tinnitus (Anonymous, 1981).

Duckro et al. (1984) defined as "complex chronic tinnitus" those forms of tinnitus with concomittant psychological problems, of considerable degree. We have decided to use this term because we believe that it makes the clinician more aware of the variety of causes and effects of tinnitus than the more common term "decompensated chronic tinnitus".

When a tinnitus patient seeks medical treatment, he is initially asked what is wrong with him. He then describes his symptom, which is consistently or inconsistently perceived as ringing, murmuring, hissing, whistling, whirring, buzzing, humming etc. Only then does the true answer follow: quiet and stillness are absent! He can only withdraw himself from these noises cognitively when external noises mask the tinnitus. Situations which are normally experienced as pleasant stillness (for example, relaxation at home after work, going to bed, waking up in the morning, meditation in a quiet room, etc.) are often threatening situations which are experienced as very aversive by the patient. The seriously affected patient develops psychologically relevant affective and phobic disorders. A large portion of patients treated by us describe threatening suicidal crises in retrospect. 21% of a random sample of 138 patients indicated that their lives are not worthwhile any more because of their tinnitus, 45% agreed with this opinion in part and only about one third regarded their lives as still worthwhile (Goebel & Hiller, 1992).

How tormenting tinnitus can be is described by famous people such as Martin Luther (1483-1546), Jean-Jacques Rousseau (1712-1778) and Francisco Goya (1746-1828). For 50 years Friedric Smetana (1824-1884) suffered from a tinnitus similar to a waterfall with occasional ringing "containing most often the highest tones of the fourth octave" (Feldmann, 1989). In the winter of 1876, Smetana, who was already deaf, composed a string quartet entitled "From my Life", in which the last movement expresses the tinnitus and its complex effects on life exceedingly well. In a letter to the violinist he clearly indicated that the high E, which was to describe his tinnitus, was to be played in an especially piercing manner. From a contemporary medical point of view, Smetana's tinnitus could be diagnosed as the result of untreated syphilis (Feldmann, 1964).

7.3 Pathophysiology

Recently numerous insights have been won in the fields of physiology and pathophysiology (Feldmann, 1987; Goebel, 1989a; Lenarz, 1989; also see Chapter 1).

Pain research, with the development of the gate control theory, has contributed to an understanding of the complexity of tinnitus (Melzack and Wall, 1965). Tonndorf (1987) relied on this theory and was able to treat various explanations of tinnitus as hypothetically identical (Fig 7.1).

According to Tonndorf, thick,

rapid-conducting afferent nerve-fibres of the internal hair cells lock a hypothetical 'gate' and thin, slow-conducting afferent nerve-fibres of the external hair cells unlock this 'gate'. The difference in the velocity of impulse conduction between the afferent A-β-fibres of the internal hair cells and the afferent C- and A-γ fibres of the external hair cells and the different amount of individual nerve fibre types may lead to a decrease of the inhibiting effect of the substantia gelatinosa (SG) when interaction is disturbed and cause tinnitus due to increased stimulation of the transmitter cell (T). When this hypothetical gate is locked, tinnitus is perceived less; in the case of uninhibited stimulation, tinnitus is perceived more.

The afferent path of the 8th nerve leads to the auditory path, which then leads to the brain stem via polysynaptic connections and from there to other parts of the brain (centres of speech, optic system, autonomous nerve system, the cognitive system, the emotional system, the sensory system, the co-ordination centre of the neck-, head- and mastication-muscles) (Melzack, R., Casey, K. L., 1968). The COGNITIVE SYSTEM, situated in the cortex, analyses the tinnitus stimulus

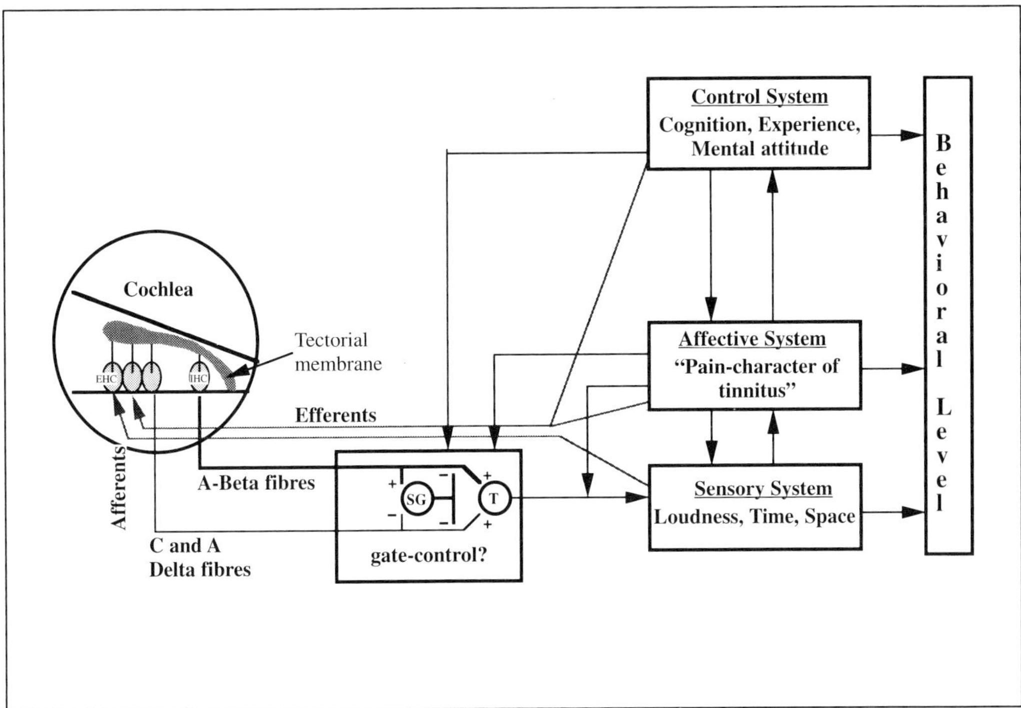

Fig. 7.1 Hypothetical multifactorial psychophysiological tinnitus model: Tonndorf's analogy and reference to Melzack's Gate Control Theory (1968); Conceptualization of a tinnitus model with peripheral and central determinants of tinnitus perception and tinnitus control; SG = Substantia gelatinosa; T = Transmission of SG to central structures; IHC = internal hair cells; EHC = external hair cells.

according to possible interpretation as disorder, prior experience, symbolic meanings, controlability, and assesses the results. It also controls the resulting data and behaviour and interacts with the emotional and sensory systems.

The EMOTIONAL SYSTEM (limbic system) contributes to the perception of uneasiness, torment, rage, etc. and mobilizes biological defences as well as reactions of the organism, with the aim of quelling the tinnitus. The SENSORY SYSTEM (cortex) is responsible for the localization of the stimuli in respect to location, time and volume (Fig. 8.1).

Another modulation is caused by higher central structures: efferent paths exist which can stimulate the external hair cells of the cochlea directly and thereby enable a change in the length of hair cells. This leads to relevant changes of the organ of Corti and via this path presumably also to the modulation of cochlear tinnitus (see Chapter 1). This is the hypothetical explanation of how momentary concentration, distraction, suggestion and anxiety can influence the modulation of the intensity of tinnitus.

The complex co-ordination of these mechanisms (together with the different functions of the transmitter substances, which are not discussed further here) results in observable behaviour on the motor, verbal and physiological level.

This multi-faceted model leads to a better understanding of the effect of tinnitus — masking, membrane-stabilizing drugs, electrical stimulation and above all the influence on tinnitus of cognitions, emotions, behaviour, etc. Given the aim of further clarification of the pathophysiology and further improvement of the treatment of tinnitus, it is only sensible to include the medical and psychological results of pain research.

On the one hand, the gate control theory has made an important conceptual contribution to basic research of pain, and has been partially verified in numerous experiments of classical psycho-physics. On the other hand, numerous neurophysiological findings could not be explained by this theory. As the differentiation and hierarchic organization of the these systems is controversial and could only be replicated in clinical practice (esp. in treatment of chronic pain) with great difficulty (Geissner, 1990), we prefer to use a more process-oriented approach to tinnitus management in respect of psychodiagnostics and therapy.

7.4 Reasons for the development of a psychological concept of treatment

When we first made contact with the board of directors of the German Tinnitus League (DTL) in 1986/87 and carried out literature research, the following situation became evident:

With few exceptions, no case reports about the psychological treatment of complex chronic tinnitus existed at that time in Germany. As the few descriptive publications (Wimmer, 1983) did not stand up to scientific review, we had to develop and evaluate a new treatment concept based on international experience and results (Jakes et al., 1986a; Scott et al., 1985; Sweetow et al., 1984).

Our experience in the psychological treatment of chronic pain disorders since 1985/86 (Goebel et al., 1989; Goebel, 1989b; Fichter & Goebel, 1989) was useful, a conclusion we shared with other authors (Duckro et al., 1984; Scott et al., 1985; Sweetow, 1986 etc.). As a medical-psychosomatic clinic, which is known throughout Germany as the largest treatment center for patients with anorexia and bulimia, no comparable contact existed with an ear, nose and throat (E.N.T.) department, as was the case in the United States, England and Sweden. Due to efforts together with the German Tinnitus League, mutual research in association with the German Organization for Otolaryngorhinology and co-operation with the health and social insurance organizations, our clinic rapidly earned the reputation of being specialized, so that we are already able to review the data of ca.400 (1991) tinnitus patients (1995: 1400 patients).

Initially the patients were treated individually in the ward for chronic pain. Experience gained in this ward encouraged us to treat the tinnitus patients together with pain patients, so that at this point 10-15 tinnitus patients participate continuously with 13-18 pain patients in a 6-12 week in-patient treatment program. Those components of therapy which are indicated for both disorders are carried out together. More specialized therapy modules such as counselling, body perception, diary groups, etc. are symptom oriented. Tinnitus patients feel more at home among pain patients than they do in a general psychosomatic ward. Both patient groups have had similar painful experiences in respect to diagnosis and therapy prior to admission. Both perceive themselves as primarily not psychologically ill and have begun to take note of the fact that the aim of therapy is acceptance not cure prior to admission, due to information brochures and interviews. Finally, a considerable desire exists among both patient groups for more medical as well as psychological information about their disorder and both groups feel similarly victimized (threatened dismissal and unemployment, misunderstandings with family, friends and colleagues). Finally, both symptom groups include many patients whose lives were significantly more goal-oriented than oriented to emotional needs. Because of their medical problem, they had little or no contact with psychological aspects of their disorder (for further parallels or differences, see Table 7.1).

7.5 Psychotherapeutic considerations for the treatment of complex chronic tinnitus

Although tinnitus is a serious medical problem, in which numerous patients subject themselves for years to various diagnostic and therapeutic measures which are not indicated, world-wide there are only relatively few research groups who have done intensive research on this disorder. Only a few empirical studies in Germany were concerned with psychological inter-relationships and different methods of psychotherapy (Wimmer, 1983; Hollweg, 1989; Ganz, 1986; Greuel, 1988). Research concerning the effects of behavioral therapy has not been published with the exception of studies by Gerber (1986) and v. Wedel et al. (1989), which report on unsatisfactory results of biofeedback and relaxation techniques. It appears that there is still widespread resignation among physicians and patients tend to resort to alternative healing methods which they have to finance to a great extent themselves. This is surprising because important progress has been made, particularly in the last few years, not only concerning the pathophysiology of tinnitus but also fundamental considerations concerning effective treatment.

7.5.1 Therapy

Patients with intolerable tinnitus as the principal complaint are often a complex puzzle for the otologist. If the examination shows no considerable pathological findings

Table 7.1 Similarities and differences between tinnitus and pain (according to Goebel et al, 1991a)

Medical level:	
afference pattern	++
modulation of afference by "gate control"	?
symptom persistence caused by afference lesions	++
sympton persistence caused by central lesions	++
existence of efferent adaptation mechanisms	++
symptom persistence caused by efferent lesions	++
symptom persistence caused by functional disorders (bruxism, cervical spine syndrome)	++
lack of objective specification of the chronic syndrome	++
effect of local anesthetics	+
effect of antiarrhythmic agents	+
effect of magnesium	+
effect of anti-epileptics	+
effect of psychopharmaceuticals	+
effect of electrical stimulation/iontophoresis	+
effect of acupuncture	++
Behavioural level:	
operant conditioning process	++
psychological communication disorder ("not hearing")	++
behavior disorder	++
flight and avoidance behavior	++
retreat behavior	++
disturbance in concentration	++
disturbance in sleep	++
Cognitive level:	
sustained passive behavioral strategies	++
symptom as enemy	++
devaluation of self-esteem	++
thinking in either-or categories	++
predominantly pathophysiological understanding of the disease by the specialist and the patient (linear-causal)	++
restricted somatic approach = nothing was found = psychogenic	++
placebo-effect	++
Emotional level:	
emotional modulation	++
depressive reaction, suicidal tendencies	++
pathological grief (depression)	++
loss of integrity	++
loss of self-esteem	++
paranoid reactions	++
anxiety reactions	++
neurotic reactions	++
pathological SCL-90-R-ratings	++
pathological FPI-R-ratings	++
Psychosocial level:	
resulting problems in marriage/family	++
resulting problems in career/household	++
disability problems	++
Psychotherapeutic level:	
prejudices of the specialist and the patient toward psychophysiological methods of therapy	+
primarily difficult access to disease using depth psychology	++
psychosomatic aspects	++
therapy goal of multidimensional understanding of symptom	++
therapy goal of disease management	++
therapy goal of symptom tolerance	++
therapy goal of symptom acceptance	++
therapy goal of change in behavior	++
therapy goal of building responsibility for self	++
therapy goal of stress management	++
therapy goal of promoting self-assurance	++
therapy goal of identification of stress	++
therapy goal of psychological improvement of communication	++
therapy goal of reduction of alcohol abuse	+
therapy goal of reduction of drug abuse	+
effect of hypnosis	++
effect of relaxation	++
effect of music therapy	+
Differences between tinnitus and pain	
Medical level:	
"sensory organ"	– –
organ structure ennervated by efferents (external hair cells or musculature/sympathetic nervous system)	– –
organic communication disorder (hearing disorder)	– –
over-cautiousness	– –
effect of analgesics	– –
vicious circle of afferent-efferent neural connections	?
Behavioral level:	
obvious over-cautious behavior	–
accepted disorder for the environment	– –
symptom understood by the environment	– –
hostility of the environment towards the patient (hearing disorder)	– –

+ = partial similarities; ++ = clear similarities
– = partial differences; – – = clear differences

and the usual therapy does not lead to success, it is important to change the strategy, relying on the active co-operation of the patient. Therapy which enables the patient to learn to live with tinnitus is of prime importance. This fact can be equated with the fact that treatment is indicated which primarily helps the patient to cope with the problems which derive from the disorder. Psychological methods of treatment help to attain this therapeutic goal (coping), and also have highly specific effects directly on the course of the disorder.

After a thorough differential diagnosis, physiological, technical and physiotherapeutic methods predominate in the initial stage of tinnitus treatment (see Chapter 1). It would be beyond the scope of this chapter to discuss the effectiveness of these types of therapy. It also appears that a considerable psychological influence exists in the sense of a placebo effect as an additional effective factor in the operative field as well as in technological methods of treatment (Duckert and Rees, 1984; Thomson et al., 1983; Erlandsson et al., 1987b), even though this is not explicitly mentioned. For a series of causes of tinnitus (sudden deafness, cervicogenic tinnitus, idiopathic tinnitus) methods of treatment such as relaxation, biofeedback, hypnotherapy, hypnosis and crisis intervention are also viable additions to therapy in the *acute stage*. We, as well as other researchers (e.g. Greuel, 1988), have observed this in individual cases. Acute tinnitus should be diagnosed quickly and should be medically treated including various holistic approaches.

Management of *chronic* tinnitus requires more serious consideration. If a complete cure can no longer be the primary therapeutic goal, strategies must be developed mutually with the patient which consider the degree of annoyance and discomfort, as well as the personal perception of the tinnitus. This means that the patient himself increasingly becomes the main focus of therapy, starts to feel responsible again for his life and actively co-operates. The otologist, on the other hand, should not feel obliged to agree to all the suggestions made by the patient, especially when he is not convinced of their effectiveness, but should rather intensify the exchange of those ideas which deal with improved coping capabilities (Sweetow, 1986).

Medical training concentrates mainly on the treatment of acute tinnitus, and therefore constantly leads to a repetition of the same approach toward examination and treatment. Not only the otologist needs training and continuing education in order to prevent the patient who is suffering from a chronic tinnitus from becoming fixated on passive expectations concerning therapy. The purpose of patient guidance in the case of chronic tinnitus must be to motivate the patient to accept a greater responsibility in coping with tinnitus (more support, less treatment).

7.5.1.1 Management of disturbances caused by tinnitus (coping)

After psychosomatic research concentrated on the clarification and relief of stress in various disorders in the 1960s, coping research, e.g. research concerning the management of a disorder, has become increasingly important in the fields of medical psychology and psychosomatics. Especially the research group of R.S. Lazarus was acknowledged for the fact that it emphasized the process aspect of disease management compared to the traditional dichotomy of the stress reaction, e.g. the division between physiological and psychological components (Lazarus and Folkmann, 1984a, and b).

The traditional clinical theory is based on psychoanalytical ego psychology with its hierarchical structural concept of ego activity, leading from normal to severely pathological manifestations. According to this theory, disease management works best in persons with so-called 'mature ego-processes', whereas persons more concerned with defending themselves from neurotic ego-processes have greater difficulties. The worst adaption occurs in persons with very weak egos (borderline-structure). House (1981) considered the effectiveness of biofeedback in relation to personality traits (Minnesota Multiphasic Personality Inventory, MMPI) and postulated that relaxation techniques were ineffective for seriously disturbed patients, although exceptions were found in a few cases. Muthney (1989), from the point of view of ego-psychology, observed that unsuccessful disease management was due to avoiding separation from a loved object, in the case of tinnitus, avoiding separation from the loved object of physical and psychic invulnerability and of peace and tranquillity (see section 7.5.2.7).

Many problems are associated, on the other hand, with this conventional approach. One of the most important is the rather static one-dimensional typology, which leaves little room for other explanations. According to Lazarus (1984) and Heim (1988), the management of disease is much more complex and variable. For example, an avoidance strategy or other defence mechanisms can be signs of a mature ego, which at one point in time are beneficial but may contribute to chronification at another point in time or under other circumstances. This means, all coping strategies can be both beneficial as well as detrimental. The new, more micro-analytical context- and process-oriented efforts emphasize four main characteristics:

— In the analysis of strategies for disease management, the situation is first identified and then evaluated in relationship to its meaning for physical and psychological integrity.

— As a process, the coping strategy changes in the course of time and experiences change within the context of new situations. Acts and thoughts are to be viewed as a result of the active interplay between the individual and his environment (transaction).

— The coping strategies should be constantly reviewed and, if necessary, corrected because of the continuously changing conditions (chronification).

— Caution is required toward the tendency to classify coping processes according to the categories 'good or bad'. Rather, they should be seen individually in conjunction with the prevailing personality and possibilities as well as various situational aspects at a given time. Also to be considered are the type and degree of the disturbing effects, the social ability and the overall physical health of the patient.

Lazarus and Folkmann (1984 b) defined a stressor such as tinnitus as being of an external physical type as well as of an internal psychosocial type (independent variables). This leads to a more or less specific psychological and physical reaction, the startting point for the actual method of disease managment or coping. The coping process itself is influenced by the rather static variables which refer to personality as well as the dynamic variables which refer to situation (transaction model). This approach implies that disease management (intervening variable) does not run strictly in one direction, but rather in a circular movement and continuously assesses the personality-related and situational variables in order to achieve an optimal adaptation (independent variable) (Fig. 7.2).

Disease management (as a process, not a personality trait) is the result of the individual effort and exertion of the patient, not the result of his personal qualities. The coping process requires constant management and should not be understood as mastering a problem so as to avoid a rating according to categories of good or bad *per se*.

It is therefore important in the

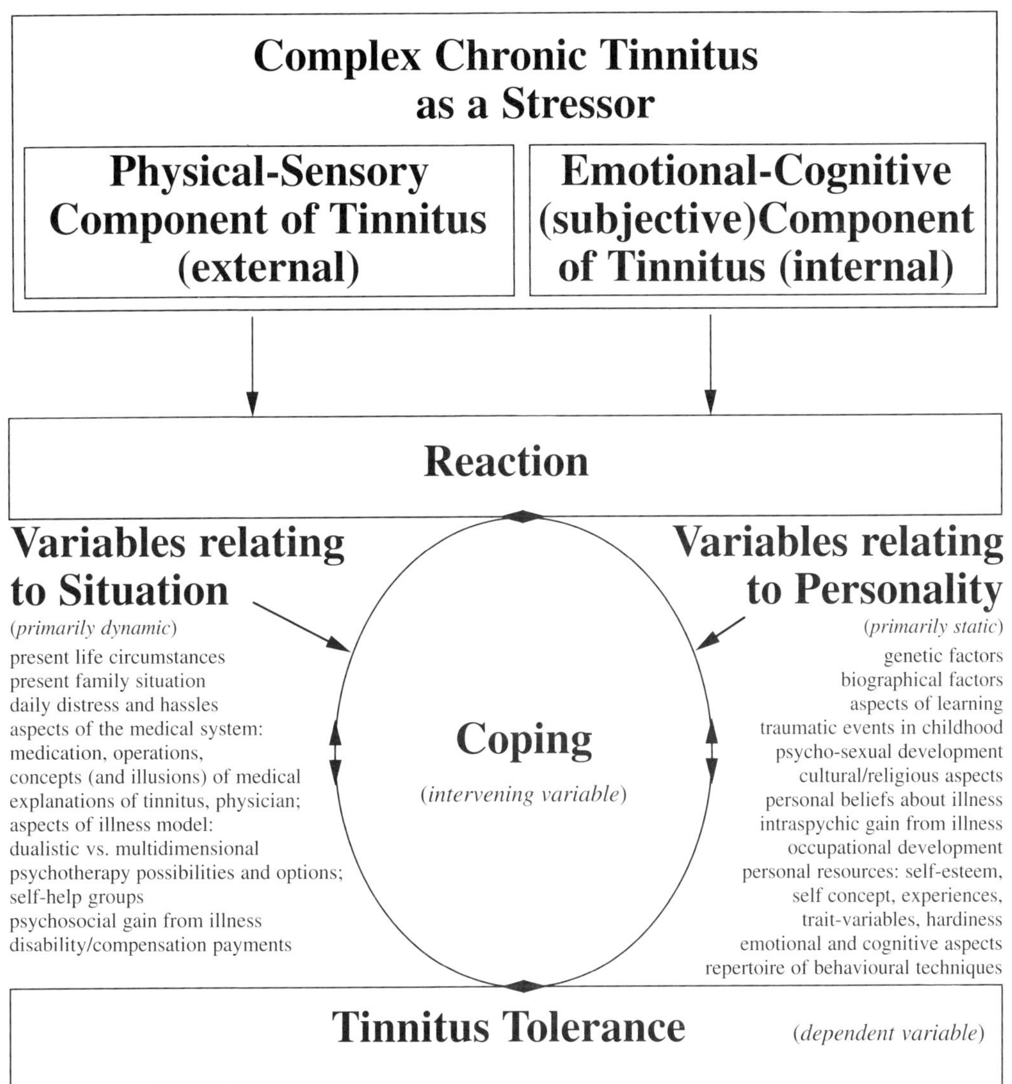

Fig. 7.2 Coping with tinnitus: Transposition and modification of the dynamic, process-related transaction model of Lazarus and Folkmann (1984) to the problem of complex chronic tinnitus; coping occurs circularly and continuously assesses variables which refer to situation and personality.

planning of the treatment of complex chronic tinnitus to integrate physiological behavior-oriented, emotional, cognitive and social factors in the analysis of etiology and course of the disorder.

As it is no longer relevant to differentiate between an organic and psychological etiology in chronic tinnitus, it is necessary to strive for the integration of psychotherapy and biomedicine in diagnosis, treatment and rehabilitation of the chronic tinnitus patient. Different monotherapies which were implemented and evaluated in the last decade (see Chapter 5), had only limited value. For this reason we proceeded from the beginning to use a treatment model derived from interactive treatment models of other disorders (Goebel, 1989 b; Fichter and Goebel, 1991).

7.5.1.2 Goal of therapy

Two coping strategies can be derived from the above observations:

Emotional-cognitive coping strategies include methods intended to change present feelings (e.g. helplessness, tension) and/or the significance of tinnitus as well as the perception of the relationship to the environment. These include distanciation (for example, 'I will continue living my life, even if the tinnitus bothers me') and positive new assessments (for example, 'I believe that I will overcome this' etc.). If one can experience the disorder less as a 'disturbing enemy' for example, the emotional crisis can be alleviated and includes dealing with different emotions such as sadness, anger, shame, guilt, anxiety, etc. (see Fig. 7.3) during psychotherapy.

By influencing the environment and individual behavior directly, problem-oriented management changes the actual perception of adaption itself. This includes confrontational management (for example, 'I won't allow myself to be brought down by tinnitus and I'll fight for my goals'), looking for social support (self-help groups, contact with similarly affected patients, directing attention of others to the pressures of a hearing impairment, etc.) self-control (for example, preservation of one's dignity, not sharing every feeling with others) and taking over responsibility for the course of treatment as well as problem-solving (for example, establishing progressive steps for management of tinnitus attacks, in the form of an emergency plan).

Of importance are the reduction of behavior involving flight and avoidance, direct communication (for example, not only relying on the disorder as a justification for additional consideration, self-assertiveness training), avoiding the misuse of tinnitus as a scapegoat and general stress management strategies (for more information, see Figure 7.3).

Both coping strategies overlap with therapeutic goals which are effective on the "external" psychophysiological level (relaxation, biofeedback, hearing aids, etc.) and in general are not as strictly subdivided as they appear in the diagram. They interrelate and interact. Thus, relaxation can be effective as an emotional coping strategy as well (systematic decrease of tinnitus discomfort) and can also be applied to the communicative (internal) level (for example, to tell one's colleagues that 15 minutes of rest is necessary). Finally, a relaxation exercise also changes one's own behavior, because rest periods are consciously included in the course of a day (problem-oriented coping).

Coping strategies should be of an individualized nature and can be functional (beneficial) or dysfunctional (detrimental), depending on the stage of the disorder. Typical wishful thinking in complex tinnitus, for example, is that the tinnitus will disappear in the near future and is dysfunctional as it does not allow the development of alternative problem solving. Unrealistic optimism in the acute stage of tinnitus can be dysfunctional because it makes a thorough differential diagnosis and treatment difficult. In the chronic stage, a positive new assessment, on the other hand, is a functional management possibility because it promotes the feeling of self-esteem and the courage to work on new coping strategies.

The decision in favour of a more emotion-oriented or a more problem-oriented management strategy can vary from situation to situation. A realistic attitude is the use of emotion-oriented coping strategies for the acceptance of tinnitus as a long-term goal;

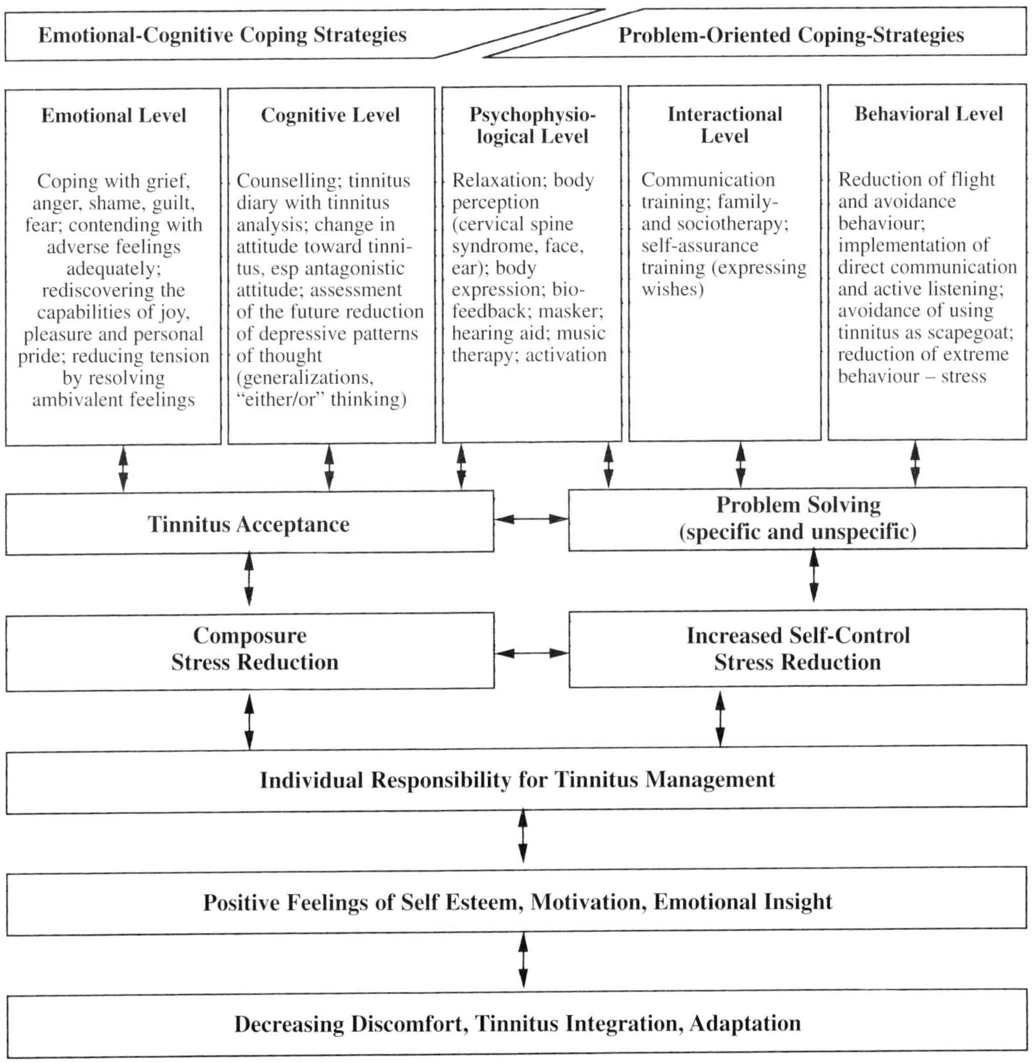

Fig. 7.3 Psychotherapy goals of tinnitus: through emotional-cognitive or problem-oriented coping strategies. The therapeutic goal of tinnitus integration should be strived for utilizing psychological interventions on various levels and the patients' active cooperation.

a strategy or problem-oriented attitude does not lead in the long run in the opinion of the majority of chronic tinnitus patients to an acceptance and adequate integration of the disorder. On the other hand, one cannot help warning against undue generalization in respect to 'good' and 'bad' coping because medical progress involves continuous re-orientation.

We know from many case histories the fatal influence a restricted somatic understanding of disease in the sense of a dualistic disease model causes; a dualistic model of disease, e.g. the division of body and soul, has been present in medicine since Descartes (1596-1650) and frequently stands in the way of an appropriate integration of tinnitus. Psychological problems which lead to a deterioration of complaints frequently increase because only the somatic aspects of a disorder are treated. The patient tends to perceive himself as ill in a purely somatic context because medicine tends to take only those patients seriously who present themselves as physically ill. Lacking somatic findings, which is often the case with both tinnitus and pain, the patients are repeatedly put on sick-leave or they are dismissed from the somatically-oriented health care system with the remark, 'You are not ill, there is nothing we can do to help you.' Offended or suspicious, the patient allows himself to be examined by other experts, and is therefore increasingly fixated on a somatically-oriented disease model. Even the use of tranquillizers and sleeping pills — which are undoubtedly beneficial in the acute stage — can be a form of treatment which makes a problem-oriented goal of therapy difficult in the long run and can increase feelings of dependence and helplessness as well as substance-dependence.

In conclusion, strategies have to concentrate on a more active self-responsible management (internal control), not a passive expectation of a solution (external control). According to Lazarus and Folkmann (1984 b), it appears that this is one of the most favorable pre-conditions for the development of an adequate management of a chronic condition.

7.5.2 Psychotherapeutic procedures

7.5.2.1 Counselling

Comprehensive information about causes and effects of tinnitus already improves the relationship between patient and therapist and leads to a correction of misconceptions and detrimental attributions (McFadden, 1982; Druckro et al., 1984; Scott et al., 1985; Sweetow, 1986; Hallam, 1987; Hallam et al., 1988; Jakes et al., 1992; Goebel, 1989 a; Goebel et al., 1991 a and b). But counselling alone is not psychotherapy. A number of psychological strategies are available which help the patient to accept his tinnitus as a disability in the initial stages of the disorder and induce the patient to develop an active attitude quickly, so as to prevent passive expectations with respect to a complete remission. Strategies of information and orientation which have been thoroughly devised can be as effective as relaxation methods (Jakes et al., 1986 a).

Because the majority of our patients know very little about their disorder and have no idea how important psychotherapy is, we inform them before admission about our treatment concept (letter or preliminary interview), recommend contact with the German Tinnitus League, with other tinnitus patients or regional self-help groups and recommend a self-help book (Hallam, 1989; Tonnies, 1991). Our aim is to help the patient to spend his time in a meaningful way before admission, and we hope this leads to an initial change from a previous one-dimensional model to a multi-dimensional understanding ("My tinnitus problem is also dependent on my emotional state of mind and my personal perception" etc.). Finally, the patient should try to learn a relaxation method before admission as a preparation for in-patient treatment.

An information group, which takes place once a week after admission, has the following goals: to increase motivation for group therapy and to minimize educational and informational components in favor of psychotherapy in a group setting. We have observed that tinnitus patients (as well as pain patients) are often afraid of psychotherapy as a means of influencing a symptom on an emotional basis because they are afraid of being perceived as exaggerating deceivers. This has to be dealt with immediately, especially if the patients are fixated on a dualistic tinnitus model, because it makes access to psychological methods considerably more difficult. In the information group, we explain to the patients a simplified model of the gate-control theory (the effect of efferent pathways on the cochlea and the complex relationships of the central nervous system). This often relieves the patients because they can now accept as normal what they previously experienced as a discriminating neurosis. At this point the patients begin to perceive emotional and somatic factors as a single interrelated complex and find rapid access to family- and work-related problems or daily hassles, which were avoided initially because they were afraid of being perceived as malingering or neurotic. The active participation of the patient concerning therapy goals and effectiveness of psychological aspects in the treatment of complex tinnitus increases the patient's belief in this treatment concept, and, as a result, the patient is more inclined to practise and develop coping strategies (Goebel, 1989 a, 1991 b) (Fig. 7.2).

7.5.2.2 Prien's tinnitus diary

An important and established part of behavioral medicine is the individual observation of symptoms in the form of a diary ('self-monitoring'). Diaries are personal reports about individual observations of the course of chronic symptoms and associated aspects. In the behavioral-therapy oriented treatment of chronic pain we and other therapy centres have evaluated the effectiveness and practicality of self-monitoring (Keeser et al., 1989), and have included diaries as an important part of therapy as a result (Tursky et al., 1982; Fordyce, 1976; Jakes et al., 1986 b; Gerber & Diener, 1987; Goebel, 1989 b; Dobbek et al., 1990). Since 1987 we have used the pain diary developed by W. Keeser because of its specificity.

All patients judge daily tinnitus loudness, tinnitus discomfort, mood, strain (stress), ability to control tinnitus (influence on tinnitus discomfort, coping) using a visual analog scale on a printed form, and finally rate personal opinions about their therapy results (development of their responsibility for the therapeutic course and its evaluation). Furthermore, the patients note daily amount of sleep, duration of tinnitus tolerance per day and the entire duration of tinnitus tolerance (amount of sleep plus duration of tolerance) (Figs 7.4 and 7.5).

The values of the above-mentioned variables are then recorded graphically so that — as is the case with a temperature curve — the development of the individual variables can be observed in the course of therapy (see appendix).

Furthermore, a space is provided on a daily protocol for recording individual opinions about tinnitus (e.g. "Will I ever make it?") and feelings that are associated with tinnitus (e.g. 'helplessness'). In therapy attention is given to how the individual opinions and feelings change and which promoting and non-promoting thoughts appear continuously, in order to discuss them in individual or group therapy (Fig. 7.5).

Finally, space is available on the protocol for recording coping strategies and evaluating the strategies in respect to duration, loudness and discomfort of tinnitus. An analysis of beneficial and detrimental strategies can be made and, as the need arises,

TINNITUS DIARY Name: ______________________ Date: __________ Time: ________
(Please complete every evening)

Roseneck Clinic, 83209 Prien, Telephone 08051-6010

1. **LOCATION OF TINNITUS:** Where did you hear the tinnitus today? Please mark the corresponding area of the body in Figure 1.

Figure 1: Location of tinnitus (indicate the exact region of tinnitus)

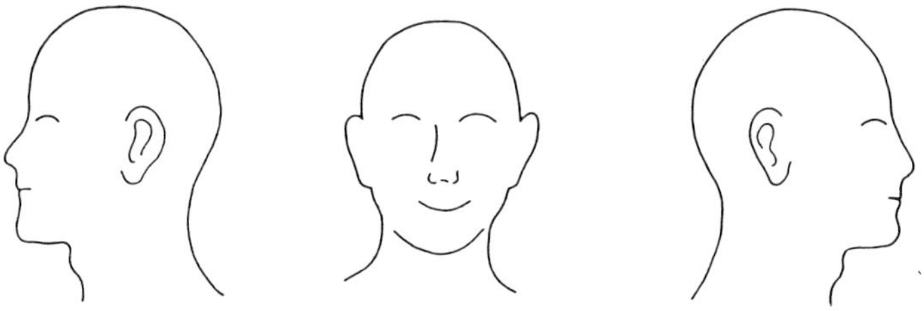

2. **TYPE OF TINNITUS:** Was today's tinnitus (indicate the corresponding)

continuous, steady, constantly present?	yes ( )	no ( )
rhythmic, periodic, occasionally worse?	yes ( )	no ( )
brief, momentary, intermittent?	yes ( )	no ( )

3. a. **TINNITUS PERCEPTION:** How much have you perceived your tinnitus compared to yesterday (mark the corresponding square)

considerably more often	more often	just as often	less often	considerably less often
☐	☐	☐	☐	☐

3. b. **TINNITUS TOLERANCE TIME:** Please estimate the time in the course of the last 24 hours during which you perceived the tinnitus as tolerable or did not notice it at all and add up the total amount of time. Please note that you do not notice the tinnitus during sleep, for example, or do not perceive or "forget" it during a loud and interesting activity/conversation (eg. 6 hours sleep + 3 hours tolerable tinnitus = 9 hours)

☐ + ☐ = ☐

hours of sleep **hours of tolerance per day** **total hours**

4. **TINNITUS LOUDNESS:** How loud was your tinnitus today? Please indicate your tinnitus loudness with a vertical line on the line between 0 (not perceivable) and 100 (extremely loud).

0 ———————————————— **100**

5. **TINNITUS DISCOMFORT:** How irritating/disturbing/uncomfortable was your tinnitus today? Please indicate your tinnitus discomfort with a vertical line on the line between 0 (none at all) and 100 (extremely strong).

0 ———————————————— **100**

6. **MEDICATION:** Did you take medication today? Yes ( ) no ( ). If yes, list only prn medication (medication as needed) in in-patients treatment; in out-patient treatment list total medication!

Time of intake	**Type of medication**	**Amount**

Fig. 7.4 Prien's tinnitus diary (front page) with the variables, tinnitus quality (location, type), tinnitus perception (compared to the previous day, tinnitus tolerance time, analog scale 4 tinnitus loudness, analog scale 5 tinnitus discomfort) and list of medication.

7. **How many hours did you "lose" today because of your tinnitus?**
(only for out-patient patients)
At work ____________ At housework ____________ At recreation ____________

8. **EPISODES OF TINNITUS:** When was your tinnitus worst today? ____________

How long did this tinnitus phase last? ____________ Where were you at this time? ____________

What did you do during this time? ____________

Who was with you? ____________

What preceded the tinnitus episode? ____________

How did you **feel** during the serious episode of tinnitus (**emotions**)? ____________

What did you **think** during the serious episode of tinnitus (**thoughts**)? ____________

What did you **do** to relieve the tinnitus? Please indicate in spaces a-f

(a) ____________ (b) ____________

(c) ____________ (d) ____________

(e) ____________ (f) ____________

How effective were these measures?
(indicate the corresponding letters (a-f) from above in the boxes!)

	intensity	duration	discomfort
did not help at all			
helped somewhat			
helped considerably			
helped a lot			

9. **How was your mood in general during the day?** Please indicate your mood again with a vertical line between 0 (very bad) and 100 (very good)

0 ———————————————— **100**

10. **How "stressed" (burdened, agitated) did you feel today?**
(0 = not at all, 100 = very much)

0 ———————————————— **100**

11. **Which events were a burden today?** ____________

____

Did the tinnitus get worse because of these stressful situations? Yes ( ) No ( )

12. **Did you have the feeling today that you could influence the tinnitus yourself (control)?**
(0 = not at all, 100 = very much)

0 ———————————————— **100**

13. **How convinced are you that the therapy will be successful?**
(0 = completely unsuccessful, 100 = very successful)

0 ———————————————— **100**

Fig. 7.5 Prien's tinnitus diary (reverse side) with tinnitus analysis (situation, trigger, mood and emotions relating to experienced tinnitus), coping strategies and their efficiency; variables mood (analog scale 9), distress (analog scale 10), general irritation, feeling of tinnitus control = coping (analog scale 12) and feelings concerning success of therapy (analog scale 13).

possibilities for correction can be discussed (Fig. 7.5).

This type of documentation promotes critical self observation (the knowledge of objective correlations between external and internal events), enables a modulation of perception and an examination of experienced coping strategies. Active self-observation especially helps the patient to assume responsibility for the course of therapy and leads to an emotional and cognitive restructuring.

The promotion of the patient's ability for introspection is furthermore improved during mutual discussion in the "tinnitus diary group", where the patients discuss their own observations and share insights. The diary also helps the individual therapist to construct a behavioral analysis of the individual tinnitus problem and is an evaluation instrument concerning the course of therapy. Working with a diary is very worthwhile (Goebel, 1989 b; Goebel et al., 1990; Goebel et al., 1991 b) and has also been used by other authors as a therapeutic element (Sweetow, 1984; Duckrow et al., 1984; Scott et al., 1985). An important difference is that our diary is more detailed in respect of effectiveness of therapy and motivation. As soon as patients understand the diary as an important contribution to a successful therapy, they are sufficiently motivated to keep a diary continuously. Experience shows that patients who do not keep a diary profit little from a psychological treatment. It takes only little time to record the variables on the analog scale, and we believe this to be obligatory. Later the protocol of thoughts, feelings and coping strategies are included.

An important educational element is the differentiation between tinnitus loudness and tinnitus discomfort, as well as the understanding of control over tinnitus (coping). The confrontation with these variables tends to lead to the realization that, in tinnitus of the same loudness, it is possible to change the degree of tinnitus discomfort, which is then rated as control over tinnitus.

The correlation between emotional mood, stress and tinnitus discomfort can also be recognised quickly and individual coping strategies can be developed as a result.

Heated discussions arise concerning the variable "Attitude toward the success of therapy". At the beginning of therapy the patients still expect a decrease in the volume of tinnitus and rate the success of treatment as practically zero, although there have been clear improvements in the variables of amount of sleep, duration of tinnitus tolerance, mood and stress, as well as the ability to concentrate ("I can read a book again"). Such erroneous beliefs about the course of therapy and false self-evaluations are then recognized and modified by discussing the course of therapy individually. This may then lead to an enormous increase of motivation with respect to attainable therapy goals.

7.5.2.3 Integration of emotional and cognitive elements of therapy

Severe chronic tinnitus is frequently combined with depression to the point of suicide (House, 1981; Tyler & Baker, 1983; Hallam, 1989; Harrop-Griffiths et al., 1987; Halford & Andersson, 1991) (also see chapter 4). The therapeutic goal in individual and group therapy in these cases is above all to facilitate coping with the disease, improving activity level, and cognitive restructuring as an element in disease management.

Grief is an important part of therapy because it is an essential emotional process that helps to cope with a disease properly. In the psychoanalytical sense, grief is the reaction to loss of a loved object (e.g. in the case of tinnitus, physical integrity, composure, etc.) and enables the grief-stricken to disengage himself (Muthny, 1989; Palm et al, 1989).

Grief as an emotion has phenomenologic similarities with depressive despondency, with disinterest, lack of drive, psychological and psychomotor inhibitions, negative cognitions, and disorders of the autonomous nervous system. Persisting depressed mood over years, however, can be classified as pathological grief or depression (Kokott, 1982). The therapeutic approach in this case corresponds with the therapy of depression.

An effective therapy of depression may also include family therapy e.g. working together with the family, relatives or close friends of the depressed tinnitus patient, because they tend to react aggressively to constant complaints about tinnitus, especially if hearing impairment and recruitment is also present (Schönweiler, 1986). The components of tinnitus, including relaxation exercises, body perception exercises and self-assertiveness training, contribute to an increase of self-esteem.

Insights drawn from the course of the diary, experience and imitation of the behavior of other patients (model learning) and increased hope which arises when the patient witnesses promising developments of other patients are also essential. The therapeutic relationship has a significant effect because patients often feel accepted once again, although they are disabled.

Analysis and psychotherapy frequently neglect the importance of phobic symptoms during the course of complex chronic tinnitus (Harrop-Griffiths, 1987; Halford & Andersson, 1991) (also see Chapter 4). Many patients have withdrawn from situations associated with noise or simultaneous conversations (for example, they do not attend concerts anymore, give up playing an instrument, etc), and as a result they give up a considerable part of their previous quality of life as well as recreational potential. Increasingly, the avoided situations become sources of anxiety and panic. We have experienced patients who only go outside wearing ear protection, spend most of their time at home, and have switched off their telephone and doorbell. Such a development requires a therapy which coincides with the therapy of anxiety neurosis (Rief & Kohli, 1991). Some of our patients participate in an anxiety management program in our clinic which gives our patients the necessary support to expose themselves to above mentioned aversive situations once again (exposition training).

Another element of phobic developments is related to situations associated with silence or stillness. For example, many patients listen to music coming from loudspeakers which they have installed in every room of their home constantly and panic when they are in quiet surroundings. Even in this case, exposition training is an important component of therapy, as it convinces the patients of their capability to cope with such critical situations. In these "exposition exercises for stillness"; the patients are asked to distanciate themselves from tinnitus (distraction) as well as consciously to perceive it (exposition) in order to strike up an "inner conversation" with it ("listening to, instead of listening away"). There is also enough time, in such a session, to record tinnitus loudness, tinnitus discomfort, emotional mood, thoughts, or to "correspond" with the tinnitus in letter-form (see Chapter 13). It is important to discuss the experience in a follow-up individual therapy session or group therapy, and to motivate the patient to undertake additional "tests of courage" (e.g. continue exposition training).

7.5.2.4 Group and individual therapy

Because all patients participate in individual and group therapy, they must be able to communicate to a certain degree. If necessary a hearing aid is tested in close cooperation with a hearing aid technician. We have sound-proofed a group-therapy room in order to eliminate to à certain degree the effects of recruitment and other disturbances. In group therapy 10-14 patients who suffer from either tinnitus or chronic pain syndrome take part. Techniques from cognitive therapy (see Chapters 6 and 8–11) as well as elements from Gestalt therapy, bioenergetic therapy and psychodrama are used (Wimmer, 1983). Group therapy lasts 90 minutes and takes place twice a week. Two therapists (a clinical psychologist and a doctor with psychotherapy training) guide the group and are also responsible for the individual therapy of each group member. Group therapy begins with a "here and now" round in which the participants report briefly on their momentary physical condition and mood as well as their expectations concerning the course of the group or subjects of interest.

After the first round, a subject is chosen which is then worked out mutually. Emotional and physical perceptions, group cohesion and the active participation of individual patients are promoted, giving (other) group members the opportunity to profit by model-learning. Educational elements are omitted from group therapy because they predominate in specific information groups (see section 7.5.2.1). Role play in the form of a dialog with the tinnitus, an element of psychodrama and Gestalt therapy is similar to the dialogue in letter-form with tinnitus (see Chapter 13). In role-playing, the patients play scenes they expect to be confronted with after discharge (problems with colleagues or superiors, probable tensions with the partner or other family members or friends, situations where the patient profits from self-assertiveness training).

The group setting is open, that is, new patients in the group introduce themselves and their problems, patients who are about to be discharged bid farewell and report on their previous progress relying on feedback from the rest of the group. During individual therapy, the behavioral analysis is made and therapy-goals are formulated using results from the tinnitus diary and other components of therapy (for example body perception, physical therapy, art therapy etc.)

7.5.2.5 Integration of depth psychology components of therapy

The integration of components of depth psychology and behavioral therapy has been practised in the United States since the 1950s. Accordingly, research concerning theory and clinical practice has increased (Arkowitz & Messer, 1984). In Germany this integration has taken place in the treatment of eating disorders (Fichter & Goebel, 1991; Roderich & Haisch, 1991). With respect to the treatment of complex chronic tinnitus, only one German study is familiar to us in which an exercise program composed of elements of behavioral medicine in combination with Gestalt therapy and bioenergetics was evaluated (Wimmer, 1983, see Chapter 13). In 1989, we integrated art therapy into our behavioral medicine treatment concept of complex chronic tinnitus (Palm et al., 1989).

Since the founding of our clinic, the integration of depth psychology-oriented therapies (psychodrama, Gestalt therapy, bioenergetics, psychoanalysis, etc.) are part of the behavioral-medicine concept of treatment. The therapist in charge of group and individual therapy refers the patient who needs more support regarding introspection or emotional coping, to an art therapy group.

7.5.2.6 Integration of psychophysiological components of therapy

Research regarding the possibilities and the effectiveness of relaxation techniques and biofeedback in the treatment of tinnitus are numerous and are summarized elsewhere (Chapters 5 and 10, Kirsch & Blanchard, 1987; Kirsch & Blanchard, 1989). We concentrate on Jacobson's progressive muscle relaxation (Jacobson, 1929) so as to enable the patient to learn relaxation in the supine as well as sitting position. This facilitates implementing relaxation in as many situations of daily life as possible. We understand relaxation to be a form of stress reduction, as well as a specific tinnitus coping strategy (Lindberg et al., 1988; Kirsch & Blanchard, 1987).

To help motivate and support the learning of relaxation methods, we incorporate EMG or skin-resistance biofeedback. Using this method the patient recognises that psychological factors can influence muscle tension (cervical spine and jaw region). We also have the opportunity to examine whether the patient can relax, which is just as difficult for tinnitus patients as for patients who suffer from chronic pain syndromes (Goebel, 1989 b).

It is often very difficult for tinnitus patients to learn a relaxation method because the tinnitus often becomes the center of attention especially if the patient practises relaxation in quiet surroundings. We advise the patient to improve their daily exercises by masking the tinnitus with meditative music or natural sounds (home-made recording). As treatment advances, the goal to be strived for is to acquire the ability to concentrate completely on the relaxation exercise despite quiet surroundings by a gradual reduction of the masking sounds. Imagined scenes are added to the relaxation exercises, which modulate the quality and nature of the tinnitus (e.g. a murmuring tinnitus is equated with a waterfall or mill, or diving into or floating in a stream). Such focusing of concentration contributes significantly to the ability of active tinnitus control and has been tested for its effectiveness (see Chapter 9).

7.5.2.7 Integration of body-oriented therapies

The integration of body-oriented methods in the treatment of complex chronic tinnitus is still in an experimental stage compared to the established behavioral medicine treatment programs in chronic pain syndromes (Goebel, 1989 b). We assume that poor posture and functional disorders of the cervical spine (Biesinger, 1989) and the jaw (Erlandsson et al., 1987b) can modulate tinnitus (see Chapters 15 and 16). On the other hand, tinnitus itself can lead to secondary muscle tension in these areas, leading to a fatal vicious circle (Fig. 7.6). Finally, we frequently notice that the sensory quality of tinnitus also is changed by lymphatic-drainage therapy of the face and neck region. Additional methods of body-therapy need to be developed, because many types of body therapy have ignored the head and neck region (e.g. Feldenkrais method).

In a special tinnitus-perception group, various exercises are carried out which consist of different components of breathing-therapy, body-perception (Feldenkrais/ Hetz), isometric exercises, dance therapy and self-massage. These components have a physiological as well as psychological effect-because they are often experienced as an additional beneficial method of improved coping and the patients are advised to combine these exercises with relaxation methods.

7.6 Treatment results

7.6.1 Description of the random sample

Two hundred and twelve patients with tinnitus were treated in our clinic from 1987 to the end of 1990. Of 45 patients with

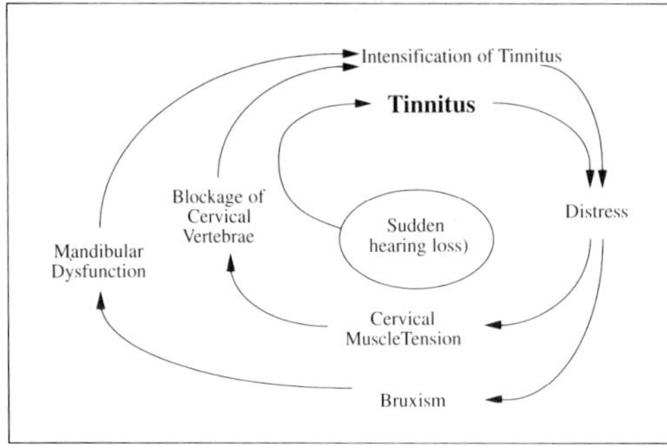

Fig. 7.6 Possible vicious circle of tinnitus in tempero-mandibular joint disorders/bruxism and/or cervicogenic influences. Tinnitus itself (eg. following an accident) can initiate a viscious circle as a stressor, but also variables which are independent of tinnitus (emotional, personal and psychosocial factors etc) can cause or intensify tinnitus.

compensated tinnitus forms, 40 were treated for other psychosomatic disorders, and 5 who had a decompensated chronic tinnitus at the time of registration, had improved to such an extent by the time of admission that their tinnitus could be considered compensated. Patients with acute tinnitus (tinnitus duration of less than 6 months) and malignant causes of tinnitus were excluded from the study.

Of the remaining 155 patients 10 left during the first 5–10 days because a persistent therapeutic concensus could not be attained for various reasons.

The different causes of tinnitus, which partially overlapped (multiple diagnoses), are seen in Table 7.2. The column "others" pertains to a second diagnosis as well as rare diagnoses including noise trauma = 14; Menière's syndrome = 13; otosclerosis = 6; otitis media = 5; cholesteatoma = 2; idiopathic tinnitus forms = 20 (Table 2).

Twelve percent of the patients were aged 20 – 39, 42% were 40 – 49, 34% were 50 – 59 and 12% were between ages 60 and 72. Further details about the distribution of age, sex, tinnitus localization and other findings, as well as details about hearing disturbances, dizziness and pain syndromes are available in Table 7.2. Hearing impairment was assessed when a hearing loss of more than 25 db in a frequency below 3000 Hz and/or a hearing loss of over 35 db in a frequency above 3000 Hz occurred (Reich & Johnson, 1984). Four percent of the patients were treated with a masker, which partially masked their tinnitus, 4% regularly wore their tinnitus instrument and 8% were treated with a hearing aid for one or both ears to compensate the tinnitus or hearing loss.

It is noteworthy that in monoaural tinnitus, the left side was affected more often. This phenomenon coincides with epidemiological data (Coles, 1984), and has also been observed in chronic pain syndromes (Merskey & Watson, 1979).

The psychological diagnoses were made in all patients according to the diagnostic statistical manual of mental disorders (DSM-III-R) (APA, 1987) and the results are presented and discussed in Chapter 4.

7.6.2 Treatment results

The control group consisted of 79 patients who had written a tinnitus diary from the time of initial contact with the clinic (registration) over a period of 14 days (short version; 100-mm visual analog scale; 0 = nothing; 100 = extreme; see appendix). The average waiting period before admission was about 6 months. The mean values of the variables of tinnitus loudness, tinnitus discomfort, mood, distress and feeling of control (coping) were compared with the mean values of the first 2 weeks of treatment. An increase from 22 – 27 only for the coping variable ($p < 0{,}001$) and a slight decrease, from 50 to 47 in the distress variable ($p < 0{,}001$) were found. Closer examination of the individual

Table 7.2 Results of a random sample of 155 patients with complex chronic tinnitus (for additional information, see text)

			Women		Men	
	N	Age mean (SD)	%	Age range	%	Age range
Diagnosis: Complex chronic tinnitus	155	48 (9.9)	35	28.67	65	22-72
1. Sudden hearing loss	37	54 (10.4)	43	24-65	54	22-55
2. Noise trauma	18	46 (9.3)	11	44-52	83	20-61
3. Mandibular joint dysfunction, bruxism	28	49 (9.5)	36	24.63	64	42-69
4. Cervical spine syndrome	56	49 (10.5)	32	41-67	68	23-72
5. Others (see text)	35	50 (8.6)	46	35-67	54	31-61
6. Drop out	10	45 (9.2)	40	22-60	60	35-55
Diagnosis: Compensated chronic tinnitus	45	48 (8.9)	38	33-64	62	26-69

	Tinnitus localization			Duration since diagnoses (years)	
	Both sides %	Left %	Right %	Mean (SD)	Range
Diagnosis: Complex chronic tinnitus	60	26	10	5.8 (6.1)	1-32
1. Sudden hearing loss	46	38	14	5.2 (5.5)	1-28
2. Noise trauma	56	22	17	7.2 (9.2)	1-32
3. Mandibular joint dysfunction, bruxism	71	25	11	5.5 (5.2)	1-20
4. Cervical spine syndrome	59	29	13	4.4 (5.3)	1-29
5. Others (see text)	66	23	11	6.7 (5.3)	1-20
6. Drop out	40	30	30	7.3 (6)	1-7
Diagnosis: Compensated chronic tinnitus	62	22	16	6.7 (7.2)	1-30

	Slight/ serious hearing loss %	No hearing loss %	Dizziness %	Affective disorders %	Anxiety disorders %	Chronic pain %
Diagnosis: Complex chronic tinnitus	77	23	46	69	26	39
1. Sudden hearing loss	89	8	41	51	16	30
2. Noise trauma	89	6	67	78	33	61
3. Mandibular joint dysfunction, bruxism	75	25	32	75	25	54
4. Cervical spine syndrome	73	27	46	45	18	48
5. Other (see text)	83	17	51	60	31	51
6. Drop out						
Diagnosis: Compensated chronic tinnitus				67	22	53

diaries indicates that these changes are caused by initial effects of therapy (Fig. 7.7).

Over the course of treatment a clear effect of therapy was demonstrated in the evaluation of available tinnitus diaries ($n = 138$): an average decrease in tinnitus loudness from 71 to 63 ($p < 0{,}001$), decrease in tinnitus discomfort from 66 to 52 ($p < 0{,}001$) and additional decrease in general stress from 47 to 40 ($p < 0{,}001$), the ability to control tinnitus (coping) increased from 27 to 40 ($p < 0{,}001$) and was reflected in an increase of the average mood value from 55 to 61 ($p < 0{,}001$) (Fig. 7.7). For better understanding of the effect of therapy, the reader must know that patients who usually describe their tinnitus as compensated as a rule rate loudness and discomfort of tinnitus with a value of less than 50!

In 30% of our patients, a decrease of tinnitus loudness of more than 20% resulted between the time of admission and discharge; 56% of the patients assessed a decrease in tinnitus discomfort of more than 20% and 62% rated the coping variable as improved by more than 20% (Fig. 7.8).

An evaluation of the tinnitus diary according to the etiologic subgroups (sudden deafness, temporomandibular joint disease/ bruxism, cervical spine syndrome and noise trauma) is shown in Fig. 7.8. It demonstrates that the most favorable treatment results were found in patients with sudden deafness (lowest non-responder proportion). Of those affected by sudden deafness, 11% had no improvement. Of those affected by noise trauma, at least 24% showed no improvement.

The observation that over 60% of those who suffered from sudden deafness as compared with those affected by noise trauma, attribute the triggering of their symptoms to psychological factors (Kropp and v. Rad, 1988) explains the increased motivation for a psychological treatment method. Those affected by noise trauma (predominantly men and soldiers) are only sufficiently motivated for psychotherapy when they have suffered severely in the past. They also have great difficulty accepting a psychologically-oriented tinnitus-therapy because they are considerably more sceptical in regard to interrelationships between a somatogenic tinnitus and psychological factors. Patients with sudden deafness are also more easily motivated to begin psychological therapy from a prophylactic point of view than patients with noise trauma, whose prophylactic measures are restricted to ear protection and are preoccupied with lawsuits for years with the aim of having their tinnitus acknowledged as an occupational disease and as a disability.

One year after the conclusion of therapy 70 patients were asked to keep a tinnitus diary for a period of 1 week, Sixty-three patients provided answers (rate of return = 90%). No significant changes resulted in the values for subjective loudness of tinnitus; the values remained as was previously the case, significantly improved in comparison with the beginning of therapy ($p = < 0{,}001$). A significant stability was apparent in the degree of tinnitus discomfort and ability to control tinnitus (coping). Mood and general stress, on the other hand, had moved closer to the values at the beginning of therapy (Figs. 7.7 and 7.8); this agrees with the findings of Lindberg et al. (1987, 1988).

All in all, the values of the tinnitus diary show a long lasting specific effect on the tinnitus compared to an insufficient effect on the variables of mood and distress. This calls for necessary out-patient care of the most seriously affected in terms of stress management and treatment of depression, as has already been provided in the form of booster sessions by other authors (see Chapter 9).

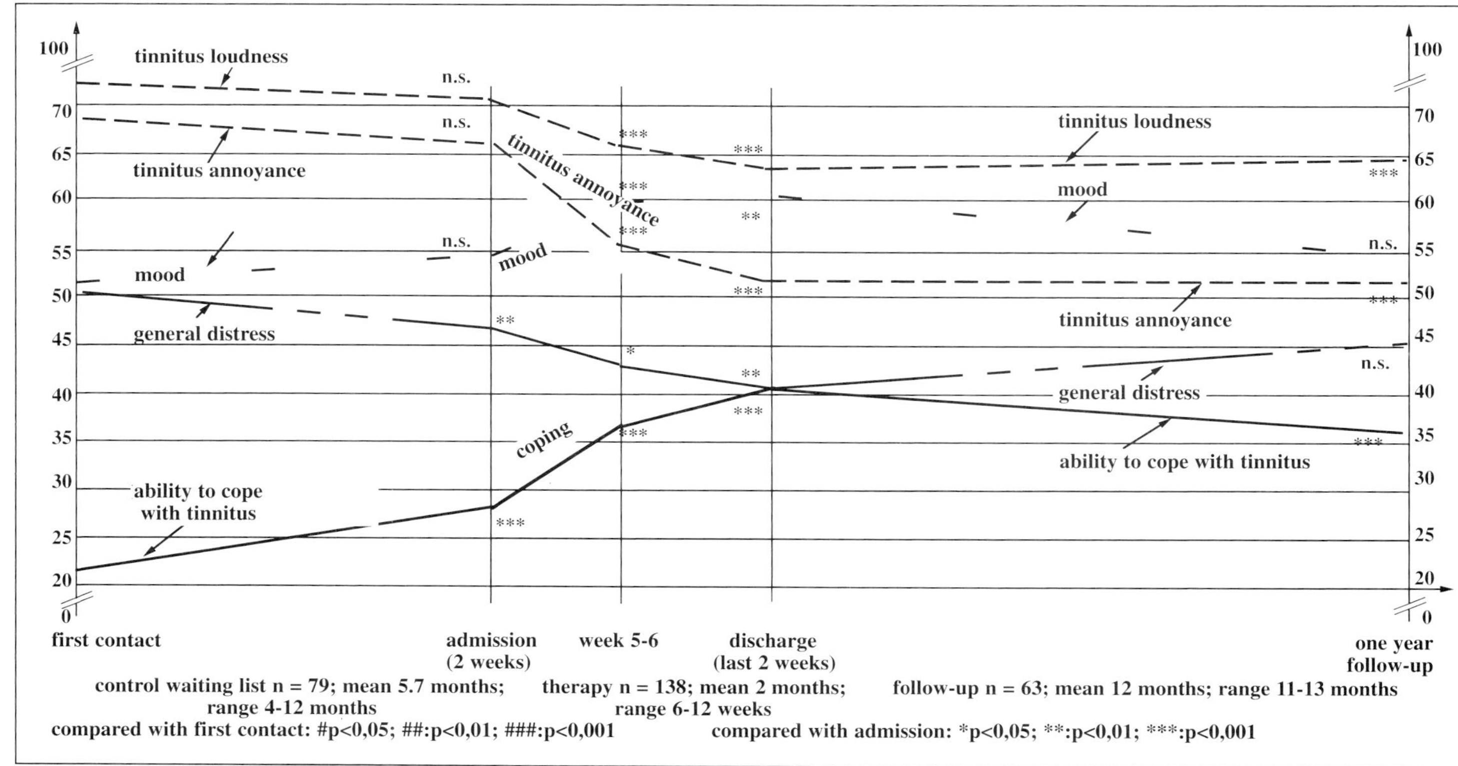

Fig. 7.7 Results of behavioral-medicine oriented treatment of 138 hospitalized patients with complex chronic tinnitus in comparison with a control group (waiting list before admission group) and 1 year after treatment (follow-up). The variables, loudness of tinnitus, discomfort from tinnitus, mood, distress and assessment of degree of successful tinnitus management (tinnitus control, coping) were recorded using the Prien tinnitus diary which was kept daily. The means of each period of 2 weeks were also assessed, the computation of the significance value was compared with the means of the first two weeks after admission (t-test for associated random samples: *: $p<0.05$, **$p<0.01$; ***$p<0.001$).

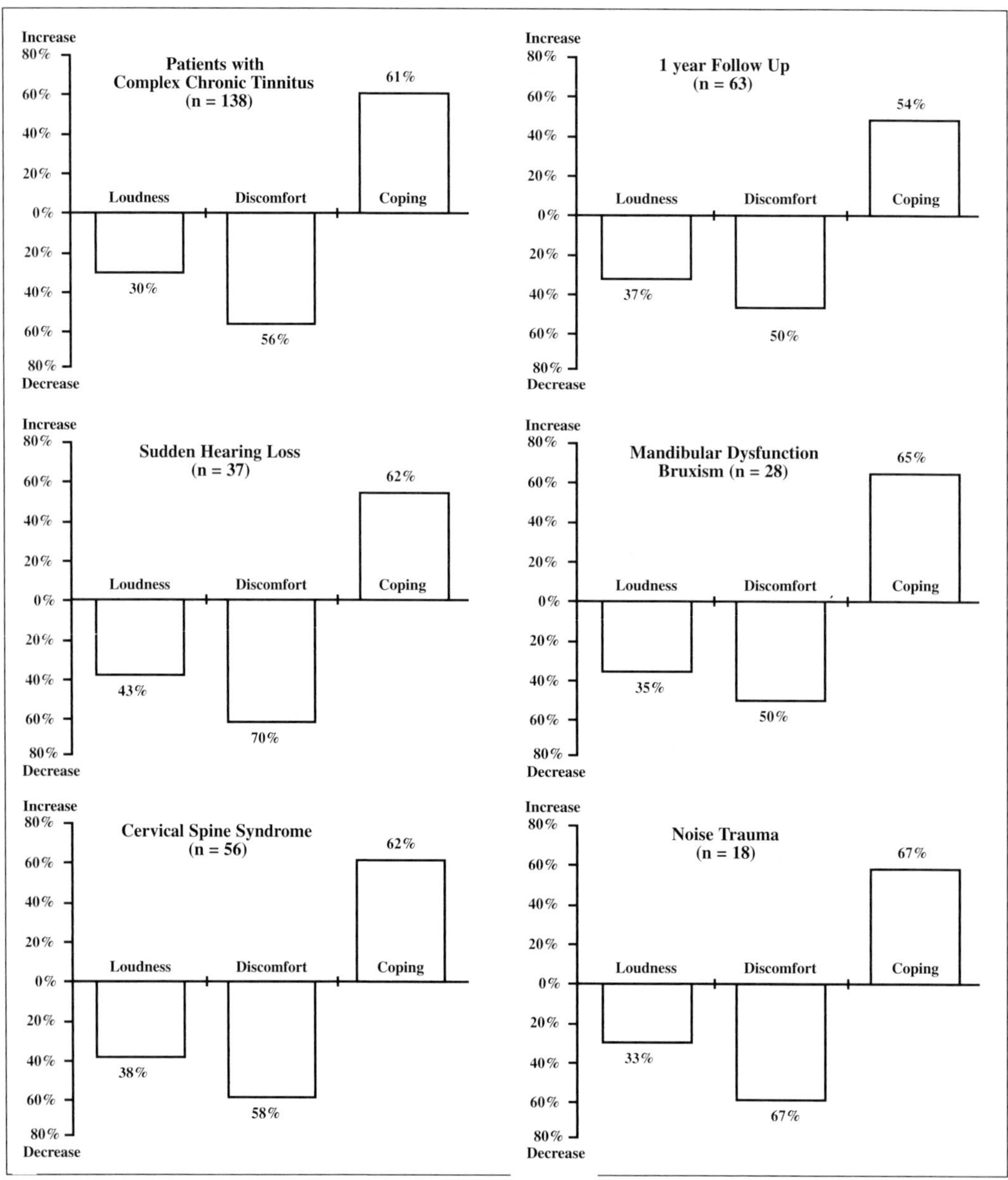

Fig. 7.8 Results of behavioral medicine-oriented treatment of 138 hospitalized patients with complex chronic tinnitus and etiologic sub-groups. The percentages give information about the number of patients who, during the course of therapy achieved a decrease of the variables tinnitus volume and tinnitus discomfort of ≥ 20% or an increase in the variable tinnitus control (coping) (means of the first 2 weeks in comparison to the 2 final weeks of treatment). The means which were determined 1 year after the conclusion of therapy in a follow-up study were compared with the means of the first two weeks.

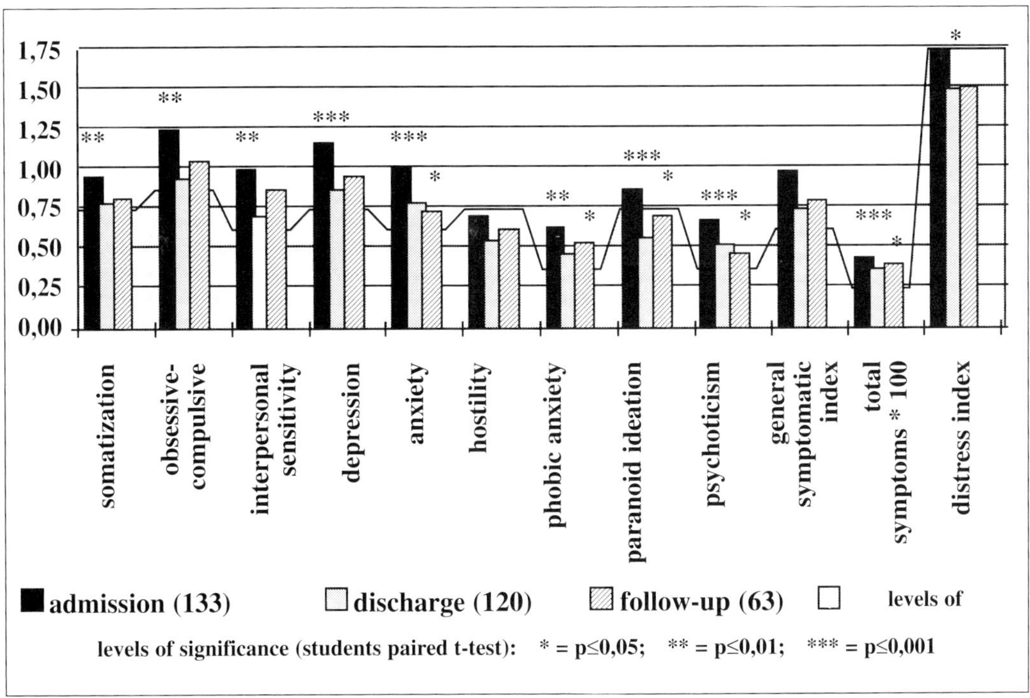

Fig. 7.9 Symptom checklist (SC L-90-R) (Derogatis, 1989): Results of the behavioral medicine-oriented treatment of 133 hospitalized patients with complex chronic tinnitus, the means of the evaluation at admission compared to the means of the evaluation at discharge and the means 1 year after the end of therapy (follow-up study). The significance value was computed using the t-test for associated random samples.

7.6.2.2 Psychological test methods

The Derogatis (1974, 1986) symptom checklist (SCL-90-R) was used for evaluation of additional symptoms. At the beginning of therapy in almost all parameters, pathological values were found which had largely become normal by the end of treatment (Fig. 7.9).

One year after conclusion of the treatment, the values for the parameters, anxiety, phobic thoughts, paranoid thoughts, psychoticism and total symptomatology were found to be significantly improved compared to the beginning of therapy. The values for obsession, social insecurity and depression, however, increased again on average, but remained far below the initial value (Fig. 7.9).

In order to obtain information about personality traits in addition to clinically relevant symptoms, the Freiburger Personality inventory (FPI-R) was used (Fahrenberg et al., 1984). This test helps to obtain information about opinions, emotions and behaviour which are directly related to the tinnitus and also increases the degree of insight into the general psychopathological impairment and personality traits/variables of tinnitus patients.

We found that at the beginning of therapy the mean values for social insecurity, agitation, stress, somatic disturbances, as well as emotional lability were not normal. The patients described themselves on the average

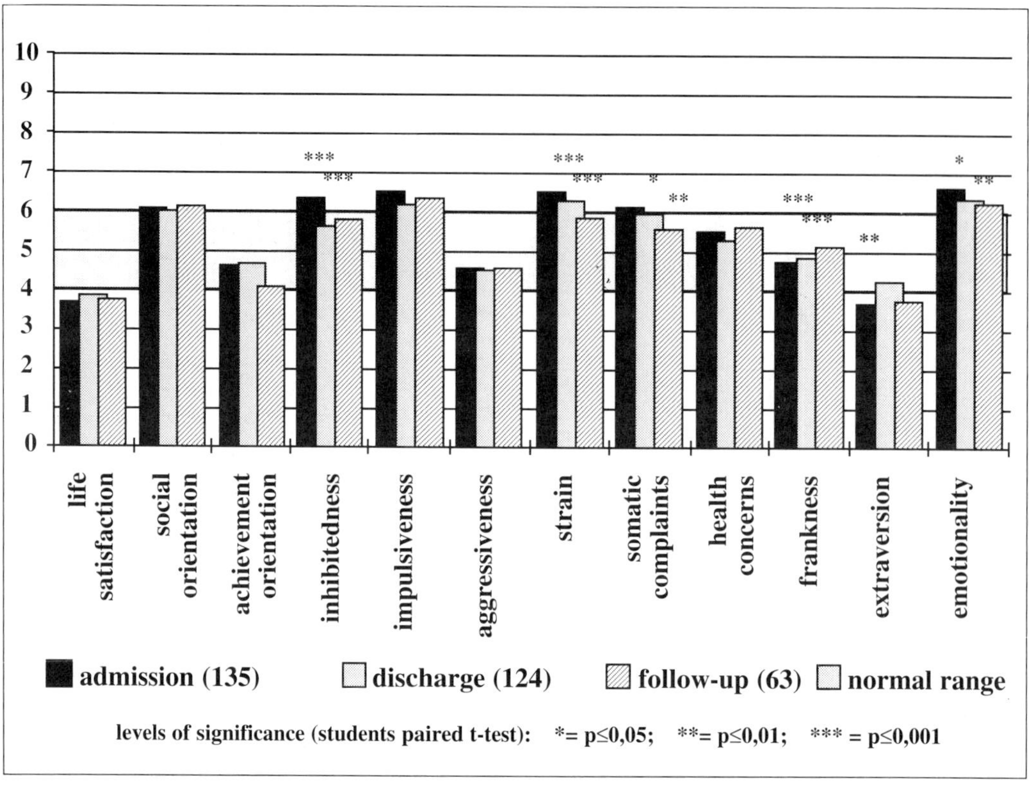

Fig. 7.10 Freiburg Personality Inventory (FPI-R) (Fahrenberg et al., 1984) Results of the behavioral medicine-oriented treatment of 135 hospitalized patients with complex chronic tinnitus. The means of the evaluation at admission compared to the means of the evaluation at discharge and the means 1 year after the end of therapy (follow-up study). The significance value was computed using the t-test for associated random samples.

as dissatisfied and introverted (Fig. 7.10). Due to therapy, the stress and somatic disturbances scales approached normal, even after a period of 1 year. The values of the extraversion scale had again approached the value at the beginning of therapy, which points to the necessity of further outpatient care, at least for the most seriously affected.

7.6.2.3 Global assessment

The global assessment of the effects of therapy by therapists and patients at the time of discharge was about 15% significantly improved (best possible assessment), 20–26% clearly improved (second best possible assessment) and 35–36% slightly improved (third best possible assessment). In 9–23%, no improvement was registered and in approximately 3–4%, the overall situation deteriorated during the course of therapy due to another attack of sudden deafness in three patients or unknown factors (Fig. 7.11).

The nonresponder rate (no improvement of the tinnitus specific variables of loudness, discomfort and coping ≥ 20% on the 100 mm analog scale) was 17%.

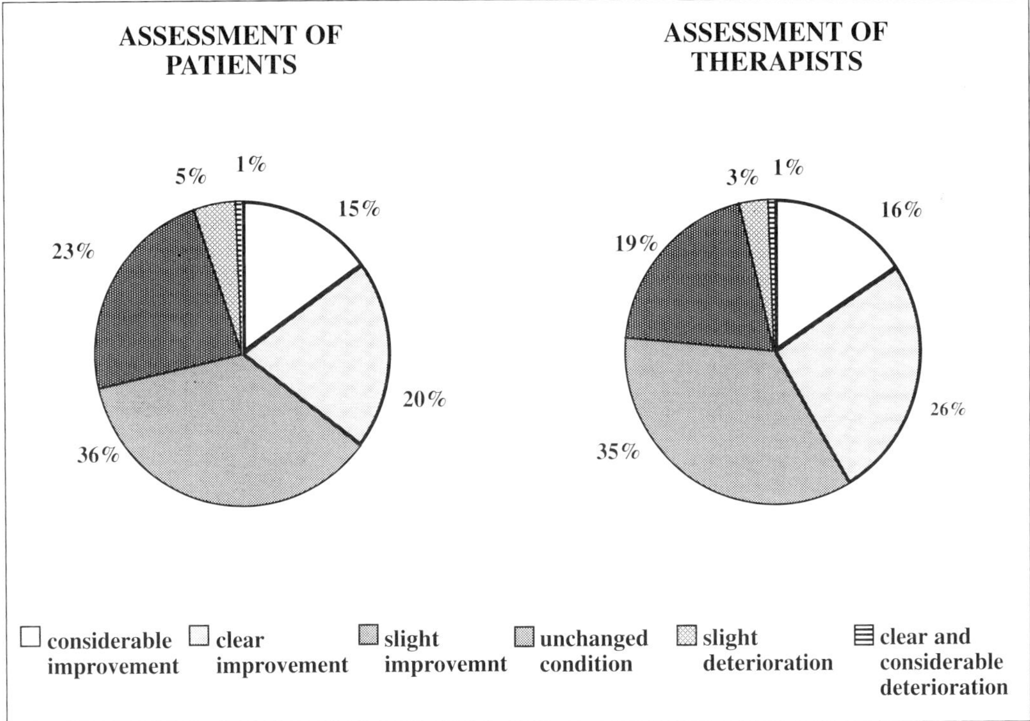

Fig. 7.11 Assessment of therapy results by patients (n = 130; tinnitus questionnaire at the time of discharge) and therapists (n = 145; case-documentation). The patients assess the results of therapy (71% — slight to considerable improvement) somewhat more critically than the experts (77% slight to considerable improvement). The assessments, which were made independent of each other, coincided to a high degree.

7.7 Conclusions

Our treatment concept of complex chronic tinnitus has proved itself to be effective. The specific therapy effects achieved are stable even after 1 year. Other multimodular cognitive therapy programmes (Jakes et al., 1986 a; Lindberg et al., 1987; Lindberg et al., 1988; etc) have attained a comparable success rate in controlled studies, which persisted in over 60% of the patients even after the conclusion of therapy. A multi-modular integrative behavioral-medicine treatment, influences problems resulting from tinnitus, such as somatization symptoms, depression and anxiety. Decisive for a successful course of therapy is individual planning of the goals of treatment on the basis of a comprehensive behavioral analysis and the corresponding integration of behavior-oriented, cognitive, emotional, psychophysiological and body-oriented treatment concepts. Better results are achieved in an in-patient clinical setting, or an out-patient clinical setting, than in a normal medical practice where the therapist is faced with difficulties concerning organisation and cost-coverage by health insurance. Further efforts are still needed to reinforce the treatment modalities that have been developed thus far and to establish them in other centers. A positive development is the increased cooperation of otolaryngology specialists whose national and international congresses show an increased interest in subjects concerning the psychological management and therapy of chronic tinnitus patients (Feldmann, 1987). Ca. 20% of the topics of the 4th International Tinnitus Congress in Bordeaux (1991) were devoted to psychological subjects and the cognitive treatment of complex chronic tinnitus!

We plan to examine the effectiveness of our therapy concept as a whole as well as its separate components and in combination with masking (Retraining-Therapy; see p. 38). Comparative studies are necessary with the aim of improving treatment according to possible differences in psychopathology and etiology. This includes the development and evaluation of a specific tinnitus questionnaire for Germany (Hiller & Goebel, 1992; Goebel & Hiller, 1992/1995; Hiller et al., 1994).

7.8 References

Anonymous (1981): In: CIBA Foundation Symposium, 85. Pitman Books Ltd. London, 300-302.

APA (1987): Diagnostic and statistical manual of mental disorders, 3rd edition, revised. American Psychiatric Association, Washington DC.

Arkowitz, H. & S.B. Messer (1984): Psychoanalytic therapy and behavior therapy. Plenum Press, New York, London 1-30.

Biesinger, E. (1989): Funktionelle Störungen der Halswirbelsäule in ihrer Bedeutung für die Hals-Nasen-Ohrenheilkunde. In: *Ganz, H. & W. Schätzle,* (Ed.): HNO-Praxis Heute, 9. Springer, Berlin-Heidelberg.

Coles, R.R.A. (1984): Epidemiology of tinnitus: (1) Prevalence. Journal of Laryngology and Otology, 98, (Suppl. 9), 7-15.

Derogatis, L.R., R.S. Lipman, K. Richels, E.H. Uhlenhutz, L. Cori (1974): The Hopkins symptom checklist (SCL): A self-report-symptom interview. Beh. Sci., 19: 1-4.

Derogatis, L.R. (1986): Symptom checklist, 3. Auflage. Beltz-Test, Weinheim.

Dobbek, Th., O.B. Scholz, C. Gärtner (1990): Schmerztagebücher und Patienten-Compliance. Verhaltensmodifikation und Verhaltensmedizin, 2: 137-149.

Duckert, L.G., T.S. Rees (1984): Placebo effect in tinnitus management. Otolaryngol. Head Neck Surg., 92: 697.

Duckro, P.N., C.A. Pollard, H.D. Bray, L. Scheiter (1984): Comprehensive behavioral management of complex tinnitus: A case illustration. Biofeedback and Self-Regulation, 9, (4), 459-469.

Erlandson, S., A. Ringdahl, T. Hutchins, S.G. Carlsson (1987a): Treatment of tinnitus: A controlled comparison of masking and placebo. British J. of Audiology, 21: 37-44.

Erlandsson, S., B. Rubinstein, S. Carlsson, A. Ringdahl (1987b): Biofeedback and stomatognathic treatment. A prospective study of tinnitus patients, pp. 389-392.

Fahrenberg, J., R. Hampel, H. Selg (1984): Das Freiburger Persönlichkeitsinventar (FPI-R). Handanweisung. Hogrefe, Göttingen.

Feldmann, H. (1964): Die Krankheit Friedrich Smetanas in otologischer Sicht auf Grund neuer Quellenstudien. Mschr. Ohrenheilk. u. Laryngo-Rhinol, 98: 209-226.

Feldmann, H. (Ed. 1987): Proceedings III International Tinnitus Seminar Münster, Harsch Verlag, Karlsruhe.

Feldmann, H. (1989): Kulturhistorisches und Medizinhistorisches zum Tinnitus aurium. Harsch Verlag, Karlsruhe.

Fichter, M. & G. Goebel (1989): Konzeption einer verhaltensmedizinischen Behandlung chronischer Schmerzsyndromme. Prax. Psychother. Psychosom., 34: 205-213.

Fichter, M. & G. Goebel (1991): Anorexia und Bulimia nervosa: Symptomatik, medizinische Komplikationen, Ätiologie und Behandlung. Internist, 32: 38-49.

Fordyce, W.E. (1976): Behavioral methods for chronic pain and illness. C. V. Mosby, St. Louis.

Ganz, F.J. (1986): Ohrgeräusche. Tinnitus-Sprechstunde. Georg Thieme Verlag, Stuttgart-New York.

Geissner, E. (1990): Psychologische Schmerzmodelle. Einige Anmerkungen zur Gate-control-Theorie sowie Überlegungen zu einem mahrfaktoriellen prozessualen Schmerzkonzept. Der Schmerz, 4: 184-192.

Gerber, W.-D. (1986). Hals-Nasen-Ohrenerkrankungen. In: *Miltner, W., Birbaumer, N., Gerber, W-D.* (Eds). Verhaltensmedizin. 345-354. Springer, Berlin-Heidelberg-New York-Tokio-Hong Kong.

Gerber, W.D. & H.C. Diener (1987): Verlaufsprotokolle zur Schmerztherapie: Das Tübinger Schmerztagebuch. Manuskript zum ersten Workshop über "Qualitätssicherung in der Algesiologie", Mainz.

Goebel, G. (1989a): Tinnitus. In: *Hand, I. & H.-U. Wittchen* (Eds). Verhaltenstherapie in der Medizin. Springer, Berlin, Heidelberg, New York, Tokyo, Hong Kong, 207-228.

Goebel, G. (1989b): Verhaltensmedizinisches Behandlungskonzept psychosomatischer Erkrankungen am Beispiel des chronischen Schmerzsyndroms. Ärztezeitschr. f. Nat. u. Reg., 8: 587-599.

Goebel, G., W. Keeser, C. Wildgruber, L. Baldhuber, B. Faust, M. Fichter (1989): Die stationäre verhaltensmedizinische Behandlung chronischer Schmerzen. In: *Laireiter, A., H. Mackinger* (Eds). Verhaltensmedizin — Gesundheitspsychologie. Mackinger-Verlag, Bergheim, 63-79.

Goebel, G., M. Lederer, W. Rief, M. Fichter (1990): Integrative multimodale verhaltensmedizinische Behandlung des komplexen chronischen Tinnitus. (Behandlungsergebnisse und Langzeiteffekt.) 61. Kongreß der Deutschen HNO-Gesellschaft, Würzburg.

Goebel, G., W. Keeser, M. Fichter, W. Rief (1991a): Neue Aspekte des komplexen chronischen Tinnitus. Teil I: Überprüfung eines multimodalen verhaltensmedizinischen Behandlungskonzepts. Psychother. med. Psychol., 41: 115-122.

Goebel, G., W. Keeser, M. Fichter, W. Rief (1991b): Neue Aspekte des komplexen chronischen Tinnitus. Teil II: Die verlorene Stille: Auswirkungenund psychotherapeutische Möglichkeiten beim komplexen chronischen Tinnitus. Psychother. med. Psychol., 41: 123-133.

Goebel, G. & W. Hiller (1992): Psychische Beschwerden bei chronischem Tinnitus: Erprobung und Evaluation des Tinnitus-Fragebogens. Verhaltenstherapie, 2: 13-22.

Goebel, G., W. Hiller, K. Frühauf, M.M. Fichter (1992): Effects of in-patient multimodal behavioral treatment on complex chronic tinnitus. A controlled one-year follow-up study. In: *J.-M. Arant, R. Dauman* (eds.): Tinnitus 91, Kugler Publications, Amsterdam: 465-470.

Greuel, H. (1983): Suggestivbehandlung bei Hörsturz. HNO, 31: 136.

Greuel, H. (1988): Viel um die Ohren. VDG-Verlag. Chronischer Tinnitus.

Halford, J.B.S., S.D. Anderson (1991): Anxiety and depression in tinnitus sufferers. Journal of Psychosomatic Research, 35: 383-390.

Hallam, R.S. (1987): Psychological approaches to evaluation and management of tinnitus distress. In: *Hazell, J.* (Ed.) Tinnitus. Churchill, Livingstone, Edinburgh, London, Melbourne, New York, 156-175.

Hallam, R.S. (1989): Living with tinnitus. Dealing with the ringing in your ears. Thorsons Publishing Group, London.

Harrop-Griffiths, J., W. Katon, R. Dobie, C. Sakaie, J. Russo (1987): Chronic tinnitus: associtaion with psychiatric diagnosis. Journal of Psychosomatic Research, 31: 613-621.

Heim, E. (1988): Coping und Adaptivität: Gibt es geeignetes oder ungeeignetes Coping? Psychother. med. Psychol., 38: 8-18.

Hiller, W. & G. Goebel (1992): A psychometric study of complaints in chronic tinnitus. Journal of Psychosomatic Research, 36 (4): 337-348.

Hiller, W., G. Goebel, Rief, W. (1994): Reliability of self-rated tinnitus distress and association with psychological symptom patterns. Br. J. Clin. Psychol. 33: 231-239.

Hollweg, W.H. (1989): Streik im Innenohr. Hörsturz, Morbus Menière und Tinnitus aus psychosomatischer Sicht. Unimed Verlag, München.

House, P.R. (1981): Personality of the tinnitus patient. In: Ciba Foundation Symposium, 85, Pitman Books Ltd., London, 193-203.

Jacobsen, E. (1929): Progressive relaxation. Chicago Press.

Jakes, S.C., R.S. Hallam, S. Rawilchmann, R. Hinchcliffe (1986a): The effects of reassurance, relaxation training and distraction on chronic tinnitus sufferers. Behav. Res. Thera., 24, 5: 497-507.

Jakes, S.C., R.S. Hallam, C. Chambers, R. Hinchcliffe (1986b): Matched and self-reported loudness of tinnitus: methods and sources of error. Audiology, 25: 92-100.

Jakes, S.C., L. McKenna, R.S. Hallam, R. Hinchcliffe (1992): Cognitive therapy in chronic tinnitus. Cognitive Therapy and Research, 6: 67-82.

Keeser, W., G. Goebel, H. Abeken, H. Schneidzik, C. Wildgruber, M. Fichter (1989): Zeitreihenanalytische Auswertungen von Tagebüchern bei der stationären verhaltensmedizinischen Behandlung von chronischem Schmerz. Kongreß der Deutschen Gesellschaft für Verhaltensmodifikation, München, Ludwigs-Maximilians-Universität.

Kirsch, C.A. & E.B. Blanchrad (1987): A multiple-baseline evaluation of the treatment of subjective tinnitus with relaxation training and biofeedback. Biofeedback and Self-Regulation 4: 295-312.

Kirsch, C.A. & E.B. Blanchard (1989): A review of the efficacy of behavioural techniques in the treatment of subjective tinnitus. Annals of Behav. Medicine, 11: 58-65.

Kokott, G. (1982): Psychiatrische Aspekte bei der Entstehung und Behandlung chronischer Schmerzzustände. Der Nervenarzt, 53: 365-376.

Kropp, U.A.K., M. v. Rad (1988): Psychosomatische Aspekte des Hörsturzes. Psychother. med. Psychol. 38: 407-412.

Lazarus, R.S. & S. Folkmann (1984a): Stress, appraisal and coping. Springer, New York.

Lazarus, R.S. & S. Folkmann (1984b): Coping and adaptation. In: *Gentry, W.D.* (Ed.). Handbook of Behavioural Medicine. Guilford Press, New York, pp. 282-325.

Lazarus, R.S. & S. Folkmann (1987): Transactional theory and research on emotions and coping. European Journal of Personality, 1: 141-169.

Lenarz, T. (1989): Ohrgeräusche. Pathophysiologie, Diagnostik und Therapie. Deutsches Ärzteblatt 2, 3: 1246-1253.

Lindberg, P., B. Scott, L. Melin, L. Lyttekens (1987): Long-term effects of psychological treatment of tinnitus. Scand. Audiol. 16: 167-172.

Lindberg, P., B. Scott, L. Melin, L. Lyttkens (1988): Behavioral therapy in the clinical management of tinnitus. British Journal of Audiology, 22: 265-272.

McFadden, D. (1982): Tinnitus: facts, theories and treatments. National Academy Press, Working Group 89, National Research Council, Washington.

Melzack, R., P.D. Wall (1965): Pain mechanisms: a new theory. Science, 150, 971-979.

Melzack, R., K.L. Casey (1968): Sensory, motivational and central control determinants of pain: a new conceptual model. In: *Kenshalo, D.* (Ed.): The skin senses. Thomas, Springfield S. 423.

Mersey, H. & G.D. Watson (1979): The lateralisation of pain. Pain, 7: 271-280.

Muthny, F.A. (1989): Krankheitsverarbeitung bei chronisch körperlich Kranken. Prax. Psychother. Psychosom., 34: 64-72.

Palm, C., G. Goebel, H. Abeken, M. Bräuherr (1989): Gestaltungstherapie bei chronischem Tinnitus als integrativer Therapiebestandteil in einem verhaltensmedizinischen Behandlungskonzept. Poster, 60. Kongreß der Deutschen HNO-Gesellschaft, Kiel.

Reich, G.E. & R.M. Johnson (1984): Personality characteristics of tinnitus patients. Journal of Laryngology and Otology, 98 (Suppl.): 228-232.

Rief, W. & G. Kohli (1991): Die Angstattacke. Von einem organmedizinischen Krankheitsmodell zu einem psychophysiologischen Verständnis. Psychomed., 3: 83-86.

Roderich, H. & I. Haisch (1991): Die Integration von verhaltenstherapeutischen und psychoanalytischen Therapieelementen bei der Gruppentherapie von Adipositas-Patienten. Psychother. med. Psychol., 36: 132-141.

Schönweiler, R. (1986): Ohrgeräusche: Ursachen, Bewertung und Therapie. DMW 111: 1489-1494.

Sweetow, R.W. (1984): Cognitive behavioral modification in tinnitus management. Hearing Instruments, 35: 14-19.

Sweetow, R.V. (1986): Cognitive aspects of tinnitus patient management. Ear and Hearing, 16: 390-396.

Scott, B., P. Lindberg, L. Lyttkens, L. Melin (1985): Psychological treatment of tinnitus. An experimental group study. Scand. Audiol., 14, 4: 223-230.

Thomson, J. (1983): Menière's disease: a 3 year follow-up of patients in a double-blind placebo-controlled study on endolymphatic sac shunt surgery. Adv. Oto-Rhino-Lar., 30: 350-354.

Tönnies, S. (1991): Leben mit Ohrgeräuschen. Ein Selbsthilfebuch. Ansanger Verlag.

Tonndorf, J. (1987): The analogy between tinnitus and pain: a suggestion for physiological basis of chronic tinnitus. Hearing Research, 28: 271-275.

Tursky, B., L.D. Jammer, R. Friedmann (1982): The pain perception profile: a psychophysical approach to the assessment of pain report. Behavior Therapy, 13: 376-394.

Tyler, R.S., L.J. Baker (1983): Difficulties experienced by tinnitus sufferers. Journal of Speech and Hearing Disorders, 48: 150-164.

Wedel, H.v., U. Strahlmann, P. Zorowka (1989): Effektivität verschiedener nicht medikamentöser Therapiemaßnahmen bei Tinnitus. Laryngo. Rhino-Otol., 68: 259-266.

Wimmer, J. (1983): Hilfe zur Selbsthilfe. Ein Therapie- und Übungsprogramm für Patienten mit subjektiven Ohrgeräuschen. Inaugural-Dissertation Ludwig-Maximilians-Universität, München (Prof. H.H. Naumann).

Appendix 1 — Example of a tinnitus diary

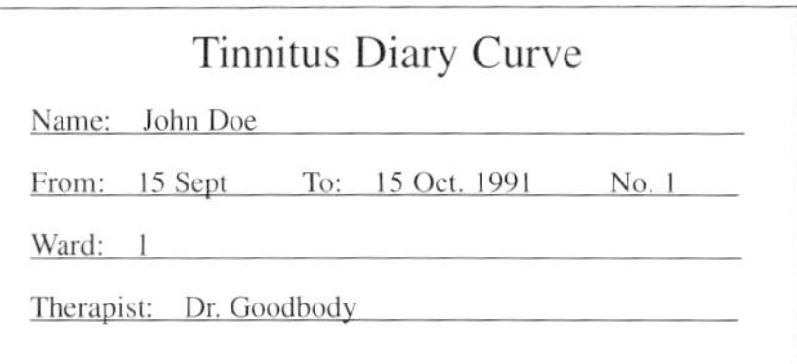
Tinnitus Diary Curve

Name: John Doe

From: 15 Sept To: 15 Oct. 1991 No. 1

Ward: 1

Therapist: Dr. Goodbody

The diary curve including the pages of the diary is a part of your medical hisotry. Please give your therapist these documents at discharge.

Please transfer the values for the pages of your daily tinnitus diary to the corresponding curve.

Begin with day 1

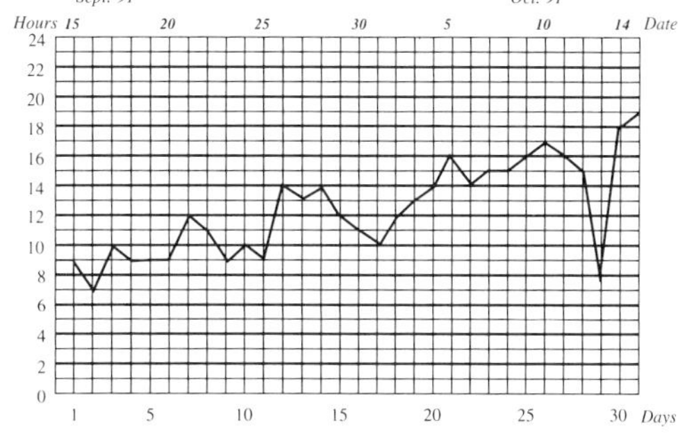

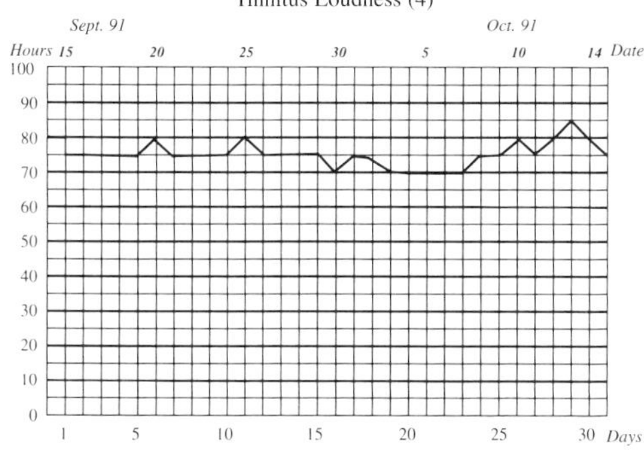

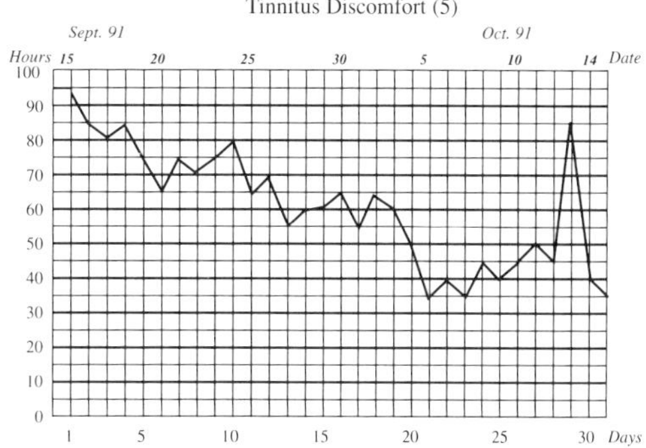

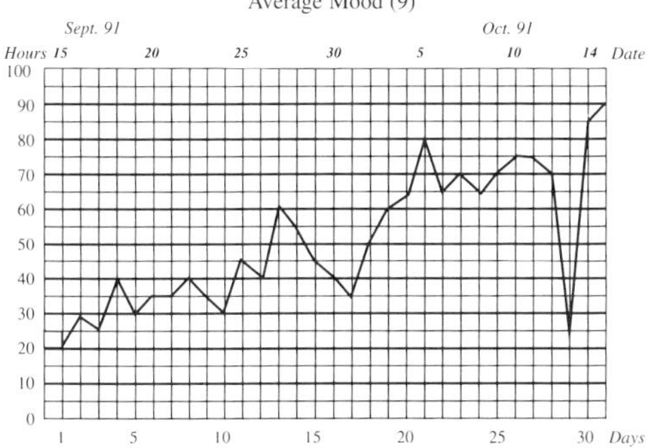

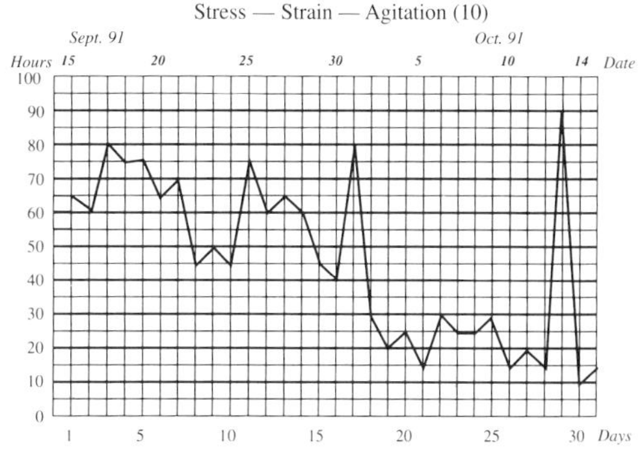

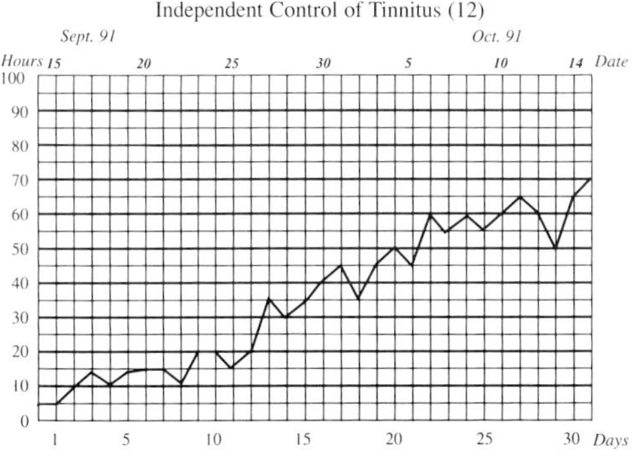

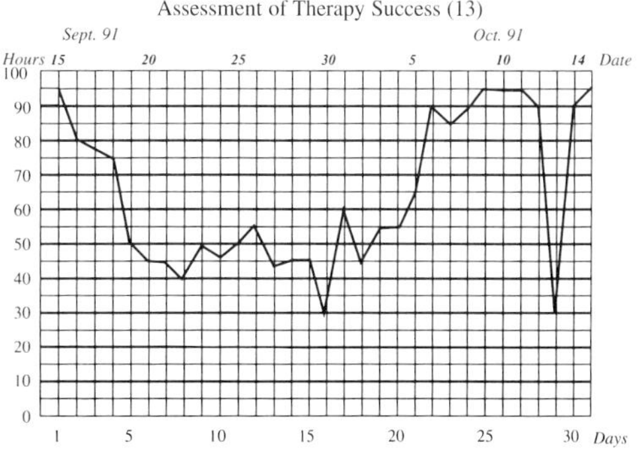

Appendix 2 — Introduction to and examples for a tinnitus diary

a) With the help of your accurately recorded activities, it becomes apparent how you plan the course of your day. A wrong schedule often leads to stress (eg. if too many unpleasant activities follow each other, although this must not be the case. Too much unplanned time can also lead to stress.) We can plan mutually when time-outs or certain activities should take place and how you can integrate them into your daily routine.

b) In the space "What am I thinking" we can mutually examine when negative thoughts cause pain or tinnitus, stress or other emotions and develop other cognitions (in a positive sense).

c) In the space "What do I feel?" you can analyze which feelings are important for you but perhaps do not crop up any longer. You also see whether you can differentiate feelings in general. If not, you can obtain a list of emotions from us and we can then decide what you can do in order to experience as many positive feelings in one day as possible (pain or tinnitus is more easily "tolerated" in a positive mood).

d) With the help of your assessment of certain situations, emotions and feelings, you can work out those factors which decrease with pain or tinnitus volume or the discomfort from tinnitus or pain. These factors will guide you in the direction of positive changes.

e) Pain killers, tranquilizers or alcohol as a drug? The wrong type of drug, taken at the wrong time and in a large dosage is harmful. We will plan a sensible drug regimen mutually.

Daily record (tinnitus)

Date: *6/28/91* Day: *Friday* Name: *John Doe*

Time	What do I **do**?	What do I **think**?	What do I **feel**?	Tinnitus volume in %	Tinnitus discom-fort in %	Medication Alcohol. What? How much?	Comments
7-8am	Personal hygiene, back exercises	The cool rain is pleasant: only a little tinnitus	good contentment	50	50	1 cup coffee	
8-8.45am	Breakfast	Everything is so quiet today	indifference	50	50		
8.45-10.30am	Group therapy	The others have more problems than I	partial sympathy	50	50		
10.30-11.30am	Reading the newspaper	Not much new in the world	contentment	50	50		
11.30-12.30pm	Lunch Measure blood pressure	The food is good Blood pressure OK	contentment and peace	50	40		
12.30-2pm	Sleep	A little sleep cannot hurt	contentment and peace	50	50		
2-3pm	Social worker	This help is good	trust	50	50	1 cup coffee	
3-4pm	Progressive muscle relaxation	Tension and relaxation in balance	warmth weightlessness	40	40		
4-5pm	Jogging	Nice landscape on lake, jogging helps	freedom, happiness, relaxation	40	40		
5.30-6pm	Dinner	I don't like this sausage	uneasiness	40	50		
6.30-9.30pm	Explain the course of therapy to another patient	Not too much at once	solidarity	30	30		
9.30-11.30pm	Reading in bed	I have read better books!	contentment and peace	30	30		

Daily record (tinnitus)

Date: *7/1/91* Day: *Sunday* Name: *John Doe*

Time	What do I **do**?	What do I **think**?	What do I **feel**?	Tinnitus volume in %	Tinnitus discom-fort in %	Medication Alcohol. What? How much?	Comments
7.30-9am	Breakfast, personal hygiene	Tinnitus is stronger	anger	70	70	2 cups coffee	
9-10.30am	Wrote letters	Bad weather, good for writing letters	peace, composure	65	65		
10.30-11am	Jogging, shower	It is also fun to jog in the rain	contentment	60	60		
11.30-12.30pm	Lunch	Soon I will take a nap	contentment	60	60		
12.30-2.30pm	Reading the newspaper	Today currency union in Germany, a beneficial development	feeling of solidarity with the GDR	60	60		
2.30-4.30pm	Relaxation exercises, sleep	Nothing	relaxation	50	50		
5-7pm	TV: soccer	It would be nice if Germany won	pleasant excitement	50	50	1 glass of tea	
7-9.30pm	Bicycling	The weather could be better, landscape is nice	contentment	50	50		
9.30-10pm	At the pub	Soon a nice Sunday will be over	contentment	50	50	½ litre beer	
10-11pm	TV: soccer	This game is exciting	Tired	50	50		

Appendix 3 — List of emotions: feeling: I feel

abandoned
bored
accepted
moved
anxious
frightened
stunned
aggravated
warm-hearted
astonished
worried
restless
understanding
acknowledged
ashamed
humbled
aggressive
embittered
burdened
hesitant
quiet
able
responsible, informative
trustworthy
confused
satisfied
in love
conquered
destroyed
beaten
lonely
without comfort
despondent
encouraged
disinterested
scatterbrained

dissatisfied
discouraged
unaccepted
denied
dispensable
disheartened
impolite
shocked
tearful

contemptuous
debased
composed
tormented
ecstatic
proud
excited
embarrassed
empty
enthusiastic
jealous
euphoric
excited
cheerful
friendly
frustrated
wild
worthless
thankful
happy
terrible
helpless
hopeless
modest
humbled
injured
equal
inadequate
incompetent

insecure
meaningless
jealous
gratified
loved
unhappy
miserable
misunderstood
used

disowned
nervous
rigid
passionate
happy

overwhelmed
proud
humbled
confused
regretful
rejected
refused
bloated
excited
eased
bemoaned
sad
satisfied
sensuous
cheerful
erotic
frightened
surprised
in suspense
threatened
stirred up
trusting
uncertain
uncooperative
understood
difficult
unhappy
unloved
upset
revengeful
unforgiving
desired
worthless
valuable
enraged
yearn
torn-apart
humbled
pleasant
disgusting
painful
disappointed
delighted
inferior
in the mood for fun

Chapter 8

Experience of group cognitive therapy with tinnitus sufferers

R. S. Hallam

Department of Psychology
University College London
Gower Street London WC1
and
Royal National Throat, Nose
& Ear Hospital
330 Gray's Inn Road
London WC1

Abstract

Group cognitive therapy has recently been evaluated in a tinnitus clinic in London and compared with aural masking, placebo masking and no treatment. Reasons for adopting the cognitive therapy approach are described. The way in which patients were selected and treated over 5 group sessions is described and illustrated. Group cognitive therapy produced greater amelioration of emotional distress and negative thinking at three months follow-up. Our chief evaluation instrument, the Tinnitus Questionnaire, is provided along with norms and scoring key.

8.1.0 Introduction

Clinical psychologists have worked for a number of years in an outpatient tinnitus clinic in London where an evaluation of group cognitive therapy for chronic tinnitus sufferers was recently conducted (Jakes, McKenna, Hallam and Hinchcliffe, submitted). This chapter explains our reasons for adopting the cognitive approach, describes the main elements of the therapy, and summarises our results. A shortened version of the Tinnitus Questionnaire (Hallam, Jake and Hinchcliffe, 1988), used in this evaluation, is appended to the chapter for readers who may wish to use it in their own research or therapy.

8.1.1 Reasons for adopting a cognitive approach to therapy

Several considerations led us to converge on this approach.

8.1.1.1 Theory of complaint:

Our theoretical model of complaint had been guided by the notion of habituation of attention (Hallam and Rachman, 1984). The central hypothesis is that tinnitus noise is equivalent, psychologically, to an external noise to which attention may or may not be given. Just as repetitive external sounds which lack signal properties are eventually ignored, it is assumed that tolerance of tinnitus can develop on the basis of a similar process. The literature on stimulus orientation and on the cognitive process of attention can therefore be used as sources of hypotheses relevant to the nature of tinnitus complaint. Initially, we focused on facilitating habituation through changing the context in which patients listened to their tinnitus. The procedure we tried at first in 1981, on a pilot basis, was to match carefully the patient's tinnitus, using a sound synthesizer, and to play back the sound in bursts over a 30 minute session. This procedure mimics laboratory studies showing habituation of the orienting reaction to external sounds. This technique produced no effect whatsoever on within session ratings of the quality of the noise or its intrusiveness. However, we did find some between session change in tinnitus ratings. We had relaxed patients prior to these habituation series on the assumption that habituation proceeds more quickly in states of lowered arousal. We attributed the between session changes to relaxation rather than to the habituation technique, and went on to conduct a trial of relaxation training (Jakes, Hallam and Hinchcliffe, 1986). Later it became apparent that cognitive therapy could be useful as a means of altering the signal properties (meaning) of the tinnitus sounds and thereby facilitate habituation of attention in a manner consistent with our general model.

8.1.1.2 Experience with relaxation training

We evaluated the effect of five sessions of progressive muscular relaxation in patients who had been distressed by tinnitus for at least 18 months (Jakes et al 1986). Without going into the details of this study, there are two findings that interested us. First, patients' emotional distress declined significantly over a two week baseline period prior to receiving relaxation. We attributed this improvement to the effect of an information booklet which was intended to give a psychological framework for understanding tinnitus complaint and to provide reassurance about the cause and prognosis of the problem.

Second, when asked following relaxation training what had been the most helpful part of the treatment, patients emphasised contact with the therapist and the adoption of a "changed attitude" to their tinnitus. Except in a few cases, relaxation was not perceived as the main cause of improvement. These observations are admittedly open to differing interpretations, but it was our distinct impression, working as therapists, that a cognitive-perceptual change was a more likely explanation of benefit than was the acquisition of new coping strategies. It seemed that we had given patients a new way of looking at the problem of tinnitus without deliberately setting out to do so. At this time, we also became aware of the work of Sweetow in San Francisco who was using cognitive therapy techniques to help patients view their tinnitus in a less negative light (Sweetow, 1984).

8.1.1.3 Empirical investigation of complaint

In addition to medical and audiological investigations, tinnitus patients are routinely interviewed by a psychologist to screen for significant degrees of emotional distress and other problems. Questionnaire assessments have now been developed. Patients can show a large range of difficulties, but certain problems, such as depressed and anxious mood, are commonplace, (Stephens and Hallam, 1985). The Tinnitus Questionnaire (see appendix) was developed on the basis of commonly encountered complaints and also on ideas about the cognitive basis of emotional distress derived from the ideas of Albert Ellis and Aaron Beck. Factor analyses have revealed three main dimensions of complaint (Hallam et al 1988). These analyses have also shown that irrational beliefs about tinnitus and coping strategies tend *not* to cluster into factors. However, the largest factor we have extracted, "Emotional Distress", does include items of a cognitive nature, e.g. "I often think about whether the noises will ever go away" (loading 0.69), "I feel I can never get away from the noises" (loading 0.61). The presence of depressed mood, anger and irritability are indicated by other items loading this factor. The content of the distress factor and our own clinical experience strongly suggest an association between emotional distress and patient's negative interpretations of the significance of their noises, especially what will happen to them if the noises never go away or become louder. There is often an unstated and underlying worry that the person will kill him/herself, alienate their family, spouse or partner through their unacceptable behaviour, or find it impossible to continue working. Certain negative beliefs are idiosyncratic, and may, for this reason, be missed by our questionnaire or, if detected, fail to correlate with the beliefs expressed by other patients.

The remaining two factors measured by the questionnaire are "Auditory perceptual difficulties attributed to tinnitus" and "Insomnia". An "Irrational beliefs" scale is incorporated into the questionnaire although this is not factorially derived. Scores on all four scales differentiate between patients who are attending the clinic on account of tinnitus being a problem for them and those attending the clinic for other reasons but who also happen to report tinnitus as a symptom, (Hallam et al, 1988).

8.2.0 Group cognitive therapy

Our cognitive therapy was based on the model provided by Sank and Shaffer (1984). The primary assumption of cognitive therapy is that emotional reactions to events are created not by the events themselves but by a person's interpretation of those events. In the case of depressive emotional reactions, it has been observed that they are mediated by negative interpretations of the self, the world or the future. The negative interpretation is usually unthinkingly adopted and tends to be plausible, although Beck has also emphasised that it may be based on faulty logical reasoning. The purpose of our therapy was to examine the evidence for negative beliefs about tinnitus and to dispute them using the Socratic method. We did not use experiential tasks or homework assignments to challenge patients' beliefs although it might be profitable to do so in future. The group therapy was conducted as follows:

8.2.1 Selection of patients

The patients attended a specialist (mainly tertiary referral) neuro-otology clinic. The etiology of tinnitus was variable and was not taken into consideration in selecting patients. All medical investigations and treatments, including provision of hearing-aids, was completed prior to selection. Patients were selected on the basis that (a) tinnitus was the most significant problem and had been present for at least one year (b) hearing acuity was adequate for group therapy (c) patients were suitable for aural masking (d) there was no major psychiatric disorder (e) the patient was willing and able to attend the hospital (f) the patient had not previously received cognitive therapy or an aural masker. The patients came from all social classes; their mean age was 59 years. The therapy was offered at no cost.

8.2.2 Information booklet

Patients were issued with a 3 page booklet explaining the aims of the therapy and the role of negative thoughts about tinnitus in producing emotional distress and raised awareness of the noises. It was pointed out that in order to change these thoughts, it was necessary, first, to identify them and, second, to question their helpfulness, sense and rationality.

8.2.3 Description of the sessions

Session one: The groups were composed of 5-7 patients led by two therapists (Simon Jakes and Lawrence McKenna) experienced in utilising cognitive techniques. The groups met for 5, 1½ hour weekly sessions. Assignment to groups was carried out on a random basis because the therapy was being evaluated and compared with alternative treatments.

The members were first invited to introduce themselves and to explain how their tinnitus affected them. The therapists guided the accounts towards the emotional effects of the tinnitus. As the various members described their problems, similarities and contrasts were pointed out. At the end of each account other members were invited to ask questions. The cognitive model of emotional distress was then explained using the booklet as the springboard for discussion. The ABC model (antecedents-beliefs-consequences) was illustrated by an everyday example (see Table 8.1). A prepared example, or one taken from the session, was then analysed in a similar way (see Table 8.2).

To summarise, the aims of the first session were *engagement*, *facilitation of self-disclosure*, directing the focuse of attention on the *emotional and psychological aspects*, and *explaining the ABC model* of analysis.

Members were asked at the end of the session to record details of episodes of tinnitus distress in the following week. Details of the antecedent situation and emotional consequences were requested as a minimal requirement and, where possible, members were invited to identify the thoughts that were associated with their distress.

Session two: Members reported back on their homework task and members who had completed it were praised for doing so. Examples were selected to illustrate the ABC analysis. An ex-patient who, in the past, had been very distressed by tinnitus but who had now learned to tolerate it, was invited to the second session. He gave his personal account of the development of tolerance. This encounter was important in disconfirming the almost universal prediction of the inevitability of emotional distress if tinnitus was present. Members were invited to question the ex-patient and further opportunities were exploited to illustrate the cognitive model.

The concept of disputing or challenging negative beliefs about tinnitus was

Table 8.1 Everyday example to illustrate the role of thinking in emotional response

A – Antecedents	B – Beliefs	C – Consequences
Someone pokes you in the back on a crowded metro		Annoyance
	Immediate unexamined thoughts: "Someone is not taking care." "Someone is trying to steal my wallet."	
You turn around and see that the person has a white stick		Remorse Feeling apologetic
	New thought: "This was unintentional because the person is blind."	

then introduced. The point of challenging them was by now clear to most group members; the fact that negative interpretations of tinnitus produce a vicious cycle of: tinnitus →worry→attention to tinnitus→further worry (and intrusion into normal mental activities)→further attention to tinnitus, was reiterated. Challenges were explained as questions that can be asked to dispute the reasonableness of tinnitus beliefs. A "challenge board" was set up in front of the group in which the most useful questions were identified (see Table 8.3). An example was taken, sometimes out of a role-play between the two therapists, one of whom played the role of a patient. The members were invited to select challenges that seemed appropriate to dispute a particular belief and then answers to the question were elicited. It was important to emphasise that questions were not implied criticism of a person as a whole, only a disputation of the belief. Where an example from a member was used, the person who held the belief was invited to answer the challenge, as, of course, any answer that was supplied by another member was likely to be perceived

Table 8.2 Example of an ABC analysis of a distressing episode with tinnitus

A – Antecedents	B – Beliefs	C – Consequences
You read an article suggesting that in the foreseeable future a cure for tinnitus will not be found		Disappointment Hopelessness Bitterness
	"It's unfair that my retirement is spoiled." "Medical science should have produced a cure by now."	

Table 8.3 Questions on the "Challenge Board"

What evidence do I have to support my beliefs?
How would someone else view my thoughts?
What are the effects of thinking the way I do?
Am I thinking in all-or-nothing terms?
Am I blaming myself for something which is not my fault?
Am I overestimating the chances of disaster?
Am I using a crystal ball to read the future?
Am I expecting myself to be perfect?

either as inappropriate or critical. A useful, general-purpose challenge is "What is the evidence for your belief?". With reference to Figure 2, one may ask: What is your evidence that having tinnitus is "unfair"? A claim that most people stay completely healthy as they get older can be disputed fairly readily. A claim that one *ought* to be healthy, can be countered by questioning on whose authority such rights are guaranteed? Faulty inferences can be challenged by reference to evidence or by simple logic. Adherence to inflated values attaching to aspects of oneself, the world, or the future can sometimes be disputed by following through a chain of questions concerning the basis of holding the value: "It will be terrible if this tinnitus never goes away" (What would be so terrible about that?), "My life will not be worth living, I will go to pieces" (What is your evidence that life will be worthless and you will go to pieces?) etc.

As homework assignment, members were again requested to record episodes of tinitus distress and to attempt to analyse them in the ABC format, thinking up challenges to dispute negative beliefs.

Sessions three to five: Sessions began with reports on homework assignments and provision of appropriate feedback. Clients practised challenging their negative beliefs primarily by using role-reversal. In this technique the patient explains to another group member or group leader as much as they can of an episode of tinnitus distress and their associated thoughts. The role-partner enacts the role of the distressed patient who, in turn, asks the questions to dispute the negative thinking. In this way the patient rehearses the mode of constructive thinking which, eventually, it is hoped, will supplant the negative thinking. The technique was first demonstrated by the two group leaders. The willingness of members to participate varied from group to group and role-reversal was not, of course, enforced on members who felt uncomfortable with role-playing. Members appeared to learn from observing role-plays even when they did not participate themselves. In any given role-play, group members assisted the patient by suggesting suitable challenges. The following is a transcript of a reverse role-play taken from one of the group sessions:

Therapist: It's a matter, David, of you taking on the role of Mary, and Mary, you try to challenge the thoughts again as before.

David: (playing Mary) Well, I think it's pretty depressing after all this time, to feel that I'm getting on top of one tinnitus, and then to be attacked by this second one. It's very depressing. What can I do about it?

Mary: Well, what did you do about the last one?

David: I came to classes and I rationalised, and I challenged my fears, to see if they were rational or otherwise, and with will-power and determination, I was making very good headway. But now I'm frightened again about the second attack and fear I'll never get rid of it.

Mary: Why are you frightened because you think you'll never get rid of it? Is that what you said just now?

David: Yes

Mary: But did you not know that you would not get rid of the sound that time either?

David: Yes. Well, in the beginning I was almost suicidal and I overcame that — but this second one seems to be the straw that breaks the camel's back. It's too much. I'm just managing to cope with the first one, how can I cope with the second?

Mary: I can only say that you can cope with the second one by following the same route that you followed on the first one. Why do you think that you shouldn't succeed with the second one?

David: Well, I have other problems that mount up and these problems with the first tinnitus may have been the limit I could cope with.

Mary: Well, when you first got tinnitus, you felt at that time that you would never ever live with it and cope with it and you felt desperate at that time because it was a big shock to you.

David: That's right.

Mary: You're feeling like that at this second sound are you?

David: No, depressed, not desperate.

Mary: So, why do you feel less optimistic about the second time than you were about the first? You knew you overcame that.

David: I suppose I needed time to feel more confident about the first one before the second one came.

The role-play continues on and Mary challenges David's lack of optimism and the worry that the tinnitus will remain for the rest of his life. (She is, in reality, challenging her own negative thinking).

In addition to role-play, videotaped interviews with ex-patients who had benefited from cognitive therapy, were played to the group as a basis for discussion. Some patients in group therapy rapidly endorsed the cognitive model of their difficulties whereas others were reluctant or unable to see its relevance. The group leaders attempted to direct the group to focus on the ideas and techniques of cognitive therapy as they applied to tinnitus, using an educational model. They gently deflected questions about somatic and medical aspects, which were, in any case, being dealt with by other professional staff. It became evident that some patients had psychological problems that required individual counselling which they were able to receive later. In general, it is our impression that five group sessions initiates positive change in a large minority of patients, but a longer course of therapy is required to consolidate benefits.

8.3.0 Results of group cognitive therapy

A full account of our evaluation has been submitted for publication elsewhere and only a brief summary will be given here.

Patients were randomly assigned to a waiting list control group (who received treatment after seven weeks), aural masking treatment, placebo masking (in which the masker was set just above the patients' auditory threshold), group cognitive therapy (GCT) and a combined GCT and masking group. Tinnitus measures were taken before and after a two week baseline period, after 5 weeks of therapy and at a three month follow-up assessment. Patients were contacted by telephone 1-2 years later to assess their progress. Although we had intended to evaluate tinnitus loudness and annoyance over the initial seven weeks using a self-monitoring, diary method, 40% of patients failed to comply satisfactorily, and so the main outcome measure was the Tinnitus Questionnaire (TQ) referred to earlier. The Crown Crisp Experiential Index (CCEI) (Crown and Crisp, 1979) was used to assess change in effect. Interference by tinnitus with daily activities was measured on a scale designed for an earlier study, (Jakes et al, 1986).

Analysis of group means revealed no change over the baseline period, except for Irrational Beliefs which were reduced in the GCT group only. Across all groups there was a trend towards decreasing "somatic anxiety" on the CCEI and decreasing interference with daily activities but no group by treatment interaction. We had predicted a decrease in the Emotional Distress and Irrational Beliefs Scales of the TQ following GCT and this was indeed found at the three months follow-up assessment. There were no group differences on the TQ scales post-treatment, however.

In summary, GCT does seem to produce more lasting amelioration of the emotional distress and negative thinking aspects of tinnitus than alternative forms of treatment. At the long term follow-up, 46% of GCT patients mentioned that they had benefited from the emotional support, sharing of problem, and the understanding they had received. By contrast, only 10% of patients receiving a masker mentioned it as being helpful. The specific contribution of cognitive techniques cannot be determined but further investigation of this question seems worthwhile.

Anecdotally, it was noted that some patients attributed their considerable improvement after GCT to the validity of the cognitive model and to the application of cognitive techniques.

8.4.0 Conclusion

Assignment of patients to treatments was random and so, inevitably, there was great variation in age and treatment compliance within the groups. Some patients were unable to accept the concept of learning to adapt to their noises and remained fixed on physical remedies. Some could not introspect in the required manner or did not fully grasp the cognitive model. Very few patients completed their homework task of writing down their thoughts that accompanied their tinnitus distress. These observations suggest that attention should be paid to suitability for this form of treatment.

Moreover, some patients were probably anxious or depressed for reasons other than their tinnitus. The opportunity for supplementary individual counselling should therefore be created.

Despite these reservations, group cognitive therapy appears to be a promising approach which deserves further evaluation.

8.6 References

Crown, S., A.H. Crisp (1979): Manual of the Crown Crisp Experiental Index. London: Hodder & Stoughton.

Goebel, G. & W. Hiller (1992): Psychische Beschwerden bei chronischem Tinnitus: Erprobung und Evaluation des Tinnitus-Fragebogens. Verhaltenstherapie, 2 (1).

Hallam, R.S., S.C. Jakes, R. Hinchcliffe (1988): Cognitive variables in tinnitus annoyance. British Journal of Clinical Psychology, 27: 213-222.

Hallam, R.S., S. Rachman, R. Hinchcliffe (1984): Psychological aspects of tinnitus. In: *Rachman, S.* (Ed.). Contributions to Medical Psychology, Vol 3: 31-54. Oxford: Pergamon.

Hiller, W. & G. Goebel (1992): A psychometric study of complaints in chronic tinnitus. Journal of Psychometric Research 36 (4): 337-348.

Jakes, S. C., R. S. Hallam, L. Racham S. & Hinchcliffe, R. (1986): The effects of reassurance, relaxation training and distraction in chronic tinnitus sufferers. Behaviour Research and Therapy, 24: 497-567.

Jakes, S. C. R. S. Hallam, L. McKenna, R. Hinchcliffe (1991): Group cognitive therapy for medical patients: an application to tinnitus. Cognitive Therapy and Research, 6: 67-82.

Sank, L. I., C. S. Shaffer (1984): A therapist's manual for cognitive behaviour therapy in group. New York: Plenum.

Stephens, S. D. G., R. S. Hallam (1985): The Crown-Crisp Experiental Index in patients complaining of tinnitus. British Journal of Audiology, 19: 151-158.

Sweetow, R. W. (1984): Cognitive behavioural modification in tinnitus management. Hearing Instruments, 53: 14-18.

Appendix

Tinnitus Questionnaire*

The purpose of this questionnaire is to find out whether the noises in your ears/head have had any effect on your mood, habits or attitudes.

Please mark the answer that applies to you.

Name: ______________________

First Name: ______________________

Age: ______________________

Date: ______________________

		true	partly true	not true
1.	I can sometimes ignore the noises even when they are there	☐	☐	☐
2.	I am unable to enjoy music because of the noises	☐	☐	☐
3.	It's unfair that I have to suffer from my noises	☐	☐	☐
4.	I wake up more often at night because of my noises	☐	☐	☐
5.	I am aware of the noises from the moment I get up to the moment I fall asleep	☐	☐	☐
6.	My attitude toward the noise makes no difference concerning tinnitus discomfort	☐	☐	☐
7.	Most of the time the noises are fairly quiet	☐	☐	☐
8.	I worry that the noises will lead to a nervous breakdown	☐	☐	☐
9.	Because of the noises I have difficulty telling where sounds come from	☐	☐	☐
10.	The way the noises sound is really unpleasant	☐	☐	☐
11.	I feel I can never escape from the noises	☐	☐	☐
12.	Because of the noises I wake up earlier in the morning	☐	☐	☐
13.	I worry whether I will be able to cope with this problem forever	☐	☐	☐
14.	Because of the noises it is more difficult to listen to several people at once	☐	☐	☐
15.	The noises are loud most of the time	☐	☐	☐
16.	Because of the noises I worry that there is something seriously wrong with my body	☐	☐	☐
17.	If the noises continue, my life will not be worth living	☐	☐	☐
18.	I have lost some of my self-confidence because of the noises	☐	☐	☐
19.	I wish someone really understood this problem	☐	☐	☐
20.	The noises distract me totally	☐	☐	☐
21.	There is very little I can do to cope with the noises	☐	☐	☐
22.	The noises sometimes lead to a pain in the ear or head	☐	☐	☐
23.	When I feel sad and pessimistic the noises seem worse	☐	☐	☐
24.	I am more irritable with my family and friends because of the noises	☐	☐	☐

* The original version in English as well as German can be requested from the editor

	true	partly true	not true
25. Because of the noises I suffer from tension in the muscles of my head and neck	☐	☐	☐
26. Because of the noises other people's voices sound distorted	☐	☐	☐
27. It will be dreadful if these noises never go away	☐	☐	☐
28. I worry that the noises may damage my physical health	☐	☐	☐
29. The noises seem to go right through my head	☐	☐	☐
30. Almost all my problems are caused by these noises	☐	☐	☐
31. Disturbed sleep is my main problem	☐	☐	☐
32. It's the way you think about the noise — NOT the noise itself which makes you upset	☐	☐	☐
33. I have more difficulty following a conversation because of the noises	☐	☐	☐
34. I find it harder to relax because of the noises	☐	☐	☐
35. My noises are often so severe that I cannot ignore them	☐	☐	☐
36. It takes me longer to fall asleep because of the noises	☐	☐	☐
37. I sometimes get very angry when I think about having the noises	☐	☐	☐
38. I find it more difficult to use the telephone because of the noises	☐	☐	☐
39. I am more liable to feel depressed because of the noises	☐	☐	☐
40. I am able to forget the noises when I am doing something interesting	☐	☐	☐
41. Because of the noises life seems to be getting on top of me	☐	☐	☐
42. I have always been sensitive about my ears	☐	☐	☐
43. I often think about whether the noises will ever go away	☐	☐	☐
44. I can imagine coping with the noises	☐	☐	☐
45. The noises never cease	☐	☐	☐
46. A stronger person might be better at accepting this problem	☐	☐	☐
47. I am a victim of my noises	☐	☐	☐
48. The noises have affected my concentration	☐	☐	☐
49. The noises are one of those problems in life you have to live with	☐	☐	☐
50. Because of the noises I am unable to enjoy radio or television	☐	☐	☐
51. The noises sometimes produce a bad headache	☐	☐	☐
52. I have always been a light sleeper	☐	☐	☐

* The English and Dutch version can be obtained at the
Psychological Corporation, Harcourt Brace & Company, Publishers
24–28 Oval Road
London NW1 7DX
UK

* The German version can be obtained at the
Testzentrale
Robert-Bosch-Breite 25
D-37079 Göttingen

Chapter 9

Behavioral therapy in complex chronic tinnitus: exposition and distraction: evaluation of therapy and long-term effects

Per Lindberg, PhD
Centre for Caring Sciences and
Department of Audiology,
Uppsala University

and

Berit Scott, PhD
Department of Clinical Psychology
and Department of Audiology,
Uppsala University

9.1 Introduction

The psychological implications of tinnitus have been discussed and recognized for a long time even though psychological treatment methods have been used sparsely and with varying success. As early as in the 19th century the famous French audiologist Itard discussed the psychological mechanisms associated with tinnitus (Stephens 1984). However, it was not until the middle of our century that we have any scientific reports on psychological interventions of tinnitus. There have certainly been attempts to relieve tinnitus by means of psychotherapeutic methods earlier, but these were often not as extensive as the ones considered here.

The strength of behaviour therapy at large and of behavioral medicine (e.g. Gentry, 1984) in particular, has led to an increased interest in learning theory among researchers and clinicians involved in rehabilitation of the hard of hearing. In this chapter we will present empirical support for a behavioural approach to tinnitus and describe it as used in the setting of an out-patient ward at a specialized "tinnitus clinic".

9.1.1 Psychological diagnosis of tinnitus sufferers

In connection with psychological aspects of tinnitus, the psychological profile and personality of tinnitus patients have been discussed. A number of researchers have pointed out the possibility that tinnitus sufferers have certain personality characteristics. Various scales and criteria, such as the Minnesota Multiphasic Personality Inventory (MMPI) (House, 1981; Reich, & Johnsson, 1984), the Eysenck Personality Questionnaire (EPQ), the Beck Depression Inventory (BDI) (Wood, Webb, Orchik, & Shea, 1983), the Crown-Crisp Experiential Index (CCEI) (Stephens, & Hallam, 1985), the American Diagnostic and Statistical Manual (DSM-III), and the Hopkins Symptom Checklist (SCL-90), (Harrop-Griffith, Katon, Doibie, Sakai, & Russo, 1987) have been used to establish the type of personality of a subject or the type of psychiatric disorder. However, there are some problems associated with these types of assessment that are often overlooked or ignored (McFadden, 1982). For instance, these personality inventories are not constructed for repeated measurements and for practical reasons it is not suitable to use them more than a few times on each subject. A second and more serious problem is that theoretically these methods are designed to evaluate stable aspects of the personality such as extroversion or affective traits. However, all psychological methods of treatment aimed at tinnitus strive for various forms of change in the patients' way of handling their tinnitus. This then, implies a dynamic process. It is therefore not satisfactory to use personality inventories, despite the good reliability of some of these assessments. However, these methods can be used for prediction, in determining the presence of psychiatric problems in the subjects or to compare tinnitus sufferers with patients with other problems.

The psychiatric problem most readily identified by the MMPI scale is depression. Increased ratings for neuroticism have also been shown on both EPQ and MMPI scales. Further, the results from the CCEI show depression to be the main feature, but also that dizziness together with tinnitus result in, for example, phobic anxiety and more frequent somatic complaints compared with the population norm. Harrop-Griffith and colleagues (1987) found that the depressed tinnitus patient (in accordance with DSM-III criteria) scored more somatic complaints than controls. Other authors have shown opposite results. For example, Gerber, Nehemkis, Charter and Jones (1985) found no correlation between tinnitus and the MMPI scale. Kearney, Wilson and Haralambous (1987) examined patients with headache, patients with tinnitus and a control group, with a number of scales as the Emotional Control Scale (ECS), the Taylor Manifest Anxiety Scale (MAS), the Stress Cognitions Inventory (SCI) and the Unpleasant Events Schedule (UES), as well as with EPQ and BDI. They found that patients with headache as a primary problem showed elevated scores for MAS, EPQ/neuroticism and SCI, while the scores of the control group and the tinnitus group were within the normal range.

With few exceptions (Harrop-Griffith *et al.*, 1987; Kearney *et al.*, 1987), in most of the studies undertaken to establish whether or not there is a certain personality type among tinnitus patients, no strong evidence of a particular personality type or psychiatric disorder as a cause of tinnitus has been shown.

9.1.2 Psychotherapeutic considerations and non-specific treatment methods

Some psychologically oriented treatments for tinnitus are directed towards supposedly underlying personality deficits and disorders claimed to coincide with tinnitus, or directed towards clinical manifestations such as depression or anxiety. Even though these methods are not notable either numerically or in respect to their results, they have gained attention and have influenced the thinking concerning tinnitus a great deal. As none of these therapies aims specifically at the tinnitus *per se* they must be considered as non-specific methods.

Other non-specific treatments with different theoretical backgrounds are methods like counselling, self-help groups, physiotherapy, and relaxation training either in a group setting or on an individual basis. Some of these methods are dealt with in detail in other parts of this book and is beyond the scope of this chapter.

9.1.3 Behavioral approaches to treatment

Behavioral medicine, with its integration and pronounced reciprocal relationship between behavioural psychology and several other disciplines (e.g. medicine, pharmacology, sociology), offers a new approach to the understanding of the concept of tinnitus. Tinnitus, with its physiological as well as psychological components, may be better understood and may benefit from methods and techniques offered by behavioural medicine. The assessments and interventions developed within behavioural therapy should be utilized. Another reason for viewing tinnitus within a behavioural framework is the poor relationship between the loudness and the degree of discomfort (Jakes, Hallam, Chambers & Hinchcliffe, 1985). The low matched loudness can be experienced as very annoying and vice versa.

A psychological approach to noise exposure was used by Glass and Singer (1972). They studied stress in relation to exposure to intense noise, and found that noise perceived as being out of control significantly increased the cognitive, emotional, and psychological aversiveness. Provided that tinnitus could be regarded as an external sound, the concept of control could offer a possible model for explaining the variations in discomfort from tinnitus between individuals and also the discrepancies between the tinnitus loudness and the perceived discomfort.

As tinnitus is a subjective experience, all evaluation of change must rely on the patient's own verbal report, as no other criteria are available. Within behaviour therapy, verbal reports and visual analogue scales are regarded as equivalent to all other types of measures, provided that these have been proven to be reliable and valid. The use of visual analogue scales has rapidly advanced within this field (Kazdin, 1980). This development has increased the possibilities of studying such an elusive phenomenon as tinnitus.

The etiology of tinnitus is still unknown, and since tinnitus has resisted most previous therapeutic methods, a behavioural approach to the problem seems appropriate. In order to optimize the treatment outcome, a treatment package consisting of relaxation techniques in combination with perceptual restructuring methods has been used in a number of studies. Azrin (1977) states: *"My strategy has been to use such programs unapologetically and to include as many component procedures as seem necessary to obtain, ideally, a total treatment success"*. That statement could also stand for the studies this chapter is based upon.

9.1.4 Components in behavioral treatment of tinnitus

There are a few basic components that are common to most attempts of behavioral medicine to relieve tinnitus. The most prominent is relaxation training in various forms (e.g. Ireland, Wilson, Tonkin, & Platt-Hepworth, 1985). It can be used as a goal in itself, but also as a tool to obtain better coping ability. The reason for using relaxation as one of the main components in a treatment package, is that a number of reports have described positive results with the use of this method as a coping technique, e.g. in anxiety (Suinn, 1975), chronic pain (Linton, Melin & Stjernlöf, 1985), phobias, epilepsy, headache, non-ulcer dyspepsia and panic disorder (Sjödén, 1988). Of special interest are the results obtained with chronic pain, as pain has been claimed to have many similarities to tinnitus (Aran & Cazals, 1981).

Even though it is claimed that relaxation methods such as EMG-biofeedback training aim specifically at reducing tinnitus, they can not be regarded as specific methods aimed at the tinnitus loudness or the discomfort caused by it. Bio-feedback methods for tinnitus rest on the assumption that tinnitus covaries with muscle tension. By reducing this physiological tension and getting the patient into a relaxed state it is claimed that tinnitus could be reduced (e.g. Grossan, 1976). However, in a well-controlled experimental study by Borton and Clark (1988) there was no evidence that relaxation initiated by EMG-biofeedback covaried with tinnitus.

The only documented feedback method aimed at tinnitus directly is that described by Ince and colleagues (1987). Their method, however, does not involve relaxation, but rather an acoustic technique where the patient decreases tinnitus by matching it with a decreasing external sound in whatever way is possible.

In other areas where relaxation has been used successfully there are special features which have to be emphasized (Öst, 1988). Relaxation is regarded as a skill which has to be practised regularly. During later parts of therapy it is trained in tension- and anxiety-provoking situations. It thus becomes a coping behaviour by repeatedly applying it and adjusting the relaxation to a particular problem. Later, after the termination of treatment it is of importance to make special efforts in maintaining these coping skills.

Cognitive components have always played an important role in all behavioural interventions. However, a point must be made concerning the terminology as cognitive *methods* and the term *cognitive* have been used lately in a broader sense than earlier, i.e. in cognitive behaviour therapy (Kendall & Bemis, 1986). Jakes and colleagues (1986) refer to informational and educational parts in therapy as "cognitive treatment components". Such concepts have little to do with the much broader theoretical framework for cognitive therapy even though the same techniques may be used. Our studies, which are presented below, use the same contextual framework, that is we use cognitive components as parts of a treatment package where the overall goal is behavioural change. We use the term cognitive to describe methods used by the patient to distract from or attend to other stimuli, thoughts and feelings than the disruptive ones associated with tinnitus. In another part of this book results of cognitive behaviour therapy for tinnitus is presented (*Chapter 8 by Dr Richard Hallam*).

The common goal of behavioural treatment methods is to integrate behavioural and cognitive components into a way of handling tinnitus in a non-destructive fashion that enables the patient to do something which he knows will reduce the agony. We call this controlling tinnitus by coping. This means that both behavioural and cognitive aspects of the patient's behaviour should be under scrutiny during therapy. In order to do so we are entitled to use various forms of assessments as for instance diagnostic tools in the initial behaviour analysis, during the treatment, and after termination of therapy to maintain and estimate the effects. Of special interest is a single case study by Malatesta and colleagues (1980) where intense monitoring of tinnitus made it possible to determine effects of caffeine and relaxation on tinnitus. This study implicates several things, but most important the use of multiple assessments over time and in different modes. It also shows that relaxation training can affect tinnitus if it is used as a strategy to attain control rather than being the goal of therapy itself.

9.1.5 Empirical studies of the effectiveness of a behavioral approach

In this section we will discuss some of our own experimental studies in clinical settings. The initial study (Scott, Lindberg, Lyttkens & Melin, 1985) was designed to determine the effects of a behavioural treatment package for tinnitus as compared to an untreated control group. In order to establish which long term effects could be expected from such a package the patients in this study were re-assessed approximately nine months after commencing treatment (Lindberg, Scott, Melin & Lyttkens, 1987).

The second study deals with a model for managing tinnitus in a clinical setting and how the treatment package should be integrated into the routines of an outpatient ward (Lindberg, Scott, Lyttkens & Melin, 1988). Finally the third study is concerned with the theoretical issue whether or not behavioural or cognitive coping styles should be emphasized in controlling tinnitus (Lindberg, Scott, Melin & Lyttkens, 1989).

9.1.5.1 Does behavioral treatment affect tinnitus?

In 1982 when our initial study of behavioural intervention was planned (Scott et al., 1985), no experimentally controlled outcome studies on psychological treatment were available. Results from specific psychological therapy were only presented as case-studies (e.g. Marlowe, 1973) or in studies where methodologically weak pre-post designs were used (e.g. Grossan, 1976). A natural first step towards a better understanding of the psychological treatment of tinnitus was to determine whether therapy was more effective in reducing tinnitus than no treatment at all. As some stress-related factors such as tension and sleeping disorders had been found to be associated with tinnitus in a previous study (Lindberg, Lyttkens, Melin, & Scott, 1984), behavioural techniques comprising relaxation and self-control were used.

Twenty-four consecutive patients referred for severe tinnitus participated in the study. Several of these patients had tried almost every available treatment for tinnitus (e.g. lidocaine injections, acupuncture, masking devices and physiotherapy) without any success. Various sorts of hearing impairments were represented and in all patients the tinnitus was classified as Grade II or III on the standardized scale of Klockhoff and Lindblom (1967).

The treatment consisted of ten one-hour sessions and had three main themes. First, the patients were taught progressive relaxation followed by conditioned relaxation and quick relaxation (Bernstein & Borkovec, 1973). Secondly, self-control techniques were introduced and the objective of this training was to get the patient to relocate attention away from tinnitus towards an imaginary scene or some scene incompatible with tinnitus. The final step was to let the patient practise these new skills in his or her daily life.

The results showed significant reductions in all daily self-recorded variables, except for one reflecting the patient's affective state. No effects on psychoacoustic measurements were found. Interview results showed that 14 of the 15 patients who had problems with headache, muscle tension, and dizziness reported improvement. Further, the drug intake related to tinnitus was reduced or completely terminated in seven out of nine patients.

The results indicated that the intervention as a package was effective, compared with no treatment at all. After the control group had received treatment, the results were combined for both groups, and significant reductions in all continuously recorded variables were found. This further confirms the usefulness of the treatment given.

It is generally known that the relapse figures for behavioural interventions are relatively high (Karoly, & Steffen, 1980). It was therefore of interest to establish how the effects of behavioural techniques to treat tinnitus were maintained over time (Lindberg et al., 1987). About nine months after termination of treatment, the patients were contacted and asked to monitor their problems during a week by using the same scales as previously. All patients but two complied and the long-term follow-up is therefore based on 20 patients. We found that the discomfort from tinnitus was still significantly reduced, while no such effect was present for subjective loudness. This finding was confirmed by psychoacoustic testing as there were no significant changes found between the assessments.

At the follow up visit to the clinic, patients also were asked to estimate their experience of tinnitus (i.e. their subjective loudness and their discomfort) before receiving treatment. They were further asked to rate loudness and discomfort during the previous week. Non-significant correlations were found between the estimates before and the estimation made at the visit to the clinic, while correlations between the self-recordings made the week before the visit and the recordings at the clinic, however, were significant. Finally, patients completed a semi-structured questionnaire for evaluation of the frequency of use of the trained coping technique and of their attitude towards the treatment received. The compliance was satisfactory; 16 of the patients were still using the coping technique and of these, 14 reported beneficial effects on their tinnitus.

The long-term effects of the treatment were satisfactory. However, the poor correlation found between baserates and recordings performed at the clinic highlights the importance of evaluating intervention through continuous assessments and not by relying solely on retrospective reports or interview data. Of interest is the fact that tinnitus patients did *not* overestimate their symptoms, which was the case for a group of chronic pain patients examined by Linton and Melin (1982).

In consideration of the fact that the patients included in this study had tried many other types of treatment without any lasting effect, and that all patients were severely handicapped by their tinnitus, results were encouraging and an integration of behavioural methods into routine management of tinnitus is justifiable.

9.1.5.2 Integration of behavioral treatment at an out-patient ward

In order to investigate what results could be expected if the treatment was applied in the clinical setting, a non-experimental study was conducted (Lindberg, Scott, Lyttkens, & Melin, 1988). As the treatment was carried out in the regular setting at the clinic, control over conditions such as training and practice was less feasible. The principal aim, however, was to investigate how the treatment package worked in conjunction with a routine management programme for tinnitus. The treatment was more individually applied and special efforts were made to alleviate other problems which were considered crucial for the outcome of the tinnitus treatment. In addition, tinnitus-related characteristics were examined in an attempt to find predictors of the outcome of therapy.

To monitor treatment results, daily measurements on visual analogue scales and a long-term follow-up were performed. Seventy-five consecutive patients referred for severe tinnitus took part. The majority of patients had various kinds of hearing difficulties, but seven patients with normal hearing were also included in the study. Each patient received about ten individualised, 1-hour treatment sessions. The treatment consisted of the techniques described earlier, i.e. relaxation and distraction, but was adapted to suit the individual patient's needs in coping with the total situation. For example, phobic reactions, depressed states and various somatic complaints were attended to in a more systematic manner. This extended treatment package included desensitisation, exposure and cognitive techniques.

The findings in this investigation showed significantly reduced discomfort from tinnitus as well as improved mood. The results were in accordance with out earlier findings and those of other researchers (Jakes, Hallam, Rachman & Hinchcliffe, 1986). Again no reduction in psychoacoustic measurements of tinnitus was observed.

Only one significant predictor of the treatment outcome was found as gain scores of the dependent variables were correlated with a number of background variables. Patients with a shorter duration of tinnitus showed greater improvement in discomfort and mood. This finding should be interpreted with caution. One explanation might be that patients with tinnitus of short duration are in a turbulent phase on account of the novelty of the sound, and that behavioural intervention might facilitate the adjustment of the tinnitus sound.

Among those who reported headache, dizziness, troublesome muscle tension, and sleeping disorders, improvement was found in three out of four patients. Furthermore, the relapse figures over a 3-month period were negligible, which confirms the effectivity of the treatment.

We believe that this study (Lindberg et al., 1988) demonstrates the possibility of integrating psychological treatment into a clinical setting. It shows that behavioural treatment enables the patient to control tinnitus to such a degree that it is no longer regarded as a major problem.

The question of which factors might be of importance for the natural development of tolerance or adaptation to tinnitus was raised. At the same time as our clinical study was conducted, Hallam and colleagues (1984) in England discussed psychological aspects in general and natural habituation in particular. As these authors pointed out, tolerance to tinnitus should be regarded as the normal state. It should therefore be asked what factors can possibly be viewed as obstacles to this normal process of adaptation and which factors facilitate the adaptation.

9.1.5.3 Coping with tinnitus by exposure or distraction techniques?

In a questionnaire study discussed in detail elsewhere (Chapter 1 of this book by Scott & Lindberg), it was shown that controlling tinnitus, operationalized as the subject's ability of distraction, was of great importance for the process of adaptation to tinnitus

(Scott, Lindberg, Lyttkens & Melin, 1990). The importance of masking effects from surrounding sounds was also emphasized. The help of environmental sound seems to facilitate adaptation. One possible interpretation of these results is that both functions, i.e. the importance of emotional control and the more specific external control (maskability) by environmental sounds, can be viewed as a control or a coping strategy which the tinnitus sufferer can make use of depending on the situation. Any intervention should therefore include strategies that facilitate various forms of coping. These results have not clarified the question of causality, however, and should rather be regarded as generators for further research. However, in order to establish the importance of the concept of control for the outcome of treatment, a group study involving this new control-measure, as well as a new approach to the acquisition of coping skills, was conducted (Lindberg, Scott, Melin, & Lyttkens, 1989).

The studies discussed earlier (Scott et al., 1985; Lindberg et al., 1988) had shown the effectiveness of a specific coping method involving relaxation and self-control techniques such as imaginative scenes and restructuring of the general attitudes toward the problem. To investigate the necessity of using a specific treatment, this treatment was compared with a coping method involving exposure, i.e. direct training in coping with the tinnitus itself while being exposed to tinnitus-provoking situations.

Twenty-seven patients referred for severe tinnitus took part in the study in which relaxation and exposure or relaxation and distraction were given as active treatments.

The treatment consisted of ten one-hour therapy sessions and in the first part of treatment both groups received identical relaxation training. In the second part patients were given different training. The first group received exposure treatment aimed at teaching the subjects to cope with the tinnitus itself. They were exposed to tinnitus-provoking sounds with increased acoustic intricacy, ranging from a situation with "party talk", i.e. two simultaneous conversations with four voices involved, to sounds from a crowded street with various echo effects. The remaining group received the same type of coping training as has been described earlier in this chapter.

To examine the overall effects of treatment, both treatment groups were compared with untreated controls regarding their tinnitus loudness, discomfort, and ability to cope. A significant improvement in all three measures was found in the combined treatment groups, i.e. the treated patients were less annoyed by their tinnitus, perceived it less loudly and had gained more control over the problem. However, there were no differences in outcome between the two treatment methods used. At the follow-up interview patients were asked to report any subjective changes in loudness, discomfort or coping. Again, there were no significant differences between the two treatment groups. Further, no differences in improvement were found between the two treatments regarding the interview data reflecting various somatic complaints. The conclusion is that both treatment approaches were superior to no treatment. However, the way in which the coping behaviour is taught to the patient, i.e. through exposure or distraction, did not seem to be essential for the outcome. Both treatment approaches increased control of tinnitus.

Lazarus and Folkman (1984) discuss the importance of subjective control over an aversive condition. Powerful coping behaviour includes both external and internal sources of control. The results of our work support the concept of coping outlined by Lazarus and Folkman. Having control over an aversive event such as tinnitus through internal focused modes of coping seems to be crucial for the tinnitus patient. Whether the ability to cope is achieved through exposure or distraction seems to be of no importance for the treatment outcome. Further, the effects of the treatment are generalized to other complaints such as headache, sleep disorders and tension, without any specific therapy of these complaints. One explanation is that the adaptive coping behaviour increased the patient's own capability of finding strategies to reduce these problems. In our study no direct assessments were made of the coping behaviour, i.e. no knowledge about what the patient actually did in a critical tinnitus situation was obtained. This kind of direct assessment should be considered in future research.

9.2 Behavioral treatment in clinical practice

Clinical practice regarding patients referred for severe tinnitus has developed at the Department of Audiology at the University hospital in Uppsala over the past ten years. The treatment method evolves out of a behavioral approach to tinnitus described in some detail earlier, as well as from the findings in the empirical studies. In this section we will describe how this is integrated into the total management of patients. We will also describe how the treatment is planned and conducted.

Figure 1 is a schematic description of how the patient passes through different phases of the treatment. This includes the medical and audiological evaluation, the behavioural treatment and finally the follow-up phase 6-months after the end of therapy. Figure 1 will be discussed in great detail in the following section.

9.2.1 The role of a medical and audiological evaluation

Patients with severe tinnitus sometimes fail to get a proper diagnosis and evaluation. However, being a university clinic the majority of cases are referred to us by ENT-specialists in the catchment area. Nevertheless, in order to rule out any underlying retro-cochlear pathology, a full medical and audiological examination, including brainstem-audiometry when necessary, is carried out. After this evaluation the audiologist discusses the test results with the patients. Information concerning different treatment alternatives are also given by the audiologist. In collaboration with the patient it is then decided whether further attention to the tinnitus is required. This process is, we believe, crucial, and it is not unusual for this conversation to last more than an hour. A preliminary decision on the applicability of psychological treatment is then made by the audiologist, and after a general explanation of the rationale, suitable and interested patients are referred to a psychologist for initial interviewing and further information.

A large number of patients who are referred for moderately severe tinnitus have never been given the proper information and reassurance. As this is done thoroughly by the audiologist, some patients are given an appointment within a year in order to evaluate their own efforts in dealing with tinnitus. (Referred to as Exit in figure I). We have had good experiences with this procedure and a majority of these patients with moderate tinnitus, have adjusted well to their problems upon return to the clinic.

9.2.1.1 Other treatment alternatives

It is at this stage, however, also possible to choose alternative ways of treatment. One such possibility is general

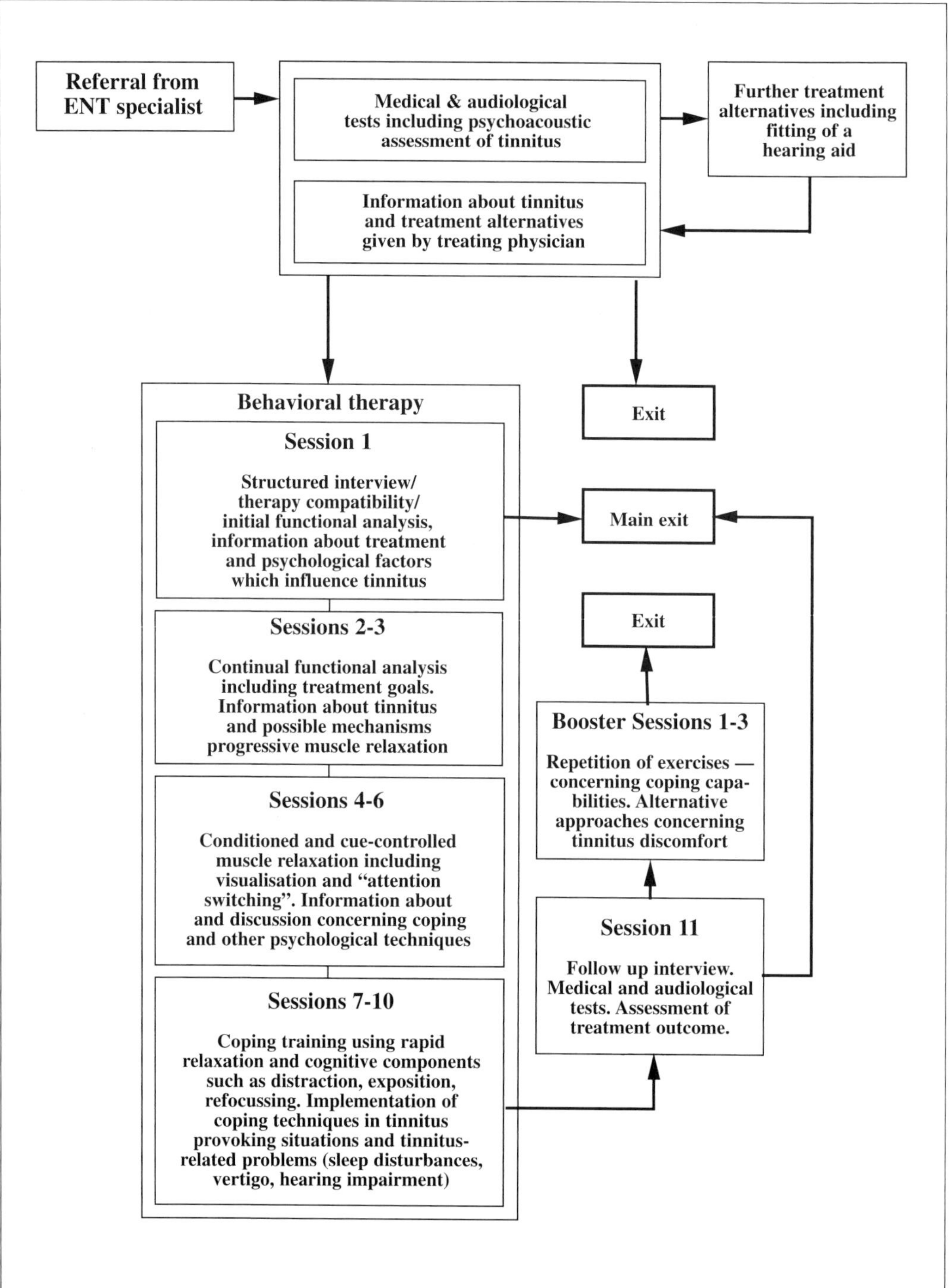

Fig. 9.1 Flowchart: Management and behavioral therapy of referred patients with tinnitus (for detailed information please refer to text).

relaxation training given by a specially trained physiotherapist. This is also used if signs of the so called Tensor Tympani Syndrome (Klockhoff, 1981) are present. This syndrome consists of increased tensor activity, tension headache and dizziness. However, results of such treatment is only sparsely documented, and should therefore only be given to patients with clear evidence of tension-related problems. Further research is desirable.

A second possibility is to use hearing-aids. This has been considered to be an initial way of using masking to reduce tinnitus. Positive results have been reported by Brooks and Bulmer (1981) and Surr, Montgomery and Mueller (1985). Logically hearing aids should be of some benefit to most tinnitus sufferers with at least moderate hearing loss, as an increased input should facilitate both psychological and physical ways of masking tinnitus sounds. However, acoustic masking therapy has many non-specific, psychological effects as well, and even researchers with long experience of tinnitus masking, claim these non-specific factors to be the dominant feature (Hazell, Wood, Cooper, Stephens, Corcoran, Coles, Baskill, & Sheldrake, 1985). This standpoint finds further support in an experimental group study of tinnitus sufferers with hearing aids where no effects on tinnitus were found, when the fitting of the hearing aid was not combined with the claim that this was a therapeutic measure destined to relieve tinnitus. (Melin, Scott, Lindberg, & Lyttkens, 1987).

Other treatment alternatives are seldom given at the Uppsala clinic. There are for instance only very few patients who are given a tinnitus masker, and only a handful have been given pharmacological therapy the past few years. The treatment of choice is behavioral treatment.

9.2.2 The behavioral treatment

To initiate the psychological treatment all patients are given a structured interview where several aspects of tinnitus and the physical proprieties of the sound is discussed. The tinnitus location, its character, and its subjective pitch and loudness are carefully discussed, as well as changes and variations over longer and shorter intervals. The main purpose of this interview, however, is to initiate a functional analysis of how and in what way tinnitus is disturbing each individual patient in their daily life. This procedure is basically the same procedure as in most behaviorally oriented psychotherapies, i.e. a behavior analysis (e.g. Sundell & Sundell, 1982).

During the interview it is decided from a psychological point of view whether tinnitus is the major otological complaint, if it has been constantly present for at least one year and finally, whether other acute psychiatric or somatic disorders are present. The final decision as to whether a patient is suited for behavioral treatment is made during this interview. We also pay special attention to explain the rationale behind this behavioral approach to the patients. As most patients fail to understand that the discomfort related to tinnitus has a psychological and cognitive origin, we believe this information is essential for further successful treatment.

The second and third sessions of therapy are mainly concerned with introducing relaxation skills. We use a modified version of progressive relaxation training (Jacobsson, 1938) as described by Wolpe and Lazarus (1966). In our version relaxation in the upper parts of the body is emphasized more than in the original version. In these sessions the functional analysis is completed and discussed with the patient, and finally realistic goals for therapy are agreed upon.

The next part of treatment (sessions 4-6) is concerned with increasing the speed with which the patients learn to relax, but also with introducing various cognitive techniques that are integrated with relaxation in order to create coping behaviour. Relaxation is first linked to the patient's breathing so that when he inhales he counts the breath and as he exhales he is prompted to say the word "relax". This is made in order to get a conditioning between the word "relax" and the relaxed state. Later, as cue-controlled relaxation is introduced in connection with cognitive techniques, it is supposed to act so rapidly that deep relaxation is reached after a few deep breaths.

A number of cognitive techniques are introduced into therapy at this stage. The most important is what we refer to as "attention switching". Initially patients are instructed to direct their attention towards a positive image unrelated to tinnitus. Later, the same technique can be applied to a neutral stimulus, in most cases a sound. This is done in a sound laboratory where several prerecorded sounds are available. The sounds are thus used to promote intentional diversion away from the tinnitus, and as patients get more skilled they can use more and more provoking sounds in this way. The patients are instructed to use relaxation as rapidly as possible in order to establish this part of coping behaviour in situations where tinnitus is especially troublesome. In doing so a continuous rapport is maintained with the patient in order to promote understanding of the psychological mechanisms that are utilized in therapy.

In the final part of therapy (sessions 7-10) more explicit coping training is performed. The sounds are used to provoke tinnitus so that patients learn to use their cognitive skills to control tinnitus discomfort. Some patients need more time to discover how to use this technique, while others can grasp it and generalize its effects after only a few training sessions. An important part of this phase of the training is to develop "portable" relaxation and coping skills. Therefore patients are encouraged to expose themselves to situations that are known for their aversiveness regarding tinnitus. Such situations are taken from the initial functional analysis and are trained and discussed in detail with the patient before they are confronted with the actual problem. Examples of such situations are acoustically and intellectually demanding situations at work, staying in environments with strong background noises etc. Patients are thus instructed and trained how to use the coping behavior in such situations and are subsequently assigned to such tasks between sessions.

Finally, in this part of the treatment special problems that may have appeared in the functional analysis are dealt with. Such problems are for instance sleep disturbances, dizziness and headache associated with tension, as well as problems concerned with the patient's capability to use his hearing ability in different situations. These related problems are often essential for a good outcome of therapy in the long run. Therapy ends after ten sessions but individual needs are considered. After termination, however, patients are scheduled for a follow up visit to the clinic. We believe that most patients need some time to establish their new strategies and attitudes towards tinnitus. During this time they are able to get in touch with the clinic, and are indeed encouraged to do so. This should also be a period which is long enough to make adjustments to their personal situation (for instance, employment questions/workload/working hours). Therefore we allow six months to pass before the treatment is evaluated for the first time.

9.2.3 The follow-up interview

Six months after completion of treatment the patients return to the clinic for the routine follow-up interview. During this visit each patient is once again interviewed by the audiologist and sees the psychologist who conducted the therapy during the earlier visits. A medical and audiological examination is performed, as well as any other psychoacoustic assessment that is necessary. The overall purpose of this visit is to find out whether any further treatment is necessary or if the patient feels that he can control his tinnitus to such an extent that further help from us is no longer required.

9.2.3.1 Evaluating treatment results

As discussed earlier there are poor correlations between the psychoacoustic assessments of tinnitus and of patients' own descriptions of their problems. We therefore routinely collect measurements of patients' subjective loudness, discomfort from tinnitus, and their coping behavior by means of self-registration made in connection with the follow up. Most patients tend to report having about the same loudness level as before treatment, but they find tinnitus less annoying at this stage.

A follow up interview of about one hour is conducted with each patient. Almost all patients report good relaxation skills under favorable circumstances, and about 75 percent claim that relaxation is used intentionally as a way of controlling tinnitus. About one third of these patients report total control of their tinnitus, while the remaining two-thirds are able to relieve their discomfort under certain more or less favorable conditions.

Other signs of successful treatment are also determined. Such changes as full employment and no sickleaves are strong indications of permanent therapy effects and an acceptable adjustment.

However, at this follow up a number of patients have either lost track of their ability to cope with tinnitus, or have not complied with the guidelines for coping which were drawn up at the completion of therapy. The latter patients are often not interested in making any further attempts to use these strategies, and are therefore often referred back to their physician. The other patients are offered a number of booster sessions.

9.2.4 Booster sessions

Booster sessions are not unusual and they often have large influence on the patients who are offered such an opportunity. Most patients who are considered for booster treatment have had good initial results, but have failed to maintain their ability because of various problems. It may well be that coming back to work on a full time basis puts a person under such strain that he loses track of his coping ability. In such cases it may only be a matter of counseling in order to solve the problem and enable the patient to do the proper adjustments to the situation himself. In other cases there may have been some change in the experience of tinnitus which has prompted the failure to comply with the original program. In these cases a few sessions in which we repeat essential parts of therapy is sufficient to re-establish successful control over tinnitus discomfort.

The essential feature in the booster treatment sessions is thus a repetition of the original treatment, and it is hardly ever necessary to reconsider the fundamental analysis which was done at the beginning of therapy.

Most patients who undergo some form of booster therapy are scheduled for yet another follow up visit. At this point the great majority of patients are able to handle their tinnitus so well that no further contact is needed unless this is due to their otological condition.

9.3 Concluding remarks

In search of an effective psychological treatment, different approaches have been proposed. Treatments aiming either at reducing the tinnitus sound itself or at problems caused by and/or associated with the tinnitus, like depression, anxiety or psychosomatic complaints. Our standpoint has been that tinnitus should be viewed as a multidimensional entity. A treatment package aiming both at tinnitus and at the problems associated with it is therefore recommended. The principle of coping with this aversive phenomenon is indirect in the sense that we do not expect to reduce the tinnitus sound itself, but rather the discomfort caused by tinnitus or associated with it. A treatment package cannot be recommended unreservedly, mainly because of the insufficient knowledge of what components are effective, or counter-productive. However, our results show that, taken as a whole, refined behavioral intervention can contribute to reducing the tinnitus significantly. Centuries have passed since the first documented treatment of tinnitus was reported on Egyptian scrolls, yet much remains to be done. However, the behavioral approach to tinnitus, comprising intervention and assessments, is certainly an important contribution to non-medical treatment.

9.4 References

Aran, J.-M., Y. Cazals (1981): Electrical suppression of tinnitus. In Ciba Foundation symposium, 85: Tinnitus, 217-225. (*Evered, D., G. Lawrenson* [Eds]). Pitman Medical, London.

Bernstein, D.A., T.D. Borkovec (1973): Progressive relaxation training: a manual for the helping professions. Champaign, II., Research Press.

Brooks, D.N., D. Bulmer (1981): Survey of binaural hearing aid users. Ear and Hearing, 2: 220-224.

Gentry, W.D. (1984): Handbook of Behavioral Medicine. New York: Guilford Press.

Grossan, M. (1976): Treatment of subjective tinnitus with biofeedback. Ear, Nose and Throat Journal, 55: 22-30.

Hallam, R.S., S. Rachman, R. Hinchcliffe (1984): Psychological aspects of tinnitus. Contributions of medical psychology. Vol 3, (Ed. *Rachman, S.*) Oxford: Pergamon Press. pp. 31-53.

Hazell, J.W.P., S.M. Wood, H.R. Cooper, S.D.G. Stephens, A.L. Corcoran, R.R.A. Coles, J.L. Baskill, J.B. Sheldrake (1985): A clinical study of tinnitus maskers. British Journal of Audiology, 19: 65-146.

Ireland, C.E., P.H. Wilson, J.P. Tonkin, S. Platt-Hepworth (1985): An evaluation of relaxation training in the treatment of tinnitus. Behaviour Research and Therapy, 23: 423-430.

Jacobson, E. (1929): Progressive relaxation. Chicago: University of Chicago Press.

Jakes, S.C., R.S. Hallam, S. Rachman, R. Hinchcliffe (1986): The effects of reassurance, relaxation training and distraction in chronic tinnitus sufferers. Behaviour Research and Therapy, 24: 497-507.

Karoly, P., J. Steffen (Eds) (1980): Improving the long-term effects of psychotherapy. New York: Gardner Press.

Kendall, P.C., K.M. Bemis (1986): Thought and action in psychotherapy: The cognitive-behavioural approaches. In: *Hersen, M., A.E. Kaxdin, A.S. Bellack* (Eds). The Clinical Psychology Handbook. New York: Pergamon Press.

Klockhoff, I. (1981): Impedance fluctuation and a "Tensor Tympani Syndrome". Proceedings of the Fourth International Symposium on Acoustic Impedance Measurements, Universidade Nova de Lisboa (pp. 69-76).

Klockhoff, I., U. Lindblom (1967): Menière's disease and hydrochlorothiazide (Dichlotride®) — a critical analysis of symptoms and therapeutic effects. Acta Otolaryngologica (Stockholm), 63: 347-365.

Lazarus, R.S., S. Folkman (1984): Coping and adaptation. In: *Gentry, W.D.* (Ed.). Handbook of Behavioral Medicine. New York: Guilford Press.

Lindberg, P., L. Lyttkens, L. Melin, B. Scott (1984): Tinnitus — incidence and handicap. Scandinavian Audiology, 13: 287-291.

Lindberg, P., B. Scott, L. Lyttkens, L. Melin (1988): Behavioural therapy in the clinical management of tinnitus. British Journal of Audiology, 22: 265-272.

Lindberg, P., B. Scott, L. Melin, L. Lyttkens (1987): Long-term effects of psychological treatment of tinnitus. Scandinavian Audiology, 16: 167-172.

Lindberg, P., B. Scott, L. Melin, L. Lyttkens (1989): The psychological treatment of tinnitus: An experimental evaluation. Behavior Research and Therapy, 27: 593-603.

Linton, S.J., L. Melin (1982): The accuracy of remembering chronic pain. Pain, 13: 281-285.

Linton, S.J., L. Melin, K. Stjernlöf (1985): The effects of applied relaxation and activity training on chronic pain. Behavioural Psychotherapy, 13: 87-100.

Malatesta, V.J., P.B. Sutker, H.E. Adams (1980): Experimental assessment of tinnitus aurium. Journal of Behavioural Assessment, 2: 309-317.

Marlowe, F.J. (1973): Effective treatment of tinnitus through hypnotherapy. American Journal of Clinical Hypnosis, 15: 162-165.

Melin, L., B. Scott, P. Lindberg, L. Lyttkens (1987): Hearing aids and tinnitus — an experimental group study. British Journal of Audiology, 21: 91-97.

Scott, B., P. Lindberg, L. Lyttkens, L. Melin (1985): Psychological treatment of tinnitus. An experimental group study. Scandinavian Audiology, 14: 223-230.

Scott, B., P. Lindberg, L. Lyttkens, L. Melin (1990): Predictors of tinnitus discomfort, subjective loudness and adaptation. British Journal of Audiology, 24: 51-62.

Sjöden, P.-O. (Ed.) (1988): Applied relaxation: Method and applications (Special issue). Scandinavian Journal of Behaviour Therapy, 17(2).

Stephens, S.D.G. (1984): The treatment of tinnitus — a historical perspective. Journal of Laryngology and Otology, 98, (Suppl. 9): 963-972.

Suinn, R.M. (1975): Anxiety management training for general anxiety. In: *Suinn, R.M., R.G. Weigal* (Eds). The innovative psychological therapies. New York: Harper & Row.

Sundell, M., S.S. Sundell (1982): Behavior modification in the human services. Prentice-Hall, Inc. Englewood Cliffs, N.J.

Surr, R.K., A. Montgomery, H.G. Müller (1985): Effect of amplification on tinnitus among new hearing aid users. Ear and Hearing, 6: 71-75.

Wolpe, J., A.A. Lazarus (1966): Behaviour therapy techniques. Oxford: Pergamon Press.

Chapter 10

Tinnitus management using stress immunization

Evelyn de Camp-Schmidt and Ulf de Camp

10.1 Summary

We report on an investigation of 44 patients who were given eight 4-hour individual therapy sessions over a period of 6 months. The patients either received a specific or non-specific treatment with either positive or neutral instruction or were put on a waiting list. Specific treatment consisted of progressive muscle relaxation in combination with EMG — biofeedback of the occipitofrontal muscle. The subjective tinnitus assessments were obtained using questionnaires and objective evaluation of tinnitus included comparisons of loudness and masking. The results showed a significant decrease of most subjective disturbance factors and tinnitus loudness in two different types of measurements, but no significant change of the tinnitus masking level. In a follow-up questionnaire after 2 years, which 22 of the patients filled out, the consistency of treatment success was evident in all variables, as well as statistically relevant.

We also report on a multi-modular tinnitus treatment concept using stress immunization. No statistically relevant data is available yet, but initial experience with approximatly 60 patients is very promising.

10.2 Introduction

Medical treatment methods often bring little relief to tinnitus patients. When we planned an investigation of the effectiveness of psychological methods in tinnitus treatment at the beginning of 1985, there were barely any references for such methods (see Chapter 5). None of the available investigations had a control group. Therefore we tried to limit ourselves to specific methods known at the time (relaxation and EMG-biofeedback) and to compare these with unspecific methods (client-centred therapy and tinnitus diary). Furthermore, a waiting list control group was essential because we wanted to examine the first results of Grossan (1976) and House (1978, 1981) and aim for more objectivity by including a waiting list group. Because of limited possibilities, our research, which was a dissertation, did not receive financial support and it took us 4½ years from the planning stage to the final evaluation of results.

10.3 Tinnitus reduction using progressive muscle relaxation

10.3.1 Design of the study and treatment setting

The first investigation included a total of 55 patients who suffered from severe chronic tinnitus of various origins. Most of them were referred by the ENT department of the Berlin-Steglitz clinic. They were placed randomly into five treatment groups. During the course of the study 11 (20%) of the patients ended treatment after one or two sessions, so that only 44 patients participated in the entire study (20 women and 24 men, ages 17–64).

The patients had suffered from tinnitus for 5 months to 11 years and it was experienced by them as being "disturbing" to "very seriously disturbing" (level 2–3). The etiology of the tinnitus was diagnosed: age related hearing loss ($n = 12$), sudden deafness ($n = 11$), occupational exposure to noise ($n = 5$), Menière's syndrome ($n = 4$), noise trauma ($n = 3$), of unknown causes ($n = 22$); in addition, there was hearing impairment from otitis media, surgery of acoustic neuroma, viral disease, and autoimmune disease (each $n = 1$). Some patients had several causes of tinnitus.

The patients were randomly placed in groups receiving specific or unspecific treatment or a waiting list control group. Specific treatment was treatment with progressive muscle relaxation in combination with EMG-biofeedback of the occipitofrontal muscle ($n = 19$) using the Zak ZAK Co. EMG feedback integrator. Unspecific treatment was a combination of tinnitus diary and client-centred psychotherapy ($n = 17$). These two groups were themselves subdivided into two groups in which two different types of instruction, which were either positive or neutral in content, induced two different expectational attitudes (compatible vs. incompatible expectational attitudes). The waiting list group ($n = 8$) received treatment only after treatment of the other groups was concluded after six months. During this interval the waiting list–control group took part only in the foreseen tests.

10.3.2 Psychological and psychoacoustic measurements

For psychological measurements subjective data was obtained by a questionnaire (see appendix) (for example, "How much did your ear noises disturb you in the recent past?" or "How loud is your ear noise now?"); the "objective" data were obtained by psycho-acoustic measurements (comparison of loudness of tinnitus with acoustic stimuli emitted by earphones of two distinct qualities: white noise or a sinus tone of comparable frequency, according to whether the tinnitus was experienced as a noise or a tone). A sinus-tone generator (Brüel and Kjaer, type 1013) and a noise generator (Brüel and Kjaer, type 1402) in combination with a calibrated earphone produced the acoustic stimuli. The stimulus had to be as similar to the tinnitus as possible in intensity as well as in frequency (tinnitus matching). This measurement was made three times during the study for each ear. In addition, in a third measurement the loudness of white noise was increased so that the tinnitus was camouflaged (masking). The questionnaire measurements were made at the beginning of each of the eight 1-hour individual therapy sessions, the psycho-acoustic measurements at the beginning of the first, fifth and eighth sessions.

A blind study was not done with the psycho-acoustic measurements. This was actually disadvantageous but we believed that this drawback would be at least partially compensated by the number of test persons.

10.3.3 Results

The result obtained by a two-factor variance analysis showed that in most subjective parameters, significant or highly significant decreases in disturbing effects of tinnitus occurred during the course of specific treatment, but not, on the other hand, in the course of unspecific treatment and in the waiting-list group. The expectational attitude had no influence on the results (Figs. 10.1 and 10.2) which makes a possible placebo effect more improbable. The "objective" parameters show a significant decrease in tinnitus intensity over the treatment period for both comparative measurements, but no significant results for masking.

The follow-up survey after 2 years showed the consistency of treatment success. The mean difference signifies numerically the difference between the initial measurement and a measurement on a 9-point scale during therapy. The course of the group means of the two variables can be ascertained in Figs 1 and 2. Therefore, for example, a value of "–2" means that the degree of disturbance/impairment of the individual subgroup has decreased by 2 points (22%) between initial measurement and subsequent measurement.

In the follow-up survey (n = 22) the patients again received a questionnaire by mail. A psycho-acoustic measurement was not made. The improvement in subjective impairment from tinnitus also remained significant in the follow-up survey (return rate 50%). The non-responders did not give any reasons for not having returned filled-out questionnaire. If one assumes the unfavorable case that the patients no longer noticed any treatment success after 2 years, one can still assume a positive influence in approximately 50% after 2 years, compared to about 65% at the end of the study. Patients were not placed into the previous subgroups in the follow-up study because all of them had participated in relaxation and EMG-biofeedback in the meantime.

10.4 Stress immunization

The results of our investigation, combined with the observation that in all cases the lack of stress management was involved in triggering or modulating tinnitus, encouraged us to plan an expanded treatment including stress immunization and other methods that had proved favorable for the reduction of stress. We would like to point out again that stress does not mean the amount of

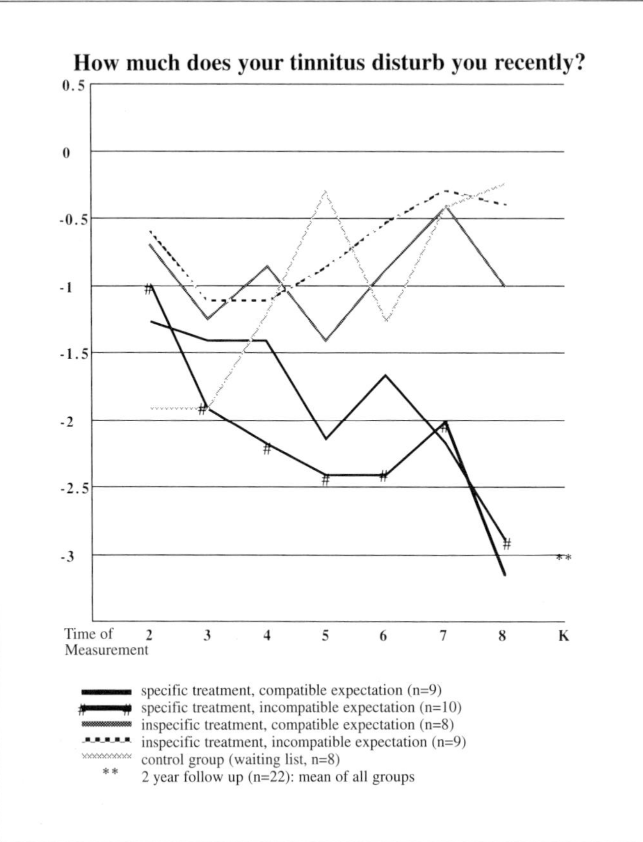

Fig. 10.1 Change of the means at various times of measurement compared to the initial value. A value under 0 signifies an improvement of the parameter, a value over 0 signifies deterioration. The difference between specific treatment on the one hand and inspecific treatment as well as the control group on the other is significant ($p < 0.001$).

impairment, but rather the problems which are not manageable or do not appear to be manageable. Table 10.1 summarizes the significant points of our treatment program of tinnitus. Of course therapy must be modified and adapted for each tinnitus patient because each one has "his" individual tinnitus and his individual problems in various areas of stress management. It must not be forgotten that many tinnitus patients suffer from impaired hearing. In severely impaired hearing the stress due to the tinnitus itself greatly increases because communication with others requires a much greater effort at concentration.

Table 10.1 Therapy components

I. Progressive muscle relaxation with EMG-biofeedback

II. Clarification of possible underlying mechanisms (counseling)

III. Development of positive thinking
   a) New cognitions
   b) Imagination techniques
   c) Pleasure and perception training

IV. Concentration exercises

V. Communication training

VI. Conflict management strategies

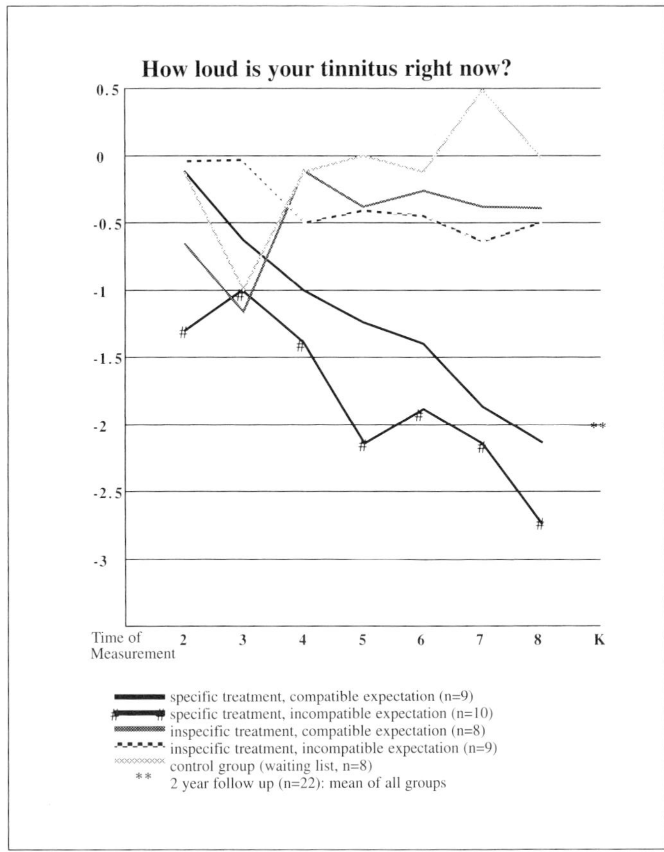

Fig. 10.2 Change of the means at various times of measurement compared to the initial value. A value under 0 signifies an improvement of the parameter, a value over 0 signifies deterioration. The difference between specific treatment on the one hand and inspecific treatment as well as the control group on the other is significant ($p < 0.001$).

For stress immunization we do not have statistically supported results yet, only experience with about 60 clients. We can only present an optimistic report of our experience here: the statistical proof of treatment results is still to come.

10.5 Observations about the components of stress immunization

10.5.1 Relaxation and biofeedback

Several important points of the treatment plan will be explained briefly. Concerning the technique of progressive muscle relaxation we give attention to the fact that contraction and relaxation of the muscles does not occur abruptly, but in waves, which is more physiological and also gives measurably better results. Due to this modification, several patients who already understood the principle of progressive muscle relaxation, but had not been able to implement it properly, were able to manage their tinnitus.

Concerning EMG-biofeedback it must be noted that this is not an independent relaxation method, but only a monitoring technique for reviewing and improving acquired relaxation techniques. Many critics of biofeedback have not observed this fact (e.g. v. Wedel et al., 1989). We did not use direct EMG-biofeedback with returned feedback through earphones. Instead we registered the integration values of the EMG-feedback device during relaxation and then discussed these values with the patient.

This procedure, e.g. "delayed" feedback, often eliminates a frequently detrimental effect: because muscle tension only decreases gradually during the first minutes of relaxation, especially achievement-oriented patients experience stress (the "task" is not being completed properly), when the effect of relaxation is not yet clearly audible in a decrease of the frequency of the acoustic feedback signals.

10.5.2 Counselling

The clarification of possible tinnitus causes and effects is important because anxiety results from inadequate information (for example, "my tinnitus will certainly get stronger from year to year"; "my tinnitus is damaging my hearing"). Adequate information reduced these fears, and realistic cognitive confrontation with the problem is possible at an early stage of management (Sweetow, 1985). In this context we also explain to the patient that tinnitus is very similar to pain (Tonndorf, 1987, Goebel et al., 1991).

10.5.3 Positive thinking

The development of positive thinking is often one of the principle objectives of tinnitus treatment. Many tinnitus patients judge themselves and their environment very negatively; this is increased by lack of information, prior experiences with physicians, lack of understanding from others and the feeling of individual helplessness. This negative thinking creates stress which again often increases the loudness of tinnitus. This is, however, a vicious circle that occurs in tinnitus often and may end in suicide. The development of positive thinking can interrupt this vicious circle (Sweetow, 1986).

10.5.4 Cognitive reassessment

Cognitive reassessment is an initial step in the development of positive thinking. Therefore, for example, the thought "My tinnitus must disappear" can gradually be replaced by "I would like to be able to cope with my tinnitus". It is also possible to change the attitude gradually: "I have tinnitus so I am seriously ill" in the direction of: "My tinnitus is my friend, it warns me if I do not cope with my stress properly," or "My tinnitus is as much a part of me as the doorplate on my door." Patients who understand tinnitus as a signal or a part of themselves have fewer problems coping with it.

10.5.5 Imagination techniques

Imagination techniques may replace the negative experience of tinnitus with positive contents. One can imagine positive situations in which sounds similar to tinnitus occur. For example, this may be a waterfall, a stream, the ocean, grasshoppers, but also, for example, a saw-mill. Another imagination technique we use is a "journey through the body" ending with positive acoustically mediated stimuli.

10.5.6 Perception training

An additional possibility of cognitive therapeutic techniques is self-awareness training. Frequently tinnitus patients pay so much attention to the ear that the other senses are often extremely neglected. In such cases we teach the patient to observe other modes of perception. In this way the sense of taste can be trained by conscious tasting and enjoyment of food. Paying attention to the smells of spices, herbs, flowers and other things can improve the perception of the sense of smell. Sleeping disturbances, which are especially frequent in tinnitus patients, can be decreased in this way by suggesting to the patient to concentrate on the smell of a little bag filled with a selection of the patient's favorite herbs instead of on the tinnitus. Tactile stimuli are also included in the training, e.g. one can "feel" various materials. The development of an individual body-feeling can also be included here. Visual stimuli naturally play an important role and the patient can consciously explore the visual impressions he has of other people, his environment and nature.

Pleasant acoustic phenomena, such as the chirping of birds, the sounds of voices or any other type of acoustic transmission of information are included in the final part of self-awareness training to distract from the negatively perceived tinnitus.

10.5.7 Concentration training and communication training

Perception training includes concentration exercises which are very important because tinnitus often inhibits concentration or at least impairs it. Thus, increased ability to concentrate reduces the disturbing effect of tinnitus.

Communication training also helps decrease fixation on hearing and is often necessary because numerous tinnitus patients suffer from communication disturbances which cause the patient to avoid communication increasingly. Stress results, because patients feel lonely, misunderstood and helpless. Training decreases avoidance mechanisms and conversation techniques such as feedback are used aiming for the goal of "comprehensive listening".

10.5.8 Conflict management training

Conflict management training can be seen in the same context as many patients have inadequate conflict management strategies. This often leads to conflict avoidance (associated with difficulties in communication and avoidance of communication). Conflict strategies include differentiation between primary and secondary conflict, the identification and expression of individual needs, a direct, matter-of-fact style of conversation, finding solutions and compromises, etc. Improved skills reduce stress considerably.

10.5.9 Reduction of stress in extreme situations

The final stage of our treatment plan is direct reduction of stress in extreme situations. According to Meichenbaum (1978), the stress-triggering situation is first defined and then rational and irrational thoughts are analyzed and assessed. In this way, anxiety is reduced by analysis, confronting irrational thoughts and replacing negative thoughts by positive self-instruction. Additional reduction of anxiety results from repeated imagination of the stressful situation, and its management, considering the most extreme possibilities as previously determined in the analysis (in vitro). As a result, the actual situation can finally be managed (in vivo).

The following case report demonstrates a typical course of treatment:

10.6 Case report

Mr. T. (56 years old) had suffered from a chronic tinnitus of unknown etiology of the left ear for 19 months. It included a variety of sinus tones with a frequency of 5.6 kHz and a loudness of 43 dB HL (the values result from a comparison between tinnitus loudness and the loudness of a similar acoustic signal, i.e. 5.6 KHz sinus tone). His suffering was intense because, as a music teacher, he had great difficulties concentrating on instruction. In addition, listening to music, one of his favourite pastimes, became "agonizing". Conflicts increased with his wife because he felt that she wasn't considerate enough. His wife thought that he over-exaggerated his suffering and his otolaryngologist had told him that his problems were psychosomatic, and that he had to accept them as they could not be influenced. All these factors increased his helplessness and his stress.

Therefore he gladly accepted our treatment plan and quickly learned progressive muscle relaxation. Thereafter he felt less helpless. The tinnitus decreased to a loudness of about 38 dB HL. Positive thinking was also successful. We relied upon the positive potential of his Christian faith and his enjoyment of work. He was able, for example, to stop negative thoughts and perform positive self-instructions of the following type: During a hike he observed his tinnitus became louder as soon as he thought about his illness and perceived the tinnitus consciously. He began to sing or recite hymns, for him a positive stimulus, as soon as he perceived negative thoughts. By doing this his hikes became more relaxing and therefore a more positive experience as the tinnitus continued to decrease in volume (rustling of leaves corresponds to about 20 dB HL, normal speech about 50–60 dB HL).

Doing puzzles for an hour each day served as concentration exercises. To improve communication, he attended communication training. He was already very satisfied with his progress when an event occurred which frightened him very much: He had an epileptic seizure (similar to the two seizures he had already experienced 3 and 15 years previously) and his tinnitus became much louder, corresponding to 53 dB HL. Analyzing additional triggers during the further course of treatment, we came across a lack of conflict management in his marriage. In order to avoid burdening his wife, who was also a teacher and frequently had back pain after spinal surgery, both he and his wife avoided conflicts. In the course of arguments he almost always gave in, and he never noticed how angry he actually was. There were problems in his sex-life as he believed he had to act as if he were a "real tough guy". His stress was greater during sex than during instruction at school. The trigger for his epileptic seizure turned out to be his sudden impotency during intercourse.

In the further course of treatment, the patient and his wife solved their conflicts mutually and, little by little, the problems in his sex-life were managed leading to reduced stress in the marital relationship. This not only diminished tinnitus volume to just under 20 dB HL, but also caused the slight epileptic potentials in the EEG to disappear.

Mr. T. feels healthy and cheerful now. The tinnitus always punctually warns him of stress situations which he hasn't coped with properly and he feels able to manage conflicts adequately. He is aware of his tinnitus but it does not disturb him any longer.

10.7 Discussion

We have achieved very good results in the management of tinnitus with our program for stress immunization. The active cooperation of tinnitus patients is required. In those patients who are not capable of active and independent cooperation or who prefer passive methods (such as, for example, acupuncture, massage, medication, etc.) an improvement can only occur if there is a change in attitude. More success is possible for patients who cooperate actively. Our study showed the advantage of a specific treatment compared to a non-specific one. The study confirms as well as disproves the results of numerous researchers who have had varying success with similar methods. Scott et al. (1985), Jakes et al. (1986) and White et al. (1986) had similar success in their treatment while Ireland et al. (1985) and Haralambous et al. (1987) did not report positive results (see Chapter 5). We noticed that in almost all investigations barely any significant changes were shown in psycho-acoustic measurements. Here we obtained similar results only in measurements pertaining to the masking curve. We had a significant loudness reduction in both types of loudness comparison, but only in the group receiving specific treatment.

A possible additional explanation is that many patients are very ambitious by nature. We have considered this fact by telling the patients that it is sufficient to adjust the volume of the matched curve "as similarly as possible" instead of "exactly". As yet we do not have a good explanation for this important difference in the psycho-acoustic measurements.

The subjective data, however, are even more meaningful; in part the improvements are highly significant. The comparable multi-modular treatments of Lindberg et al. (1987, 1988, 1989), Scott et al. (1985), Jakes et al. (1986) and Goebel (1989) coincide partly with our treatment plan because they integrate several cognitive methods. We have tried to develop a more specific treatment of tinnitus using stress immunization in the same manner and our first observations confirm this method. Our next step is a statistical evaluation of the results of our method of treatment.

10.8 References

Borton, T.E., W.H. Moore, S.R. Clark (1981): Electromyographic feedback treatment for tinnitus aurium. Speech Hear Disord., 46, 39.

Camp, U. de (1989): Beeinflussung des Tinnitus durch psychologische Methoden. Diplomarbeit am Psychologischen Institut der FU Berlin.

Goebel, G. (1989): Tinnitus. In: Hand und Wittchen (Eds): Verhaltenstherapie in der Medizin. Springer, Berlin, Heidelberg, New York, Paris, London, Tokyo, Hong Kong: 207-228.

Goebel, G., W. Keser, M. Fichter, W. Rief (1991): Neue Aspekte des komplexen chronischen Tinnitus, Teil II: Psychotherapie, Psychosomatik, Medizinische Psychologie, 41: 123-133.

Grossan, M. (1976): Treatment of subjective tinnitus with biofeedback. Ear Nose Throat Journal 55, 22.

Haralambous, G., P.H. Wilson, S. Platt-Hepworth, J.P. Tonkin, V.R. Hensley, D.H. Kavanagh (1987): EMG-Biofeedback in the treatment of tinnitus: An experimental evaluation. Behaviour Research and Therapy, 25, 49-55.

House, J.W., L. Miller, P.R. House (1977): Severe tinnitus: Treatment with biofeedback-training — Results in forty-one cases. Transactions of the American Academy of Ophthalmology and Otolaryngology, 84: 697-703.

House, J.W. (1978): Treatment of severe tinnitus with biofeedback training. The Laryngoscope, 88: 406-412.

Ireland, C.E., P.H. Wilson, J.P. Tonkin, S. Platt-Hepworth (1985): An evaluation of relaxation training in the treatment of tinnitus. Behavior Research and Therapy, 23: 423-430.

Jakes, S.C., R.S. Hallam, S. Rachman, R. Hinchcliffe (1986): The effects of reassurance, relaxation training and distraction on chronic tinnitus sufferers. Behaviour Research and Therapy, 24: 497-507.

Lindberg, P., B. Scott, L. Melin, L. Lyttkens (1988): Behavioural therapy in the clinical management of tinnitus. British Journal of Audiology, 2: 265-272.

Lindberg, P., B. Scott, L. Melin, L. Lyttkens (1989): The psychological treatment of tinnitus: An Experimental evaluation. Behav. Res. Ther., 27: 593-603.

Meichenbaum, D. W. (1979): Kognitive Verhaltensmodifikation. München, Wien, Baltimore: Urban and Schwarzenberg.

Scott, B., P. Lindberg, L. Lyttkens, L. Melin (1985): Psychological treatment of tinnitus. An experimental group study. Scand. Audiol., 14: 223-230.

Sweetow, R.V. (1985): Counselling the patient with tinnitus. Arch. Otolaryngol., 111: 283-284.

Sweetow, R.V. (1986): Cognitive aspects of tinnitus patients management. Ear and Hearing, 17: 390-396.

Tonndorf, J. (1987): The analogy between tinnitus and pain: A suggestion for a physiological basis of chronic tinnitus. Hear. Res., 28: 271-275.

Appendix: Tinnitus questionnaire

Please indicate at which point you assess yourself on the following scales:

1) How well did you hear during the last week?
I heard very well I heard very poorly

2) How often were you conscious of the ear noises?
always occasionally

3) How much did your ear noise disturb you this week?
barely very much

Please indicate the correct answers to the following questions:

4) Was your understanding of other people impaired by your tinnitus?
( ) yes
( ) no

5) Was your ability to concentrate disturbed by your tinnitus in the last week?
( ) yes
( ) no

6) Do you have the feeling that your hearing has deteriorated at this moment because of your tinnitus?
( ) yes
( ) no

7) Do you have the feeling that your tinnitus improves when you are really relaxed?
( ) yes
( ) no
( )no, it is even worse
( ) it varies

Please indicate at what point where you assess yourself on the following scales:

8) How loud is your ear noise at this moment?
very loud very quiet

9) How unpleasant is your ear noise at this moment?
very unpleasant not at all unpleasant

Please indicate the answers to the following questions:

10) How much does your tinnitus disturb you this week?

intolerable very much somewhat strongly not much not at all

11) How often did your tinnitus occur in the last 8 days?

always	very often	often	seldom	very seldom

12) How loud did you find your tinnitus this week?

intolerable	very loud	somewhat loud	quiet	very quiet

13) How unpleasant do you find your tinnitus this week?

intolerable	very unpleasant	unpleasant	somewhat unpleasant	not at all unpleasant

Name (abbreviation): . . . .

Chapter 11

Hypnotherapeutic approaches in complex chronic tinnitus

Heribert Joisten

11.1 Summary

A combination of behavioral therapy and clinical hypnosis appears to be an appropriate approach to treatment of tinnitus despite rather limited experience.

Not only a general conflict-resolving and conflict regulating alteration in behavior and adjustment is sought, but also individual possibilities for active coping with the stressful and annoying symptoms.

An outline of the behavioral therapy framework is followed by fairly extensive description of a variety of hypnotherapeutic interventions.

11.2 Introduction

Tinnitus, as a complex disturbance with far-reaching effects, requires a complex, holistic therapeutic approach. This approach must consider the individual, and his overall relationship to his social surroundings.

Behavioral therapy in combination with hypnosis seems to be appropriate as a means of eliciting the changes necessary and desired by the patient:

— *increasing the patient's level of activity and interest*, thereby diverting the patient from concentrating on his symptoms;

— *achieving self-control*, to improve self-perception and control of the triggering factors in order to alter the possibilities for positive self-reinforcement and focused attention;
— *attainment of an altered perception of symptoms* and *reduced interference from them.*

Hypnosis is not used here as an independent or isolated form of treatment, but rather as a psychotherapeutic method (Kossak, 1989) which increases the effectiveness of behavioral therapy, a more comprehensive form of treatment.

Hypnosis has long been used in behavioral therapy as a relaxation technique or as imagined representation of observed learning processes (Revensdorf, 1987).

Weitzenhofer (1972) provides a review of the combination of behavioral therapy and hypnosis, highlighting the advantages of this combination using a series of examples.

11.3 Review of literature

Literature concerning the treatment of tinnitus by hypnosis is extraordinarily rare compared to literature concerning the treatment of pain. It may be assumed that the treatment of tinnitus, despite the often stated similarities with the treatment of pain and its relatively frequent occurrence has gained little attention because very few tinnitus patients take advantage of psychotherapy. Three articles dealing with the treatment of tinnitus under hypnosis were published in the 1950s (Guild, 1959; Mihalyka and Whanger, 1959; Pearson and Barnes, 1950).

Mihalyka and Whanger (1959) describe the case of a man with objective tinnitus ("A clicking could be heard up to 2 feet from the patient's head, synchronous with the pulse, an unusual sound resembling the snapping of finger nails.")

According to the authors, the patient learned sufficient relaxation in four treatment sessions that, for the first time in 9 years, the tinnitus disappeared. The report asserts that the tinnitus returned only in conditions of extreme stress and could be modified by the patient using auto-suggestion techniques.

Pearson and Barnes (1950) describe two cases of objective tinnitus, both of which had a similar, unbelievably successful course of treatment due exclusively to induction of relaxation.

Marlowe (1973), Oystragh (1974) and Kroger (1977, 1979) describe tinnitus treatment using hypnosis in the 1970s.

Marlowe (1973) reports on two successfully treated tinnitus patients aged 25 and 46, who developed tinnitus following high frequency hearing loss due to occupational exposure to noise. Observations his patients made during treatment were integrated into the theoretical framework and Marlowe pointed out the research work of Heller and Bergmann (1953) in this context, who found that approximately 94% of persons with normal hearing experienced subjective noises in a soundproofed room. This was taken as an indication of a constantly present subliminal noise level which is normally masked by the ordinary, daily noises of the environment. Under the experimental conditions described, the external noise is eliminated to such an extent that most persons with normal hearing hear internal sounds.

In one case, after induction of hypnosis (by eye fixation and a distraction technique), Marlowe asked the patient to concentrate on the tinnitus. He gave the hypnotic suggestion that by doing this the patient would perceive a gradual decrease of the tinnitus, and while registering this effect would become more relaxed and fall into a trance. Marlowe coupled the acoustic impression with relaxation.

Marlowe's posthypnotic suggestions were aimed at inducing the patient to concentrate on the tinnitus in a similar way when falling asleep.

After 6 weeks (six treatment sessions), falling asleep was no longer a problem and difficulties due to the tinnitus during the day no longer disturbed the patient significantly.

Marlowe's second patient was given ego-strengthening suggestions following trance induction through fixation. These included the information that 94% of persons with normal hearing had subjective hearing impressions in a soundproofed room. In addition, the patient was induced to remember a favorite piece of music which he was to recall immediately following the appearance of the first signs of tinnitus. This second patient was nearly free of symptoms during the first phase of therapy (which lasted 4 weeks) but, according to the report, perceived "strange music." After 6 months he suffered only minimal tinnitus discomfort during the day, and no longer had sleep disturbances.

Kroger (1977, 1979) emphasizes the high sensitivity/reactivity of the sense of hearing in man to psychic stress and the close relationship to anxiety. He recommands that the therapist does not adopt the patient's fixation on "sounds in the head" as "tiresome, disturbing and harassing". Instead the therapist looks for stressful situational factors which trigger the tinnitus using behavioral therapy. These stimulus conditions then should be considered and altered by an appropriate hypnotic suggestion.

Whenever it is not possible to find a clear situational trigger, Kroger emphasizes this, and accentuates it using the hypnotic method of time distortion, which induces an expansion or contraction of the subjective perception of time. Kroger warns against an impatient, excessively rapid treatment and blatantly direct suggestions (e.g. "Your tinnitus will be reduced" or "It will diminish").

Instead, he recommends suggestions which include specific characteristics of the tinnitus such as frequency ("When the frequency becomes lower, it will be less disturbing").

Kroger rates the effects of relaxation and self-hypnosis very positively (improvement in symptoms greater than 60%, but does not mention criteria regarding improvement). Unfortunately, Kroger continues, many patients discontinue treatment too soon as a result of their over-optimistic expectations. Brattberg (1983) treated 32 patients. A 15-minute hypnosis session took place immediately following the initial interview with the patients and this session was tape-recorded. The patients, who were put into trance using a combination of progressive relaxation and hypnosis received the following information during this "treatment-phase":

— It is not certain that the symptoms of tinnitus will disappear.

— The conscious perception of the tinnitus may be reduced.

— This effect can be expected no sooner than after 2–3 weeks of home practice using the recorded tape-cassette.

— In the best case, the buzzing will disappear, provided that you as the patient do not make an effort to hear it.

The patients listened to their own individually prepared audio cassettes daily for 4 weeks.

Follow-up examination after 2 months demonstrated a subjective improvement in 22 patients (68.7%); especially successful patients were able to achieve a high degree of relaxation (as measured using the hand levitation test).

Crasilneck (1985) reports that patients with whom hypnosis can be induced well were able to achieve a 50% reduction of symptoms. He speculates, without further description of the therapeutic intervention, that this is caused by blocking the patient's attention (also see Brattberg, 1983).

Crasilneck also refers to Black

and Wigan (1961), who induced a temporary selective deafness for tones of specific frequencies in hypnotic trance, and urges that these considerations be included in the treatment of tinnitus (see also Feustle, 1985).

Without further detail, Jovanovic (1988) reports on a successful treatment of a tinnitus patient using hypnosis.

Hypnosis of a 75-year-old woman suffering from "buzzing in the ear" is vividly described by Erickson and Rossi (1983) (see 11.5.3).

11.4 Treatment of tinnitus patients with combined behavioral therapy and clinical hypnosis

11.4.1 Fundamental considerations

The treatment described below has been developed since 1988, and is based on clinical experience with approximately 30 outpatients. The patients were treated for periods of up to 2 years, in 4–45 sessions in a psychotherapy practice. The similarities between tinnitus and pain as symptoms were a prime consideration from the beginning (Joisten, 1991). That our patients were aware of and experienced their tinnitus on a very individual basis was particularly important for the development of our therapeutic approach.

Four main patient groups can be differentiated:

1. *Patients who are stressed by tinnitus but seek help for other psychological problems,* and who mention their tinnitus, during the initial session or during the course of treatment.

   These patients have no prior "knowledge of tinnitus", lack a prior diagnosis of tinnitus or specific information about tinnitus and ascribe it to one or numerous other symptoms. As one of many frequently stressful symptoms, tinnitus plays a minor part in their emotional experience.
2. *Patients with prior "knowledge of tinnitus" and a "tinnitus diagnosis."*

   In this group, even in the presence of additional existing symptoms, tinnitus is of such significance that they more or less concentrate on tinnitus exclusively and classify their other disturbances as a part or a consequence of their condition.

   In contrast to the first group of patients, this group is fixated on tinnitus.

   Patients in this group may be subdivided into:

2.1 *Patients who desire general psychiatric treatment.* In addition to the tinnitus, they generally also experience other symptoms, which they usually experience as resulting from tinnitus.

2.2 *Patients who desire general psychiatric treatment, and suggest hypnosis during the initial interview, at least as a supplementary treatment-modality.*

2.3 *Patients who desire hypnotherapy, exclusively, generally rejecting general psychotherapy.*

These patients usually have unrealistic, exaggerated ideas about the effect of hypnosis and expect that their symptoms will be overcome, without personal effort and active participation.

11.4.2 Fundamental considerations

Patients, with their various "tinnitus backgrounds", were and are the "scouts" who search for appropriate treatment strategies. Stimulated by the patient in his role as a teacher, the combination of behavioral therapy and hypnosis has been modified to the extent possible within the framework of outpatient treatment.

— from an exclusively symptom-oriented approach with increasing considerations of a holistic nature;
— from a relatively predominant orientation toward hypnosis to one which concentrates more on basic approaches of behavioral medicine toward hypnotherapeutic intervention;
— from a relatively uniform treatment to greater individualization;
— from initially less "homework" to more individual practice at home;
— from general relaxation with appropriate imagery to a differentiated, individualized imagery interspersed with symptom-oriented and problem-oriented suggestions.

The following factors have shown themselves to be especially relevant for treatment and therefore should be explored and taken into account in an individualized treatment scheme. This occurs during an unstructured therapy session (eg cognitive restructuring) or during hypnosis using appropriate suggestions:

— The degree of subjective discomfort from tinnitus. For example, patients experience tinnitus as more or less stressful, depend- on their familial, social or occupational position and on the degree of their external and internal isolation.
— Changes which have occurred in their daily lives due to tinnitus. For example, early retirement leads to isolation for some patients and is experienced as a punishment, while for others it signifies an opportunity, even though it is accompanied by tinnitus.
— The significance of the tinnitus as a disturbance in the patient's life varies if sufficient behavioral alternatives remain viable despite the tinnitus.
— The duration of the discomfort and disability caused by tinnitus and the prior experience concerning the previous number and types of treatment, the possible disappointments and how well they were coped with, the patient's degree of information concerning tinnitus as well as the degree of active acceptance of and coping with the disease.
— The thoughts and convictions of the patient concerning the origin and sustaining factors of his tinnitus, which may be more somatically oriented (organ defect) or of a psychodynamic nature (tinnitus as a warning signal/a punishment).
— Individual experiences with tinnitus in respect to the quality of the sound ("sounds like . . ."), particularly loudness, tonality, oscillation, variability over time and situation.
— Expectations toward therapy and the degree of influence on the disorder; expectations toward the therapist.
— Prior knowledge of psychotherapy and hypnosis; degree of cooperation and willingness of the patient to question his past within the framework of psychotherapy.

11.4.3 Course of treatment of tinnitus patients within the framework of an outpatient psychotherapy practice

1. *The biography and behavioral analysis* as well as the *VT questionnaire* and the analysis of a "life-script" as homework serve to define the tinnitus in its development, in its relation to other symptoms, critical life events, conflicts, its triggers, and situational/personal reinforcers (Fig 11.1).

The initial "homework" makes it clear to the patient that a large amount of cooperation and activity is expected of him during therapy.

2. In the *explorative, tinnitus-specific phase of therapy*, the patient is questioned about the details relevant for tinnitus therapy and information is provided about hypnotherapeutic treatment as part of a treatment regimen. At the same time, the patient is prepared for futher therapeutic steps (development of a framework suitable for the therapeutic relationship).
3. Suggestibility and cooperation of the patient for hypnotherapy are checked out using an imagery test as well as a suitable induction technique.

Trance induction can be a problem in tinnitus patients because quite a few of them are afflicted with hearing loss, which limits their ability to communicate. The classic induction of hypnosis, eg by the fixation technique or coupled to respiration (Kossak, 1989), has been found to be superior to more indirect techniques.

4. Depending on the suggestibility of the patient, various approaches to the therapeutic process are available:
   a) *Given insufficient suggestibility*, hypnotherapy is not considered further in the total context of treatment.
   b) *Given sufficient suggestibility*, hypnotic interventions are used in addition to behavioral-medicine

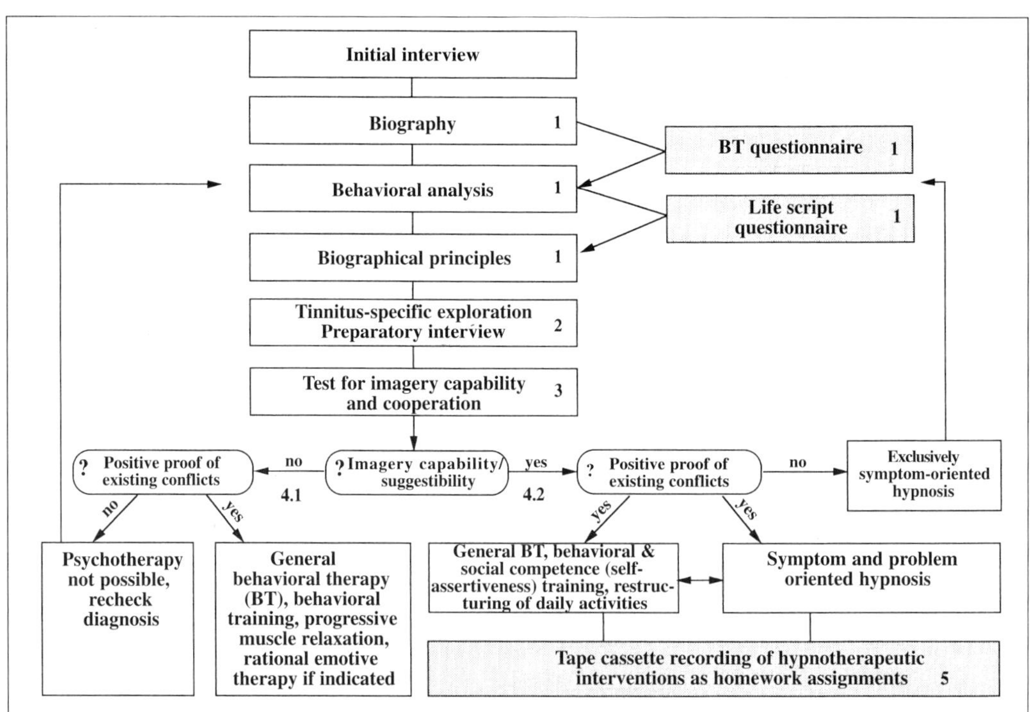

Fig. 11.1 Flow chart: phases of the treatment of tinnitus patients, using a combination of behavioral therapy and hypnosis. The shaded boxes signify homework assignments; the numbers indicate the sections in the boxed-in text. BT = behavioral therapy.

approaches (described in detail below). The hypnotic interventions are used for:

i. symptom-oriented intervention
ii. problem-oriented intervention
iii. combination of symptom- and problem-oriented intervention.

5. The *individual* hypnotherapeutic interventions during treatment are recorded on an audio-cassette during therapy and are given to the patient with the requirement that he *listens to this therapy session at least once daily at a fixed time.*

Listening to the tape *just before falling asleep* has been found to be particularly useful for the course of therapy, because especially at this time of the day the stress due to tinnitus is often nearly unbearable and leads to sleep disturbances.

This homework requires at least 20-30 minutes daily.

The audio-cassettes improve the patient's capabilities at autosuggestion and result in a self-initiated, self-responsible management of his symptoms.

11.4.4 Hypnotherapeutic intervention — different points of emphasis

11.4.4.1 Symptom-oriented hypnotherapeutic interventions

Symptom-oriented hypnotherapeutic interventions are especially relevant when:

— "psychic problems" play a minor role and this can be verified by a thorough analysis of possible causative factors — positive proof of existing conflicts.
— the patient is not able or prepared to utilize problem-oriented interventions due to an extreme fixation on his tinnitus or a lack of conflict awareness.

The symptom-oriented approach in hypnotherapy of tinnitus patients has a great similarity with the treatment of patients suffering from a chronic pain syndrome.

One of the most fascinating and controversial phenomena of hypnosis is dissociation. According to Hilgard's neodissociation theory (1974, 1979, 1989) cognitive symptoms function parallel to each other, each possessing a certin unity, consistency and functional uniformity. These symptoms, which usually interact, can also function separately.

Hilgard also postulates that a control system exists, that regulates the interactions and competitive cognitions with the aim of inhibiting a constant flow of simultaneous cognitive patterns.

A third supposition Hilgard makes is that an additional central "surveillance and control-structure" exists which regulates the interactions of the subsymptoms.

In hypnosis the therapist influences and restricts the "executive power" of the surveillance-and-control structure with the aim of modifying the hierarchy of the sub-symptoms. Certain processes are decreased, others reinforced and the subjective perception of reality is modulated.

11.4.4.2 Problem-oriented hypnotherapeutic interventions

As is the case in approximately 70% of our patients, problem-oriented interventions are preferable when a definite causal relationship can be found between a psychic conflict/a personal stress situation/ critical events and the development of tinnitus; when

— a psychological conflict can be associated with the development of tinnitus;
— spontaneous or hypnotically induced (eg through reorientation) cognitions or emotions point to the development of conflicts;
— emotions or cognitions prevent the patient from coping adequately and force him to resort constantly to neurotic mechanisms (rational emotive therapy in combination with hypnosis).

When improper processing or inappropriate assessments lead to irrational assumptions or convictions in tinnitus patients, (1989) modified rational-emotive therapy (Stanton, 1977, 1989) and ego-strengthening exercises (Hartland 1965, 1971) are available in addition to the behavioral medicine concepts of Ellis (1977), Beck (1979) and Mahoney (1979).

If the occurrence and reinforcement of tinnitus symptoms are clearly associated with situational triggers, hypnotherapy is a recommendable method (Crawford, 1983; Kossak, 1987, 1989).

Problem-oriented hypnotherapeutic interventions, have been frequently described in the general literature of clinical hypnosis (see authors noted above) but we will not go into further details at this point.

11.4.5 Symptom-oriented hypnotherapeutic interventions in the context of tinnitus treatment

Numerous possibilities derived in part from the clinical experience made in the treatment of pain are known for a symptom-oriented hypnotherapy of tinnitus. The following passage provides examples of possible interventions.

11.4.5.1 Intervention targeted directly at the symptom or its modification

Suggestions which modify the tinnitus directly and lead to its complete disappearance are poorly suited because the suggestions themselves elicit resistance in the patient. For the patient the suggestions diverge from his previous and current experiences, and are in conflict with the belief-system he has developed (Kroger 1977, 1979).

11.4.5.2 General relaxation and feeling of well-being evoked by the patient's individual imagery

This includes, for example, the suggestion of "taking a walk in the woods", which may not only include the various senses (sight, smell, taste, etc), but also emphasizes the sense of hearing specifically by concentrating on typical sounds which are associated with the situational context of the suggestion.

For example, in "taking a walk in the woods", the call of a cuckoo, the rustle of leaves, the chirping of birds or the rushing sound of a brook is highlighted by changing the pitch and loudness etc of one's voice. (Erickson 1966), thus increasing the patient's sensitivity towards ordinary, everyday sounds which "compete" with the tinnitus. As a result the patient reconstructs his "world of hearing" and copes with the symptoms adequately.

11.4.5.3 Suggestions directed at certain qualities of the experience of tinnitus

This type of suggestion in addition to pure relaxation suggestions have been mentioned most frequently in literature concerning hypnotherapy of tinnitus (Kroger 1977, 1979; Brattberg 1983; Oystragh 1974; Crasilneck 1985, among others).

These authors refer to suggestions which either mention specific aspects of the symptom (eg tone, loudness) or induce the patient to perceive the existing symptom as less harassing or stressful.

11.4.5.4 Suggestions directed at the situational context of experienced tinnitus

The patient is given the suggestion, for example, of a river boat cruise, together with that of the sound of the beat of a diesel engine, or "taking a walk in the woods" is associated with "passing a sawmill" and its screeching, high-frequency sounds. A scenario is then developed which modifies the experience of the senses on which the patient concentrated beforehand.

11.5 Interventions which modify symptoms or the experience of symptoms indirectly

The interventions described below are directed at the capacity for dissociation under hypnosis and derive to a great extent from effective hypnotherapeutic intervention used in pain control

11.5.1 "Voyage through the body"

In the "voyage through the body", the patient is induced to concentrate on other parts of his body with the aim of distracting his attention away from the site of his symptoms (the head, as a rule), as well as the symptoms themselves. Objects observed from a distance appear smaller, noises heard from a distance sound softer and modified (Joisten 1991).

11.5.2 "Hear colors, change colors"

The capability for dissociation is also used when the patient is induced to associate colors with the sounds of his surroundings, then to change these colors so that the entire experience is more pleasant (Joisten 1991). It is difficult for many patients who are fixated on their hearing, to modify acoustic impressions. By associating the acoustic impressions with a color, this fixation is "sidetracked". This transformation of sensory qualities (from seeing colours in the direction of hearing colors) has positive repercussions and patients report that their tinnitus is experienced as less disturbing.

Patients are made aware of ordinary sounds such as those of birds, cars, lawnmowers, the telephone, the rustle of leaves, the clatter of coffee cups, the slamming of doors and the running of water from a faucet. They are instructed to associate every tone and every sound with an appropriate color. Then, the preferred and rejected colors are determined. What makes colors pleasant or unpleasant is discussed, and that these colors can be changed, mixed, blended or darkened, leading to a change in their qualities. With the tinnitus classified as a color, as a rule, it has the color the patient rejects.

In one of their first homework assignments, the patients are told to practice the hearing of colors in their daily lives. Then imagery containing the patient's favorite color ("pleasant") as well as the color of his tinnitus ("unpleasant") is developed mutually.

One patient, who experienced her tinnitus as a shrill yellow and whose favorite color was royal blue, developed the imagery of a "sunset at the seaside". The yellow sun slowly turned orange and then dark red, a red which finally sank into a dark blue.

11.5.3 Metaphors

In working with metaphors, it is important to question and confront the patient with his personal belief-system concerning the tinnitus. The patient who experiences his limitations should be made aware of an expanded system of values, emotions and cognitions using a metaphor, which permits a re-orientation.

The therapeutic effect, in contrast to the technique described in section 11.4.5 above, is less direct and allows the patient more latitude. This technique includes information about hypnosis and tinnitus as a means of restructuring the patient's mental framework, a reactivation of helpful common experiences such as "everyone knows that ..." as well as a means of developing appropriate changes using adequate imagery.

As an example, Erickson (1981) used the image of a factory filled with the sound of pneumatic drills and hammers: E: I understand. I want to tell you a story now, so that you will understand me better. We learn things in very unusual ways, in ways we know nothing about. During the summer of my first year at university, I happened to pass a boiler factory. The employees worked on 12 steam boilers at the same time in three shifts. The air was filled with the noise of pneumatic hammers which forced the rivets into place. I heard the noise and wanted to find out what it was. After I discovered that it was a boiler factory, I entered it but could not understand what was spoken. I noticed that the lips of the foreman moved, but I could not hear what he said. He heard what I said on the other hand and I asked him to come outside with me so that I could speak with him. I asked him to permit me to spend a night in the factory. He thought that I was crazy! I explained that I wanted to study medicine and that I was interested in the process of learning. Finally he allowed me to stay the night and he explained my presence to the workers and left instructions for the next shift. When I woke up the next morning, I overheard the workers talking about this "crazy young man". Why did he sleep on the floor and what did he expect to learn from this? While sleeping, I had excluded the terrible noise of the 12 or more pneumatic hammers from conscious perception — and now I was suddenly able to hear the voices of the workers. I discovered that it was possible to learn to hear only certain sounds by adjusting one's ears properly. You hear a buzzing in your ears but you have not considered adjusting yourself in such a way that you will no longer consciously hear the buzzing.

11.6 Discussion

Our current therapeutic approach is characterized by important details which have been described as being advantageous in the sparsely available literature:

- Individual hypnotherapy sessions should be recorded on audio-cassettes and given to the patient as homework, as suggested by Kroger (1979) and proven effective by Brattberg (1983).

  Deviating from the method of Kroger and Brattberg, the audio-cassettes used in our approach may be reviewed, and brought up to date several times during treatment, according to the patient's progress and modified experience.

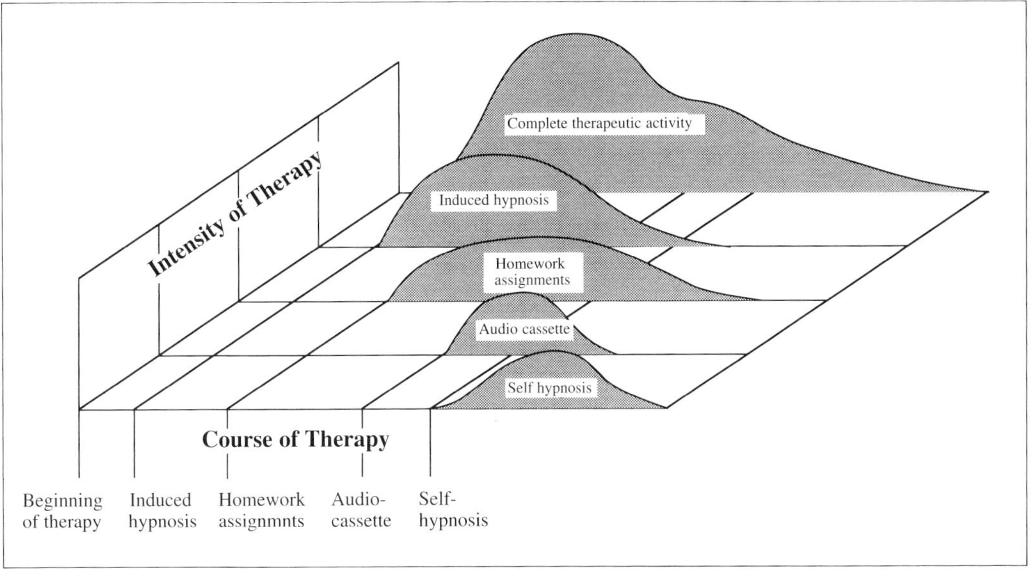

Fig. 11.2 Self-hypnosis during a treatment. Therapy begins with induced hypnosis and is accompanied constantly by homework assignments. The patient practises the individual inductions and suggestions provided by the audiocasette until therapy is completed. (From Kossak, 1986)

- It is effective to avoid extremely direct hypnotherapeutic interventions and to concentrate on the different qualities and the situational context of the experienced tinnitus as well as on an adequate metaphorical system with the aim of modifying the patient's perceptions.
- A problem-oriented approach is recommended by Kroger (1979). Interventions described by Stanton (1977, 1979) and Hartland (1965, 1971) support simultaneous behavioral-therapy interventions.

  The combination of cognitive behavioral medicine and hypnosis is described as being particularly appropriate and effective by Ellis (1984) and by Kossak (1987, 1989).
- The question which underlying mechanisms are basically effective in the combination of hypnotherapy and behavioral therapy remains unanswered and allows speculation only.

It is certain, however, that three aspects are significant:

- A distraction of attention is produced, resulting in an additional decrease or disappearance of a recalcitrant fixation on the tinnitus.
- Even non-specific relaxation leads to positive relaxation effects and inhibits anxiety. (Keen, 1977).
- By learning autosuggestion techniques, the patient increasingly experiences himself as active in the struggle with tinnitus and his environment, resulting in increased self-esteem.

The problems that tinnitus provides for the patient and the therapist have not been solved.

This chapter hopes to stimulate further development of the manifold treatment approaches. Perhaps a planned evaluation of therapy will clarify the approaches described in this chapter.

11.7 References

Beck, A.T. (1979): Wahrnehmung der Wirklichkeit und Neurose. Pfeiffer, München.

Black, S., E.R. Wigan (1969): An investigation of selective deafness produced by direct suggestion under hypnosis. British Medical Journal, 2: 736-741.

Brattberg, G. (1983): An alternative method of treating tinnitus. Intern. J. of Clinical and Experimental Hypnosis, 2: 90-97.

Crasilneck, H.B., J.A. Hall (1975): Clinical hypnosis, principles and applications. Grune & Stratton, New York.

Crawford, H.J. (1983): Enhanced visual memory during hypnosis as mediated by hypnotic responsiveness and cognitive strategies. Journal of Experimental Psychology, 112: 662-665.

Ellis, A. (1977): Die rational-Emotive Therapie. Pfeifer, München.

Ellis, A. (1984): The use of hypnosis with Rational Emotive Therapie (RET). Int. Journal of Eclectic Psychotherapy, 3: 15-22.

Erickson, M.H. (1966): The interspersal hypnotic technique for symptom correction and pain control. American Journal of Clinical Hypnosis, 8: 198-209.

Erickson, M.H., E.L. Rossi (1981): Hypnotherapie: Aufbau-Beispiele-Forschungen. Pfeiffer, München.

Feustle, G. (1985): Hypnotisch induzierte Taubheit. Eine Literaturübersicht der experimentellen Hypnoseforschung über hypnotisch induzierte Taubheit. Experimentelle und klinische Hypnose, 2: 153-165.

Fromm, E. (1978): Dissociative and integrative processes in hypnoanalysis. In: *Dengrove, E.* (Ed.): Hypnosis and behaviour therapy. C.C. Thomas, Springfield.

Greuel, H. (1989): Ambulante Behandlung von Hörbehinderungen nach Hörsturz, M. Menière und/oder artverwandtern Tinnitus. In: *Viefhues* (Ed.): Rehabilitation von Hörgeschädigten mit psychischen Störungen oder Erkrankungen, 119-127. Herne, edition bosofo.

Guild, J. (1959): Hypnosis for tinnitus. Canad. Med. Ass. J., 78: 426-427.

Hartland, J. (1965): The value of "ego strengthening" procedures prior to direct symptom-removal under hypnosis. American Journal of Clinical Hypnosis, 8: 89-93.

Hartland, J. (1971): Further observations on the use of "ego strengthening" technique. American Journal of Clinical Hypnosis, 14: 1-8.

Heller, M. & M. Bergmann (1953): Tinnitus curium in normally hearing persons. Annuals of Otology Rhinology Laryngology, 60: 73-83.

Hilgard, E.R. (1974): Toward a neodissociation theory: multiple cognitive controls in human functioning. Perspectives in Biology and Medicine, 17: 301-316.

Hilgard, E.R. (1979): Divided consciousness in hypnosis: the implications of hidden observer. In: *Fromm, E.R.* (Ed.). Hypnosis: Developments in research and new perspectives. Aldine, New York.

Hilgard, E.R. (1989): Eine Neo-Dissoziationstheorie des geteilten Bewußtseins. Hypnose und Kognition, 6: 3-22.

Jahoda, G. (1969): The psychology of superstition. Penguin, Baltimore.

Joisten, H. (1991): Hypnotherapeutische Ansätze im Rahmen der kognitiven Verhaltenstherapie bei Tinnitus-Erkrankten. In: *Fromberg, J.* (Ed.): Rehabilitation Schwerhöriger, Ertaubter und Gehörloser, 115-124. Salamanderdruck, Kornwestheim.

Jovanovic, U.J. (1988): Methodik und Theorie der Hypnose. Gustav Fischer, Stuttgart, New York.

Keen, E. et al. (1977): Emotion Brooks. Cole Publishing Company, Monterey, Calif.

McKinney, J. (1973): Problem solving strategies in impulsive and reflective second grade. Developmental Psychology, 8: 145.

Kossak, H.C. (1987): Verhaltenstherapie nächtlicher Asthmaanfälle. Kognitive Umstrukturierung unter Hypnose. Hypnose und Kognition, 4: 41-57.

Kossak, H.C. (1989): Hypnose: ein Lehrbuch. Psychologie Verlags Union, München.

Krampen, G. (1982): Differentialpsychologie der Kontrollüberzeugungen. Hogrefe, Göttingen.

Kroger, W.S. (1977, 1979): Clinical and experimental hypnosis in medicine, dentistry and psychology. Lippincott, Philadelphia.

Mahoney, M.J. (1979): Kognitive Verhaltenstherapie: Neue Entwicklungen und Integrationsschritte. Pfeiffer, München.

Marlowe, F.I. (1973): Effective treatment of tinnitus through hypnotherapy. American Journal of Clinical Hypnosis, 15: 162-165.

Mihalyka, E.E. & A.D. Whanger, (1959): Objective tinnitus aurium hypnotically treated. American Journal of Clinical Hypnosis, 2: 85-86.

Oystragh, P. (1974): The relief of symptoms by the use of hypnosis. Brit. J. of Clinical Hypnosis, 5: 38.

Pearson, M.N. & L.J. Branes, (1950): Objective tinnitus aurium: report of two cases with good results after hypnosis. J. Philad. Gen. Hosp., 1: 134-138.

Revenstorf, D. (1987): Hypnose und Verhaltenstherapie. Hypnose und Kognition, 4: 10-21.

Rotter, J.B. (1966): Generalized expectancies for internal versus external control of reinforcement. Psychological Monographs, 1: 80.

Sacerdote, P. (1982): Techniques of hypnotic intervention with pain patients. In: *Barber, J.B., C. Adrian* (Eds.): Psychological Approaches to the Management of Pain. Brunner/Mazel, New York.

Seligman, M.E.P. (1983): Erlernte Hilflosigkeit. Urban & Schwarzenberg, München.

Stanton, H.E. (1977): The utilization of suggestions derived from rational-emotive therapy. Int. Journal of Clinical Hypnosis, 25: 18-26.

Stanton, H.E. (1989): Streßreduktion durch Rational-Emotive Therapie und Hypnoseinduktion. Experimentelle und Klinische Hypnose, 5: 83-90.

Tönnies, S. (1991): Selbsthilfemöglichkeiten für Tinnitusbetroffene. In: *Fromberg, J.* (Ed.): Rehabilitation Schwerhöriger, Ertaubter und Gehörloser, 125-132. Salamanderdruck, Kornwestheim.

Weitzenhoffer, A.M. (1972): Behaviour therapeutic techniques and hypnotic methods. American Journal of Clinical Hypnosis, 15: 71-82.

Wooley, S.C. (1972): Physiologic versus cognitive factors in short term food regulation in the obese and non-obese. Psychosomatic Medicine, 34: 62-68.

Chapter 12

Art therapy in the treatment of chronic complex tinnitus and its integration into a behavioral medicine therapy concept

Christine Palm and Gerhard Goebel

12.1 Summary

Art therapy is a method based on depth psychology and is a component of our inpatient behavioral medicine treatment of chronic complex tinnitus.

We will define the principles of art therapy and its applications. Using a case history we will attempt to describe the experience and management of a tormenting tinnitus during a therapy lasting six weeks.

12.2 Introduction

A conglomerate of various symptoms as is the case in chronic tinnitus is in many cases assessed by doctors and patients as an organic condition in which psychotherapy is not applicable.

Patients with chronic tinnitus appear to have little motivation for an exclusively introspective method of treatment. As a rule, the patients who came to our clinic have made extensive use of conventional treatment without receiving the necessary support.

The first goal of an integrated treatment strategy is to establish a relationship with the patient which is conducive to psychotherapy. In addition to psychophysical and somatic treatment, the patient should receive help in improving his introspective abilities. Motivation is considerably increased using informative and cognitive components of behavioral medicine as part of our inpatient treatment (Goebel et al., 1991) (see also Chapter 7).

For years tinnitus treatment which combines depth psychology with behavioral therapy has been used predominantly in the USA (see Arkowitz & Messner, 1984). Reports of the application of art therapy have not been published to our knowledge. We became aware of this aspect in our preliminary work (Palm et al., 1989; Goebel, 1989) and believe our study is a valuable contribution to this book.

12.3 Art therapy

Art therapy is a method based on depth psychology in the form of individual or group therapy. It concentrates on elements of unconscious experience and its conscious reflection and expression.

The main focus of therapy is the experience, not the result, of a creative process and gives the patient the opportunity to develop from a passive sufferer to an active manager of his tinnitus.

According to Schrode (1983) art therapy allows emotional impulses to find their conscious experience without being censored by the super-ego. An important prerequisite is a tenable therapeutic relationship, which in art therapy includes the patient, his work, the therapist and the group. The medium of art therapy is either paint or clay, enabling the patient to express himself spontaneously. The patient's work reflects the unconscious as well as conscious elements of the interrelationships that develop during group therapy.

After the patient has finished his work, it is reflected upon and discussed with the aim of integrating the evident emotions. Emotions have received a visual form of expression and emotional aspects of the patient's personality, feelings and behavior become apparent.

With the help of the therapist and other group members the patient tries to understand his latent, i.e. unconscious feelings as they become increasingly perceptible (Schrode & Kurz, 1986). In his work the patient experiences the interrelationships between the unconscious and instinctive on the one hand and its conscious execution and perception on the other. This leads to a synthesis of the conscious and unconscious. Intensive observation and understanding promotes insight into the causes of the condition and the integration of psychological contents which were previously isolated, suppressed or unconscious. The "psychic energy" previously employed in the suppression of undesired thoughts and emotions is now available for a positive development and an active and constructive approach to life.

12.3.1 Setting

In our clinic (Roseneck Clinic in Prien, Germany), art therapy is part of our behavioral medicine oriented treatment concept which is employed on a ward which specializes in the treatment of patients with chronic pain and complex chronic tinnitus (Palm et al., 1989) (see also Chapter 7).

The art therapy group is designed for about 8 patients and takes place twice a week for one and a half hours.

Because the patients are accustomed to prestructured forms of therapy in a clinical setting, they also await a prestructured form of art therapy, but the art therapist tends to support the patient's spontaneity. (To avoid going beyond the framework of this chapter, group-dynamics in our case history are only briefly described.)

12.3.2 Therapeutic objective and problems

The primary goal of our work is to develop strategies mutually which support the patient in attaining a modified (psychological) attitude toward his tinnitus.

Working with emotional processes is required for introspection and is particularly significant in art therapy. The ability to tune into oneself is especially impaired in tinnitus patients who suffer not only from the tinnitus itself but from the loss of peace and quiet. Concentrating on inner processes leads to a more intense perception of the abhorred noise, and is a considerable problem for tinnitus patients.

The medium (e.g. paint or clay) facilitates introspection by allowing the patient to concentrate on something material and concrete. This can help the patient to actively deal with his emotional world and gives him the opportunity to express pleasant or unpleasant emotions.

This work reflects an inner emotional process, supports the patient's ability to perceive and to differentiate, confronts his emotions, and increases the degree of introspection, enabling him to depart from passive suffering and to achieve active coping.

In our treatment concept, the art therapist does not initially deal with the treatment of neurotic conflicts. The patient comes to the clinic with a somatic finding. The sympton causes considerable suffering, and the patient is concerned with getting rid of it or with finding support for its management.

The first goal of art therapy is to lead the patient toward dealing with his experience of disease (Muthny, 1989; Goebel et al., 1991). In some patients this occurs on the behavioral level during his work with the chosen medium, in other patients the conscious reflection of and confrontation with psychological mechanisms is of primary importance.

12.4 A case history

12.4.1 Development of problems

After a diving accident (barotrauma) 15 years previously, dizziness and pressure in the left ear occurred for the first time. Since then an ever increasing whistling noise developed. The tinnitus was initially perceived only on the left side and later on both sides.

The original ENT examinations found a moderate sensorineural hearing loss in high frequencies, predominantly of the left ear, possibly as a result of previous noise trauma (moderately steep decrease starting at 2 kHz up to 60 dB at 4–6 kHz in the audiogram). The tinnitus was localized at about 6 kHz and had a masking threshold on the left side of 65 dB HL. A (central) cerebral cause of tinnitus was ruled out using cranial computer tomography and BERA.

Various medications to improve circulation were unsuccessful. The patient received a tetracyclic antidepressant, occasionally also benzodiazepines, for the treatment of depression and sleeping disturbances until the time of admission.

Admission was recommended by his psychiatrist, who had diagnosed a depression and anxiety syndrome with a "psychovegetative tension syndrome" due to tinnitus. The patient was fitted with a maxillary occlusal overlay splint by his dentist because of malocclusion and bruxism. He had also learned autogenic training.

In his tinnitus diary (for more details see Chapter 7) which he submitted at the time of application, he had continuously rated the loudness of his tinnitus at 75 (0 = no tinnitus; 100 = extremely loud tinnitus) and the discomfort due to tinnitus varied between 60 to 90 (0 = no discomfort; 100 = extremely severe discomfort). Control over tinnitus (coping) was continuously rated as 0 (no control).

12.4.2 Situation at initial interview

Our tinnitus patients are hospitalized for approximately 8 weeks, and participate in art therapy for about 6 weeks.

During the initial interview, the 50-year-old patient was cooperative and described in detail his previous experiences with the health-care system, especially his exasperating contacts with several ENT specialists. With hesitation he also talked about his severe suffering which had led him to our clinic. Over the years he had suffered from increasing resignation and lack of drive. He was convinced that he had failed in life and was scarcely able to accomplish anything because of his severely impaired concentration. Falling asleep became a major problem and he often awoke after nightmares. He had retreated from his social life and this had led to family conflicts even though his wife was very considerate.

Even though he had held his job for years in his company, he was also afraid of being fired because the workforce was being reduced for economic reasons. In addition, the atmosphere at work had deteriorated and his relationship to his new and younger superior was full of tension. He was afraid that he could no longer care for his family properly.

The patient was extremely polite, but appeared tense, over-precise and over-correct. He also seemed to be extremely sensitive and emotionally unstable. He emphasized his motivation to participate in art therapy but it was not clear whether his interests were of an artistic or therapeutic nature.

The art therapist developed sympathetic feelings as well as a sincere desire to help the patient, but was also sceptical. His stubbornness and recalcitrance were a direct contrast to his overadapted behavior and this aroused curiosity as well as sympathy.

12.4.3 Basic biographical data

The patient is the first of three children (a brother is 2 years and a sister 4 years younger.)

He has no memories of his father, who was a fighter pilot in WWII and was shot down at age 30. He was six years old at that time and could remember his mother's grief after she was informed of his father's death. Later his mother had told him that she married his father because she had become pregnant unexpectedly. As the eldest, he often felt unfairly treated by his mother, who was often overworked and exhausted.

At the end of WWII our patient was 8 years old, and his family was forced to flee the Soviet-occupied zone. At age 15 he fled to West Germany and lived in a refugee camp for the first 2 years. At age 30 he married and became the father of a daughter, whom both he and his wife had expected with joy. He is a technical assistant and still finds his occupation fulfilling.

12.4.4 Presentation of the course of treatment

12.4.4.1 Description of Fig. 12.1

The drawing technique was rather unsteady but the patient seemed to be certain of the subject he wanted to portray. He drew a burning house, which has a ground floor and an attic. The fire began in the house and red smoke as well as flames blaze out of the windows and the door on the ground floor. He himself is clearly visible, standing in the attic, because he decided not to draw the wall that would have concealed him. Stairs leading down to the ground floor are missing; perhaps they were already consumed by the blaze. He cannot escape and can only rely on being rescued. Persons in a helicopter have already dropped a rescue line which he attempts to reach and one has the impression that he will be rescued.

The patient explained his drawing, saying that it described exactly how he felt. He was proud of the fact that he was able to show so clearly how his current situation threatened his life. On an unconscious level it appeared to be the case that he was also able to experience hope, the possibility of help and impending rescue.

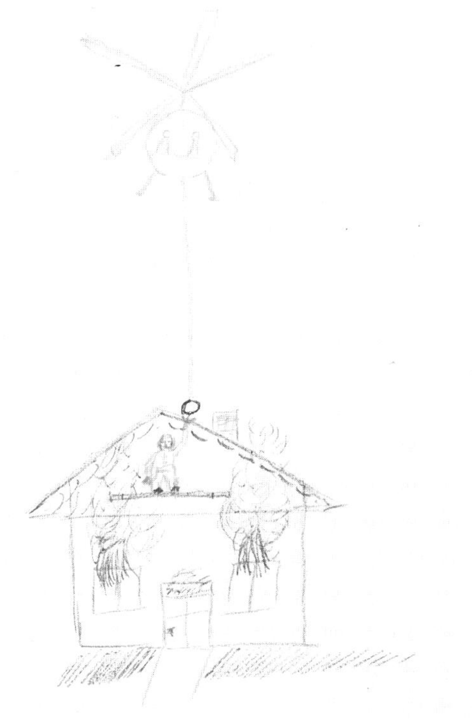

Fig. 12.1 Hoping for rescue in a life-threatening situation.

12.4.4.1.1 Observations on Fig. 12.1

The patient was candid in his portrayal of his great need as well as his hope for rescue at the time of admission.

The house, as a symbol of the surroundings in which the patient felt secure and at home, is now on fire, a life threatening situation for the figure in the drawing.

Tinnitus is experienced as a fire which suddenly burns down a life, which had been secure previously. Where peace and quiet had once existed there was now a disturbing noise that, like the destructive flames, could not be contained or controlled. Nothing can be done and without help, escape is not possible. The only imaginable escape route leads up and thus away from everything which is threatening (see Fig. 12.6). It is virtually a matter of life and death and he feels incapable of rescuing himself. Competent professional help symbolized in the drawing as the rescue crew of a helicopter, is necessary and he can only hold on tightly to the rescue line. The patient experiences himself as completely dependent.

On an objective level and therefore resulting from a conscious intention of the patient, the clinic with its specialized therapy rescues him. The competence of specialists bolsters his hope for rescue and he trusts blindly, grasping at every possible means of help. However, he appears to idealize the specialists, regards his own ability as minor and therefore remains dependent as well as convinced of his own inferiority.

On a subjective level, the picture represents the entire psychological situation of the patient. The house can be interpreted as a psychological function which, until now, offered security and stability. The fire destroys the house and is an expression of a violent turmoil of aggressive and self-destructive emotions. Destructive instinctive impulses dominate and threaten the patient who is symbolized by the paralyzed figure in the drawing. The fire apparently began on the ground floor of the house. In search of an escape route, the figure has fled to the attic.

His attempt to escape allowed the assumption that the patient was able to cope with conflicting and precarious situations in the past.

Considering the 15 years in which the patient attempted to control his tinnitus, his unshakable perseverance is apparent in his persistent pursuit of his goal.

He himself is able to mobilize an emotional function in the form of a rescue team in a helicopter. Hypothetically it may be assumed that the patient, whose father died as a fighter pilot in WWII has preserved positive unconscious impressions of his father in the form of a positively internalized father-figure and has transferred these impressions to the clinic.

Two psychological states are apparent in the drawing: a stationary state in the form of the house and a state of motion in the form of a helicopter. The patient is able to interconnect both states in his drawing.

12.4.4.1.2 Observations concerning therapeutic methods

In the drawing the patient expresses his suffering and his expectation of help. In the drawing he also shows his willingness to cooperate by allowing the figure to raise its hand to grasp the rescue line.

Therapy will consist of helping him to come into contact with his own abilities, conveying interest and understanding for his drawings and supporting individual steps of his development, i.e. attempts at increased autonomy.

The patient appeared to be able to use the drawing as an expression for his emotional situation in the sense of a message. In contrast to tinnitus which, as a subjective perception of noise, remains inaudible to others and thus incomprehensible, the patient can visualize and comprehensibly portray his experience by drawing a picture.

The patient found images which correspond to his situation. He was able to draw them and give his inner sounds a certain shape, and thus give his plight a right to exist. This drawing is a reflection of inner emotional processes and by analysing it the distressing emotions are also recognizable for the patient.

Subjective considerations concerning the drawing (e.g. father-image) were not discussed with the patient because they did not comply with his intentions. It may also be possible that he would not have been able to identify himself with this explanation derived from depth-psychology.

12.4.4.2 Description of Fig. 12.2

The patient drew a busy road. What is peculiar is the small red flower which has delicately burrowed its way through the asphalt (bottom right) and is threatened by cars which speed by.

The patient saw himself as a flowwer, the cars symbolized his tinnitus.

12.4.4.2.1 Observations on Fig. 12.2

The small flower was able to grow, so there had to be roots which could find nourishment and water in the soil under the street (in contrast to drawing 12.1 in which destructive flames blazed from underneath). The flower, as a living being, appears to be a red spark of hope in an otherwise inanimate

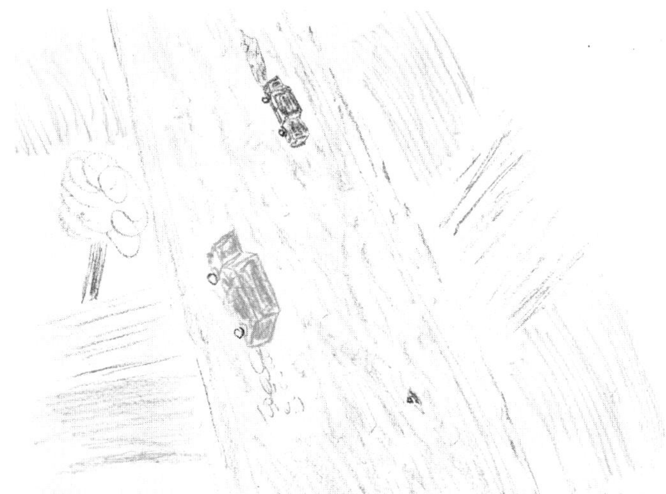

Fig. 12.2 Self-portrait as a threatened flower.

scene drawn with dull colours and seems to be small enough to duck in the cracks of the asphalt, avoiding the passing cars.

The patient is only able to survive his overwhelming tinnitus by making himself small, ducking and staying put. In relation to his biography it may be assumed that the patient, as the eldest, also had to stand still and duck often when he was treated unfairly by his mother.

On the other hand, it seemed that he had also developed abilities to cope with threats and danger (war, life in a refugee camp, disease) using adequate measures to remain hopeful.

The extent of the threat tinnitus poses for the patient is apparent in the extreme difference in size: gigantic cars threaten a tiny flower. Tinnitus is experienced as emotionally overwhelming and the goal of therapy (to be able to cope with tinnitus) appears to be unimaginable. The main purpose of life is still exclusively distinguished by a constant battle against tinnitus.

12.4.4.3 Description of Fig. 12.3

On the right side of the picture an archer is seen who is holding a bow and arrow. With intense concentration he aims at a target, which is situated on the left half of the picture. The patient comments that he remembers his neglected hobby again and wants to resume archery.

12.4.4.3.1 Observations on Fig. 12.3

The patient no longer feels like the flower, he now again feels able to be active.

Observed on the objective level, he remembers the possibility of resuming a former hobby, which he enjoyed as a recreational activity. He tries to actively counter his suffering – an initial attempt toward independence.

The drawing contains the fantasy that patience and concentration will enable him to hit the bull's eye of the target.

Referring to therapy this implies that patient practice will lead to adequate coping. ("I must only want and do enough, then I can master my fate.") The danger of resorting to familiar strategies already appears as a trap in the first drawing. Despite all attempts, the danger exists that the sought goal is not reached.

On the relationship level, the fact

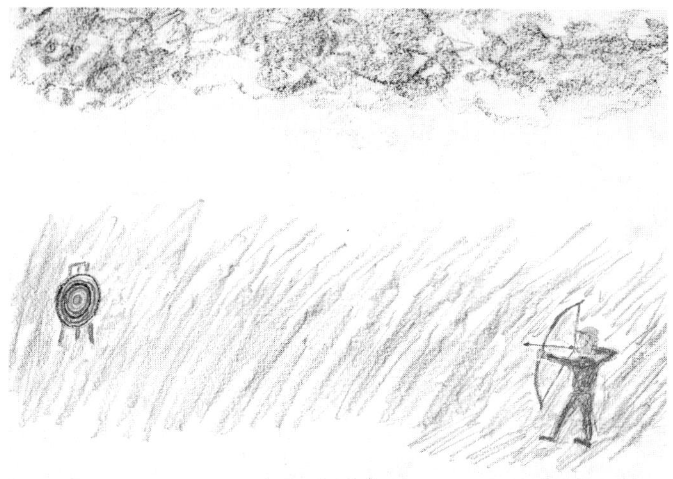

Fig. 12.3 Vitality returns/remembering a previous hobby.

that the situation appears to be controllable is significant. The patient is accustomed to working toward a definite goal. The target symbolizes a definite goal and the patient can determine the distance to the target. By externalizing the threat tinnitus poses to the patient, he can again experience himself as more active and energetic. He hopes to be able to tackle the internal dangers by increasingly mobilizing his goal-oriented capabilities. As unconscious elements such as the fire and the little plant do not appear in this drawing, situations which require more inner flexibility still tend to put excessive demands on the patient. Intrapsychically, the patient expressed these unconscious elements as the destructive energy of the fire and the threatened growth of the flower. With such a rigid attitude the patient cannot resolve his conflicts and further therapy has to concentrate on his rediscovered vital energy and less familiar as well as more flexible coping strategies.

12.4.4.4 Description of Fig. 12.4

The patient drew a clown puppet which seems to be laughing. But the smile on its face is forced and it seems to be stiff and motionless. The marionette hangs on strings but the puppeteer's hand does not appear.

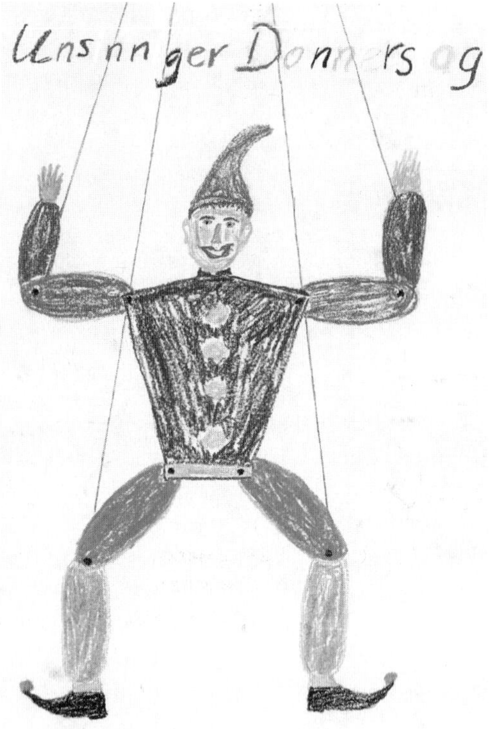

Fig. 12.4 Protest: self-portrait as a Jumping Jack "Senseless Thursday" (= Mardi Gras).

12.4.4.4.1 Course of treatment

The members of the art therapy group had decided to concentrate on a specific subject at the beginning of their session. This decision expressed resistance toward the predominating competitive atmosphere as well as the desire for a playful and stress-free atmosphere. The therapist did not make any suggestions and the patients chose their subject, the Mardi Gras.

During the succeeding phase of mutual discussion the patient spoke about his drawing for the first time thereby escaping from his "my tinnitus and me only" prison. He was able to express his annoyance concerning group pressure as well as his feeling like a puppet occasionally. He had also noticed how he actually wanted to do something else but had complied with the predominant group atmosphere. At work the situation was similar, but with tinnitus it had no longer been possible for him to work overtime as had been the case in the past.

12.4.4.4.2 Observations on group interrelationships and psychodynamics

Group pressure is a powerful and restrictive mother-figure for the patient. The patient experiences the therapist's intervention as support coming from a father-figure, which makes rebellion against the mother-figure possible.

In the drawing the patient actually turns into a dependent "Jumping Jack", but this change also implies an unconscious opposing fantasy: the wish to be the puppeteer himself and to be able to control others! Indirectly he revealed this to the other group members, who were engrossed in their Mardi Gras drawings, by calling his picture: *Senseless* Thursday! (one of the most important days during Mardi Gras in Southern Germany). He also tried to externalize his feelings of helplessness and dependence by expressing his disdain toward the other group members.

12.4.4.5 Description of Fig. 12.5

The patient drew himself standing naked under the shower with his back turned to the beholder. His hands turn the water

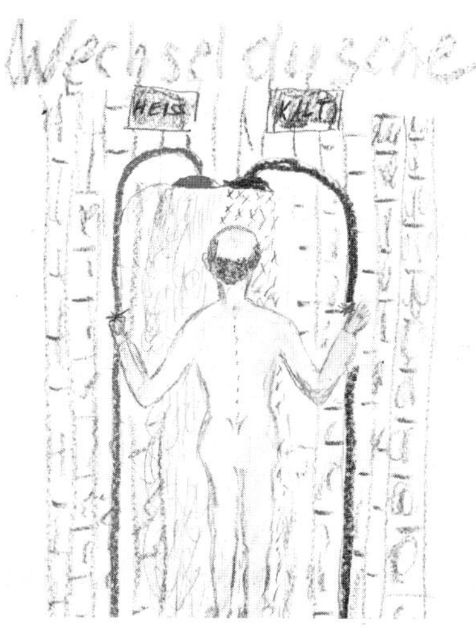

Fig. 12.5 Criticism of therapy represented by a hot and cold shower (Wechseldusche): rediscovery of possibilities for regulation.

faucets and cold and hot water showers down on him.

He mentioned his anger toward the therapists. Sometimes he felt as if he constantly "received cold and hot showers" during therapy. At the time he was running a temperature and was angry at the therapists, who considered the possibility that his temperature was the result of his emotional state.

12.4.4.5.1 Observations on Fig. 12.5

The patient turned his back on the beholder as if he wanted to say: you can get lost with your hot and cold showers. For the first time he rebelled against his "helpers". He tried to disassociate himself from his dependence and strove toward autonomy.

12.4.4.6 Description of Fig. 12.6

The patient drew himself in a hot air balloon holding a large knife in his hand with which he wanted to cut off the ballast (tinnitus) in order to float into space.

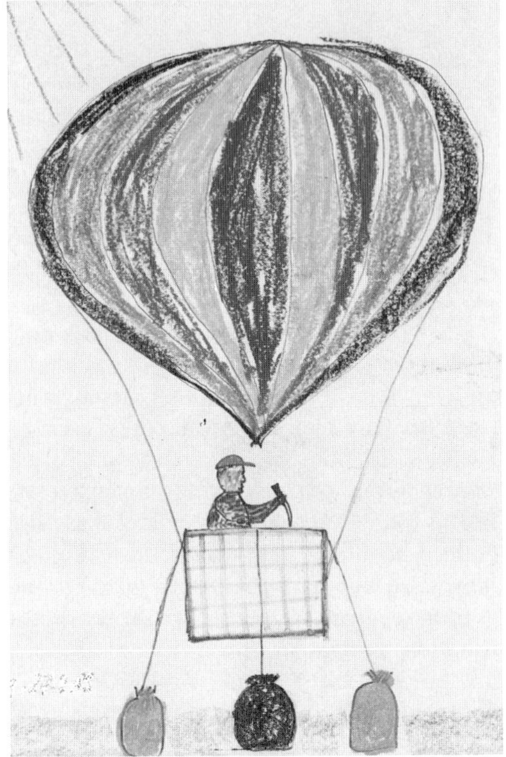

Fig. 12.6 Trying to free myself.

12.4.4.6.1 Observations on Fig. 12.6

The hot-air balloon cannot be controlled by a burner. Only the dark grey ballast serves as the steering mechanism. The patient tried to put a distance between himself and all earthly problems with the intent of being able to float pleasurably and unburdened to great heights. All ballast, everything which burdened him, was to be cut off.

Stubbornly he continued to cling to the illusion of freeing himself from his tinnitus, if necessary even aggressively and self-destructively. Thus he hoped to be free of all undesired additional complaints such as depression and feelings of inferiority. Inner psychological powers and neurotic structures however, cannot be cut off or severed.

12.4.4.7 Description of Fig. 12.7

The assignment was to find a partner in the group and draw a picture mutually. The patient chose a partner with whom he got along well. He drew himself on the left side of the drawing standing in front of a wall with a door. His hand was stretched toward the door as if he wanted to open it. The distance of the human figure to the door, however, indicated his ambivalence.

Two parts emerge in the picture: on the right side is the drawing of the partner, on the left that of the patient. Few contacts develop and the patient clearly separated himself by drawing a wall thereby rejecting his partner.

While discussing the drawing he

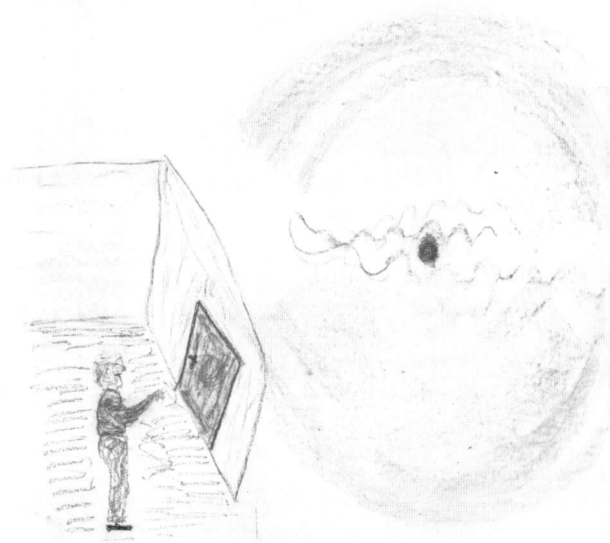

Fig. 12.7 Partner work: The door to the partner remains closed.

expressed that he actually wanted a closer relationship and that his drawing was the result of his insecurity.

12.4.4.7.1 Observations on Fig. 12.7

This subject confronted the patient with his social fears and his wishes. The tinnitus did not stand in the way of a spontaneous acceptance of a relationship, but the wall which he erected between himself and others does. Yearning, he paused in front of a door of a glowing color and felt inhibited. We were better able to differentiate between the patient's personality and the consequences of his tinnitus. The confrontation with his tinnitus slowly became less important in the course of therapy.

12.4.4.8 Description of Fig. 12.8

Working together with a partner our patient once again chose the same partner

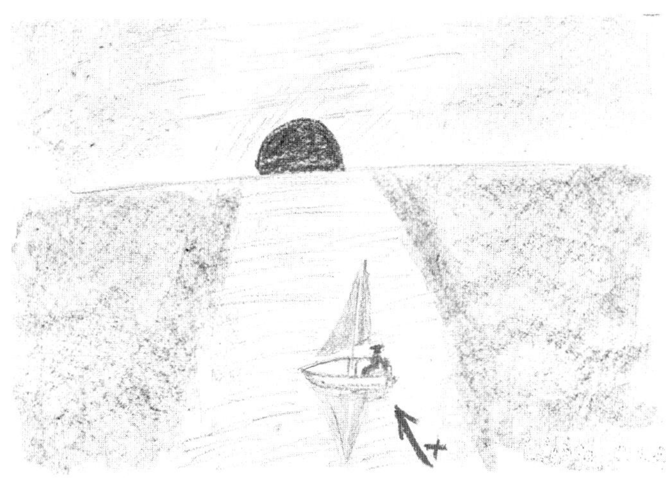

Fig. 12.8 Longing/yearning.

as before. The drawings were to be exchanged so as to give each partner the possibility to respond by drawing another picture on a new sheet of paper.

12.4.4.8.1 Observations on Fig. 12.8

This drawing was his answer to his partner's drawing, who depicted herself sitting in a boat.

Our patient placidly sailed on the open sea and waited for his partner to join him. The red symbols at the bottom of the drawing indicated that the burning red color was now more related to libidinous desires than to threatening instinctive impulses as was the case in drawing 12.7.

12.4.4.9 Description of Fig. 12.9

In the middle of the picture stood an underlined "*me*" under which an anchor sketched with powerful strokes can be seen. On the left side of the picture the patient drew a Bunsen burner, symbolizing his work. The two hearts on the right side of the picture indicated his relationship with his wife.

The patient portrayed his hopes for the future, having planned to separate his professional from private life to a greater extent, not to work overtime to such an extent and to devote himself more to his family.

12.4.4.9.1 Observations on Fig. 12.9

The emphasis of *me* was meant to express his own importance. He now filled the space which the rescue helicopter had originally occupied (Fig. 12.1). The fact that *me* appeared as a word demonstrated how unportrayable this term remained for the patient.

The anchor signified hope. The patient no longer hoped, as in the previous pictures, to be rescued by others from a house but rather sought security and support arising from the bottom half of his drawing. The anchor represented deep-rooted aspects of a stable and positive mother-figure, which he was able to use adequately when required. Cast out, the anchor stabilized and hauled in, allowed movement. As a symbol which unifies opposites, the anchor signified contact as well as detachment, stability as well as motion. The patient subdivided his drawing into two parts, work and private life. The anchor as a symbol has great similarities with the symbol of a scale and therefore could be helpful in finding well-balanced and new

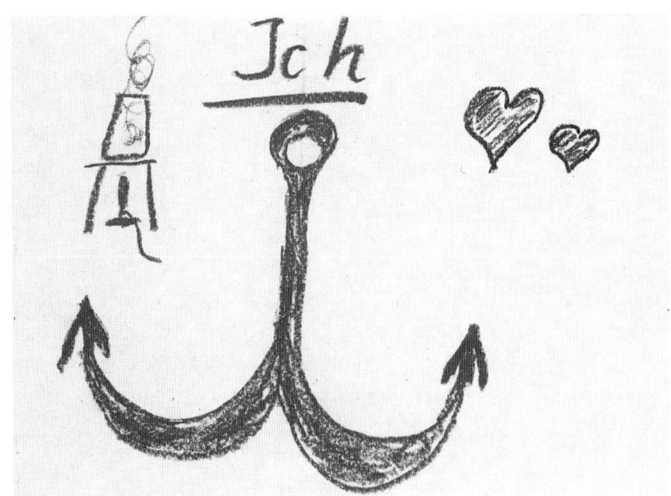

Fig. 12.9 Wishes in regard to the future (Ich = me).

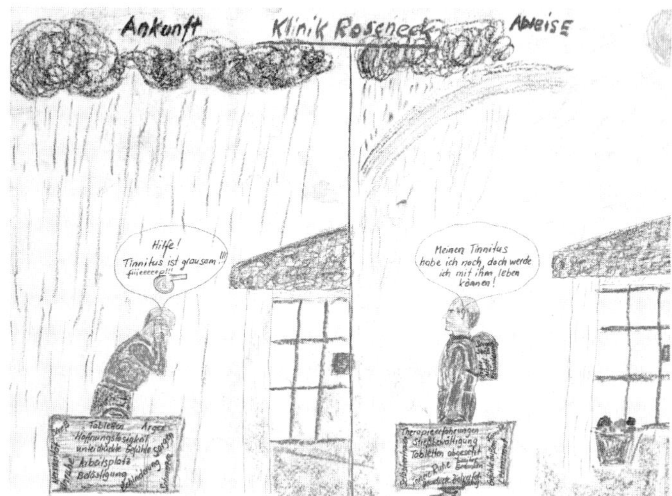

Fig. 12.10 Summary of treatment.

personal standards. The scale seemed to be tipped in favour of the side representing relationships and his private life.

12.4.4.10 Description of Fig. 12.10

This drawing did not evolve in a group context. Instead we requested our patient to concentrate on his progress in art therapy. He compared his situation at admission with his intention at the time of dismissal.

At admission (left side) he had to drop his suitcase because he needed his hands to cover his ears. He could only hear his tinnitus, a whistling sound resembling that of a fan, and could only feel the torment of his tinnitus. He perceived everything as grey and dull, and his medication no longer helped.

At the end of treatment (right side) he left the clinic standing erect with his head held up high. He was able to carry his suitcase again. Although the size and the weight remained the same, the contents had changed into something beneficial. In addition he even carried a small backpack filled with a few and less burdening future problems (see inscription).

He also took his tinnitus along, but he had found his inner peace again. Even though stress and anxiety could not be left behind, new possibilities of coping had been found.

12.5 Concluding remarks

The drawings of the patient demonstrate the development from dependence to autonomy.

In the beginning hope was still directed toward an external object (Fig. 12.1: rescue crew) but later was directed convincingly toward personal abilities and competence (Fig. 12.9: anchor). The patient was again able to carry the burden himself (small backpack) at the end of therapy and was full of confidence (large suitcase).

The course of therapy was reflected in the tinnitus diary in which a distinct decrease of tinnitus discomfort (decrease of about 45%) without change of tinnitus loudness was evident. Control over tinnitus (coping) rose from 0 to 50, the scales for depression and anxiety normalized in the symptom checklist (SCL–90–R; see Chapter 7).

One year after conclusion of therapy (follow-up study) the values of the tinnitus diary and the SCL–90–R remained stable.

Art therapy as part of the management of a complex disorder such as tinnitus may be valuable in achieving thorough disease management by allowing the patient to perceive his own emotions.

12.6 References

Arkowitz, H., S. B. Messner (1984): Psychoanalytic therapy and behavior therapy. Plenum Press, New York, London: 1-30.

Fichter, M. M., G. Goebel (1989): Konzeption einer verhaltensmedizinischen Behandlung chronischer Schmerzen. Prax. Psychother. Psychosom. 34: 205-213.

Goebel, G. (1989): Tinnitus. In: *Hand, I., H. U. Wittchen* (Eds.) Verhaltenstherapie in der Medizin. Springer, Berlin, Heidelberg, New York, London, Paris, Tokyo, Hong Kong: 207-228.

Goebel, G., W. Keeser, M. Fichter, W. Rief (1991): Neue Aspekte des komplexen chronischen Tinnitus. Teil I: Überprüfung eines multimodalen verhaltensmedizinischen Behandlungskonzeptes. Teil II: Die verlorene Stille: Auswirkungen und psychothereapeutische Möglichkeiten beim komplexen chronischen Tinnitus. Psychother. Psychosom. med. Psychol. 41: 115-133.

Muthny, F. A. (1989): Krankheitsverarbeitung bei chronisch körperlich Kranken. Prax. Psychother. Psychosom. 34: 64-72.

Palm, C., G. Goebel, H. Abeken, M. Bräuherr (1989): Gestaltungstherapie bei Patienten mit chronischem Tinnitus; Integration in ein verhaltenstherapeutisch orientiertes stationäres Behandlungskonzept. 60. Jahresversammlung der Deutschen Gesellschaft für Hals-Nasen-Ohrenheilkunde, Kiel (7-11.5.89).

Schrode, H. (1983): Gestaltungstherapie als Therapie mit bildnerischen Mitteln auf tiefenpsychologischer Grundlage. Prax. Psychother. Psychosom. 28: 117-124.

Schrode, H., H. Kurz (1986): Gestaltungstherapie. In: *Seifert, Th., A. Waiblinger* (Eds): Therapie und Selbsterfahrung. Kreuz Verlag: 139-146.

Chapter 13
Letters to tinnitus

Gerhard Goebel

13.1 Summary

A dialogue with an absent person, an object or a significant symptom is an established element of Gestalt therapy and psychodrama. The goal of such exercises is to consciously perceive attitudes and feelings about an internalized object. During therapy the patient can make himself more comprehensible to the therapist and his fantasies can be examined for irrational cognitions. An important step aiming for the integration of tinnitus takes place when the patient starts to identify himself with his tinnitus and develops fantasies in which he converses with his tinnitus either in the form of role play, role reversal or a letter addressed to his tinnitus. Identification leads to a more conscious perception of the "psychological messages" or signal functions of tinnitus, to a dismissal of the unrealistic goal of "disassociation from the symptoms" and finally to an acceptance of tinnitus as an uncomfortable but basically constructive companion in life. Examples of this psychoanalytically oriented element of therapy, which is integrated into a behavioral medicine concept, are cited. The intention is less to describe a special therapeutic technique as to increase the reader's understanding of the suffering and consternation expressed in these letters.

13.2 Introduction

A dialogue with a symptom, an object or an absent person is an established element of Gestalt therapy and psychodrama. It would go beyond the scope of this book to present the possibilities and limitations of these effective techniques (for more information see Perls, 1976; Petzold, 1978; Moreno, 1959). Within the framework of our pain treatment concept, a dialogue with pain has been used for role play in group therapy from the beginning and it has proven itself as very helpful for all participants (Goebel, 1990).

One can incorporate the therapeutic element "letter to tinnitus" at any time in psychotherapy. Some therapists recommend asking patients to write a letter at the beginning of therapy. Others, however, suggest this intervention only when patients have a more advanced understanding of their symptoms (Wimmer, 1983).

For the therapist, the letter dialogue is first of all a means to gain a better understanding of the patient's problems. It may help to establish the initial diagnosis in relation to cognitive attitudes and emotions associated with tinnitus. When a patient refuses to fulfill this component it may indicate either a still deficient understanding of psychotherapy by the patient or a premature and too rapid step taken by the therapist. We therefore suggest to practise with such a dialogue with a motivated patient during group therapy. The patient first imagines that the tinnitus is sitting on an empty chair opposite to him and he tells the tinnitus everything which is on his mind in words or gestures. He then sits on the opposite chair and imagines that he is the tinnitus himself and responds to the accusations etc. previously made (role reversal). He can also ask a fellow patient to play this role. A dialogue can then develop, which may be compared with the technique described extensively elsewhere (see Chapter 8). Depending on the situation, other group members can support the patient by positioning themselves behind him and briefly articulating their thoughts, feelings or even appeals.

Catharsis, a method of Gestalt therapy, enables the patient to have actual physical contact with his tinnitus as symbolized by a block of styrofoam or a similar object, allowing him to express his desperation and rage in front of the other group members and to find reconciliation with his tinnitus. The patient is also able to recognize in which instances he still accuses perceived causes of tinnitus falsely (noise trauma, another person etc). Another experience in psychotherapy can be that the patient realizes that the experience of tinnitus is similar to prior experiences and it may then be possible for him to reappraise his tinnitus using methods oriented to depth psychology.

For the inexperienced reader it may appear very disconcerting that it is possible to speak with a symptom. If, however, one considers how often a person speaks loudly to himself when alone, reprimands himself, curses his sprained foot or gives body parts nicknames, it can be easily understood that this is also possible during therapy. In understanding the entire person, the question also arises whether all parts of the body, all physical symptoms, and physical reactions are components of the ego. We do not like to give up pleasant characteristics, abilities and those parts of our body which are conducive to our well being, but we like to get rid of cancerous or painful body parts as quickly as possible. We prefer to distance ourselves from undesired parts of our body and experience them as strangers. On closer examination, this subdivision of body parts and symptoms is not conducive to personal integrity. One part cannot exist without the other. If I try to get rid of my tinnitus I will lose my sense of hearing. If I anaesthetize my tinnitus with alcohol I will slowly lose my intellect. Everything is connected with one's ego: my liver is me, my ear is me, my tinnitus is me. Without me my tinnitus would not exist; I would, however, gladly get rid of my tinnitus; or, for example, my stuttering or my tendency to blush, etc.

If such an exercise does not fit into individual or group therapy, we suggest that the patients communicate with their symptoms in letter-form: the patient begins by writing a letter to his tinnitus. No specific instructions are given, whether the patient uses an informal or formal address is up to him. When he has finished writing the letter as authentically as possible (including date and signature) the patient should switch positions and imagine that he is the tinnitus himself. After reading the letter from the viewpoint of the recipient (tinnitus) he responds.

Identification with an undesired object leads to surprising experiences and developments which merit further examination. Without further commentary the following examples lead to a better understanding.

The following letters, which originated in various stages of therapy, have supported and often crucially facilitated psychotherapy. It is left to the reader to form his own opinion about this; perhaps it may even prompt one or two readers who suffer from tinnitus to utilize this idea for themselves.

Twenty patients who carried out a written dialogue with their tinnitus in the course of their therapy were asked for permission to have anonymous excerpts published. All patients gave their consent and were happy that they were able to contribute to a better understanding of their suffering. Once again I would like to express my gratitude for their support.

13.3 Letters to tinnitus

13.3.1 Example 1

13.3.1.1 Information pertaining to the patient

A postman, 50 years old, raised in a strict family, an ex-athlete, married, tense family atmosphere, built two houses largely on his own. Right-sided tinnitus in the form of intermittent whistling noises for a duration of 1 year. Slight bilateral hearing impairment of the inner ear with positive recruitment. Considerable phobic and depressive reactions ("There must be something wrong"). The letters were written during the first third of therapy.

13.3.1.2 Letter to tinnitus

To my tinnitus!

You fiendish tinnitus! Who actually gives you the right to sneak into my ear? I always carried out my work correctly and conscientiously, and now you come and rob me of my sleep and my tranquillity. I just don't understand how you could do something like that to me?

Not only do you disturb me at work, you are also very annoying when I get up in the morning or go to bed at night. You are always present and you will soon bring me to despair. You make my family suffer. Because of you I don't enjoy my job any longer.

It is just about time for you to disappear again from my life.

13.3.1.3 Response from the tinnitus

Why are you complaining about me? Aren't you to blame? Day after day you slave away, work from morning until night and don't allow yourself one single minute to relax. Life is not only work! At work you also tolerate too much. If I were you I would give your boss hell and tell him that things have to change.

You are to blame for the arguments in your family because you are never satisfied with what your family accomplishes. It is about time that you change your life and thoroughly think about your past mistakes. Maybe then I will be ready to disappear from your life and you can continue living in peace again.

13.3.2 Example 2

13.3.2.1 Information pertaining to the patient

Forty-four-year-old female laboratory technician, raised by her grandparents. Suffered from intense migraine attacks for 20 years, exhausted due to additional nursing obligations in the family. Right-sided broad band tinnitus for $1\frac{1}{2}$ years following sudden hearing loss and acute cervical-spine syndrome (brain tumor suspected initially). Slight right-sided hearing impairment of the inner ear, tinnitus 5 dB SL masked only by loud environmental sounds. Considerable disturbance of concentration and sleep disturbances; considerable guilt feelings due to depression and feelings of failure. The letters were written during the second third of therapy.

13.3.2.2 Letter to tinnitus

My other me!

As you have noticed by the way I addressed the letter, you know me already.

Since the beginning of March you have almost brought me to the verge of despair with your constant roaring and whistling.

But then I experienced peace in the Roseneck Clinic. This was a disaster for you. I do not control you completely, but you are now forced to constantly make an effort. When you rage I no longer steep myself into work until I'm exhausted, but make your roaring and whistling as pleasant as possible by taking breaks. Because I enjoy the seaside, as you well know, I will perceive your roaring as the sound of the surf, and by doing so will feel like I'm on vacation.

If I become too boring for you, write about what does not suit you. We may still become as one at some time in the future.

Yours truly,
B.T.

13.3.2.3 Letter from tinnitus

Hello R!

I am quite mad at you! I had you in my grasp for half a year, when you tried to distract yourself by working incessantly. Afterwards, when you were completely exhausted, I had a grand time of it. Now you have ruined everything with your therapy in Roseneck. During the first week and at the beginning of the second week you paid attention to me, but now you start to neglect me. Despite this fact I will not lose hope.

I still don't agree with your suggestion that we should again become as one.

Maybe you will still give me a chance.

Yours,
Not another me!

13.3.3 Example 3

13.3.3.1 Information pertaining to the patient

Fifty-five-year-old teacher, raised with many siblings in a very strict and religious family, frequent anxiety as a child, married with adolescent children. Following several left-sided attacks of sudden deafness the patient suffered from a bilateral high frequency tonal tinnitus for the last $1\frac{1}{2}$ years and moderate left-sided hearing impairment of the inner ear. Bilateral fitting of a masker. Considerable phobic and depressive reactions, fear of failure at work and repeated suicidal thoughts. The letter was written during the last third of therapy.

13.3.3.2 Letter to tinnitus

You damned tinnitus!

I curse you just as I curse the devil. You have maliciously assaulted me at night for almost $1\frac{1}{2}$ years and do not let go. It's just the opposite — you have become even more intolerable. After my attacks of sudden deafness I heard roaring in my ear, which was tolerable. But that was not enough for you, you soon became worse. You developed into a high-pitched, almost intolerable whistling in my left ear. But even that was not enough. To finish me off completely you decided to take possession of my right ear. You tormented me so much that I could not sleep any more and I had a terrible depression. At times you nearly toppled me over the edge, because my depression became so severe that I was often afraid of committing suicide.

Last year, my wife, our youngest daughter and I had booked a flight to Tunisia, for an Easter vacation, which we had looked forward to for months. Because of you we had to cancel the flight, and the depression was overwhelming.

You have robbed me of a great part of my quality of life. My ears have become so sensitive that I sometimes can no longer tolerate loud, happy laughter. This has also affected my family and social life. Wherever you accompany me the atmosphere is more subdued than in the past. I can no longer listen to loud music. I used to enjoy dancing but I cannot any longer, because you live in my ears. You make my wife and children miserable. You torment me so much at work that I can no longer concentrate, even though I only work part-time. You become so intolerable that you forced me to stop working and to resort to psychotherapy.

But I won't let you beat me. I will win and I will tear you apart. I will annihilate you and your brothers so that you can't torment anyone any more! Hope never to see you again.

M.

13.3.3.3 No letter from tinnitus

13.3.4 Example 4

13.3.4.1 Information pertaining to the patient

Thirty-nine-year-old professional soldier raised in a very competitive family. Early marriage, one child, career as officer. After repeated noise trauma and repeated sinusitis, bilateral permanent high-frequency tonal tinnitus for the last 3 years, slight to moderate hearing impairment of the inner ear in the high frequency range. Considerable depressive reaction with phases of suicidal tendencies and marital problems. Letters were written during the second third of therapy.

13.3.4.2 Letter to tinnitus

Hello you nerve-racking, horrid thing!

After 3 years I have decided to write, to share with you what concerns me; yes, what actually concerns both of us.

I hated you from the beginning. I tried to fight in any way possible, tried everything. But it was all in vain! I then began to suppress you, to ignore you. This worked out well, but I became lonely. Somehow you were always at the centre of my attention. I was lonely, even though I believed that I was able to control you. But the fact is that you were about to control me! Your behavior was quite insidious, you always ambushed me. But I am not unforgiving and I want to try to get along with you.

I would like to make friends with you and don't want to ignore and suppress you. I would like to get to know you better, to recognize your habits and merits as well as your weaknesses. In return I expect you to accept me and remain silent in "normal" situations. I just want you to make yourself noticed whenever I do something you don't like. I want to learn to live with you, and to experience you as a friend.

13.3.4.3 Letter from tinnitus

Hello my friend,

You wrote a letter to me recently and clarified several things. At the end of your letter you made many promises — are you willing to keep them? I realize that you actually have progressed, but you always relapse. You want me to be a friend, but does one kick friends around, does one make empty promises and does one ignore a friend?! You still have a long way ahead of you, and it won't be my fault if you don't make it. I will wait, but — not forever!!

Your friend tinnitus!

P.S. You cannot manipulate me and you cannot impress me when you're not true to yourself. Be the way you really are, then I will like you.

13.3.5 Example 5

13.3.5.1 Information pertaining to the patient

Fifty-six-year-old employee with technical training, married. Following an explosion which caused a perforation of the ear-drum, bilateral whistling tinnitus of a progressive course with considerable fluctuation of volume. Positive bilateral recruitment. Increasing isolation and development of phobia which included other organs. Considerable loss of performance, increasing exhaustion in the afternoon, difficulty in concentration and lack of sleep. Letters were written during the second third of therapy.

13.3.5.2 Letter to tinnitus

Mr Tinnitus,

You will understand that I cannot address you as "dear sir" and especially not as "dear". An informal address just does not fit at all.

You have destroyed all of my good feelings with your cruelty! Why do you torture people so? Torment them so? Do you enjoy it? Who allowed you to leave hell and assault people? At the beginning I would have asked you "Why me?" But after I had to tolerate this torment for so many years, I would not want this to befall others. I do not have a single enemy whom I would wish this to happen to.

Sometimes I'm close to despair when I notice that your shrill noise suppresses everything and controls me completely. And you do this on purpose.

Why do you want to get me fired? To isolate me from society? To kill me? But I will not grant you this victory. If I were dead I would not have to tolerate anything. But you, as devilish as you are, would find a new victim, maybe a young person as I was at that time, and you would also make this person unhappy.

Mr Tinnitus, I declare war! And if I can't destroy you, I will confine you to a "reservation", which you won't be able to leave. I want to know what you are up to. And if you try to escape, I will call you to order. I will make sure that you do not torture and torment me more than I will tolerate!

Be assured that this is not an empty threat as I have my allies. We will keep you in check!

My allies are:

1. My supreme boss, Jesus Christ; 2. My wife; 3. Dr L.; 4. My g.p. 5. My friends.

Mr Tinnitus, I know you are thoughtless and brutal and you enjoy torture! But even so my despairing heart beseeches you to be satisfied with the suffering I can tolerate and please remain in the reservation I offered you.

Please let me know of your decision soon and consider that you have already witnessed my suffering for 3 years.

P.F.

13.3.5.3 Letter from tinnitus

You wrote to me! You should know that I am unapproachable and don't find it necessary to react to demands or requests. You overestimate yourself if you think that I have personally chosen you to satisfy my sadistic tendencies. I have nothing personal against you. But you had bad luck and I have made myself comfortable inside you and will remain there. I'm a squatter. If you know how to evict me from your dear head, then do so! But you don't know how!!

With scornful laughter I read your suggestion to confine me to your head, to confine me in a "reservation"!

Who do you think you have inside you? It's me, tinnitus, and no headache, my inconsistent colleague who comes and goes! I, however, am here to stay. Maybe, I will eventually allow my sphere of influence to be limited to your head. But that is all that I could possibly promise you. Somehow you are right, thirty-two years is a long time even for me.

But beware. Do not delude yourself!

Your tinnitus

P.S. How about giving me a description of your allies sometime?

13.3.6 Example 6

13.3.6.1 Information pertaining to the patient

Forty-five-year-old engineer raised in a strict family, as a child: anxiety, shyness and tendency to blush, 3 siblings, married, one child. Menière's disease for 25 years. Increasing right-sided roaring tinnitus for 10 years, left-sided buzzing tones following sudden deafness three years prior to admission. Right-sided hearing impairment bordering deafness, slight to moderate left-sided hearing impairment, *hearing aid* for the left ear. Letters were written at the end of therapy.

13.3.6.1 Letter to tinnitus

To my tinnitus

Tino, you mean dog, since 1963 you torment me with your roaring in my right ear. For years I could cope with you well by concentrating on my career and family.

It was 1970 when you, my little Tino, settled down in my left ear and even though you are not as loud as big Tino, you still irritate me. Until 1987 I could cope with you both somehow. But then, after my left ear became deaf, you increased to such an extent that I can barely defend myself against you. Here at Roseneck I have learned how I can handle you properly and I will begin doing so immediately.

W.

13.3.6.2 Letter from tinnitus

Dear W

Your accusations are completely unfounded. It is your fault that we were able to develop so well. Your wanting to be better than others and your constant suppression of feelings have made it easy for us to ruin your life.

Big Tino and Little Tino

13.3.7 Example 7

13.3.7.1 Information pertaining to the patient

Fifty-four-year-old language teacher, raised in poor and isolated surroundings, later ambitious professional and political career, married, one child. A serious car accident (which was not his fault) caused a fracture of the base of the skull, cerebral trauma and left-sided high-frequency tinnitus with very irritating recruitment. Protracted convalescence, disturbance of concentration and headaches due to cerebral damage and tinnitus. Development of severe phobia and depression, suicidal phases, considerable strain in the marital relationship. Letter was written during the second and last third of therapy.

13.3.7.2 Letter no. 1 to tinnitus

Aren't you ashamed of yourself? Your whistling echoes through my entire head, you fill my brain with pain, but aside from that you exhaust my brain with your endless whistling. Even if you do not consider me, it is obvious that you have no respect for what is beautiful. What do you do with a good meal? You ruin it by whistling, as if the cook had added too much salt or pepper. Wherever I go or drive, the beautiful landscape of the Chiemgau and the Alps, Salzburg, the Corbières and even the magical and quiet valley of Fonto Gazela, where eagles perch in the sun on the rock called Klamensou, this valley with its scent of sweet oleander, spicy thyme and strong rosemary: you ruin all that by whistling incessantly. You intrude on a sky glistening with light and at night on the nightingale and the trickling of a brook.

But all this is only the beginning: you stand between me and my attractive wife. You chased away everything that I loved and valued: my social life — but not my entire life up to now!

I have, however, been victorious in one instance: even if you try to take away my sleep — and in the beginning you were even successful at that, I have taken it back and up until now I have defended it well. My sleep, which comes and goes every day, does not disappoint me. How much less will that eternal sleep disappoint me, an eternal sleep where you cannot intrude.

13.3.7.3 First letter from tinnitus

You complain about me, but I am a part of you. You are the one who is whistling — you, as well as my partners, your eyes. You are still able to enjoy a good meal!

And everything you lost — did you believe you had it for keeps? The little, well-cultured and erudite games you played with your pupils and which you were so proud of because you considered no one your equal — what kind of arrogance is that! Where is your modesty? Look, I give you the opportunity to be modest again. Here you must honestly acknowledge that I have never embarrassed you — imagine if I had done so in front of your pupils, showing them what state you are in now. Well? How do you feel now? Be happy that your pupils are still impressed by you and still think you are "great" — even if this is only a thing of the past. Other teachers just leave and don't give a damn what impression they made. Just be modest and acknowledge the fact that there are even worse situations in life!

Not only do I give you modesty, but also a new life. It was probably an exciting experience flying an aeroplane over the Pyrenees or the Sahara, but be honest: a charter flight is cheaper and less dangerous. And don't forget the risky situations you experienced! You're not getting any younger and more flexible. Just think about it, perhaps I do have good intentions.

And be honest: without me, would you have even thought of devoting yourself to Esperanto as a universal language that should be taught in all schools? This is now of utmost importance for you — would that be the case without my help? I am the one you owe thanks to. Look at it this way: I have enabled you to devote yourself to what you find most important. When you try to enjoy a good meal, imagine who is *actually* accompanying you: it is what you find most important. Be happy that what you find most important follows you around everywhere and doesn't desert you! It is self-evident that when you sleep, temporarily or eternally, that you don't find anything important anymore, not even me. But as long as you are awake and alive, I am in harmony with you and what is important to you.

13.3.7.4 Letter no. 2 to tinnitus

"You must honestly acknowledge" you write. So far I agree, but honesty has to count for both of us if a sensible conversation is to develop. And I have the impression that you want to deceive me by quite awkwardly using Dr Goebel's arguments, with whom you appear to be on more friendly terms than I.

I ought to be happy that my pupils cherish me, because they could also have experienced someone completely different. Yes, but only because of you I run this risk — without you I wouldn't be in this risky situation and I would be able to continue teaching! I don't need you and such circumstances to cure me of arrogance! Even the term arrogance is an unsuitable exaggeration. By the way: will I be rid of you when I've shed my "arrogance"? You are also dishonest when you mention other teachers — after all, you know that I am in a completely different situation. If at least I had a reason to be thankful to you (for example that I don't have to bother with strenuous students), then you would have an argument that I could understand.

In response to my being a pilot, you argue solely with the aim of tipping the scales. This is not honest, but at least you found something similar to an argument which is worth discussing.

Are you trying to make a fool of me with what you said in respect to my interest in Esperanto? The degree to which you see yourself as the catalyst of my interest is pure bluff. After all, you know that I did not need any additional encouragement in this respect before you came and began to torment me. One can't even say that you — by keeping me away from my work — have given me the opportunity to study this language properly: see how slow my progress is and how much you interrupt my efforts! In the past I could have done well — teach and learn Esperanto — and I would have felt satisfied; you know that!

And now the greatest nonsense of all: Even when your whistling ruins my every pleasure you want me to accept as a fact that you are not an austere prude, that you are the one who encouraged my interest in Esperanto. Don't you see that I could immediately get permission to teach Esperanto at my school from the Senate of Berlin — due to my social contacts — and that this would be the best, most effective method to promote Esperanto? But you ruined all my chances of succeeding with this endeavour. The tragic irony is that just as I started to learn Esperanto, I lost the opportunity to propagate it. And this personal achievement is barely worth anything. You are proclaiming my achievements as your own. And I, stupid ass that I am, even listen to you and am convinced for a while that you may be right. But that is due to the influence of Dr. Goebel with whom you seem to be on good terms.

You want to be a part of me? You crashed into me in the form of a car and had to fracture my skull to trespass.

What also betrays you is the fact that you wisely avoided addressing subjects I have not mentioned to you until now. Who caused such desperation that I was ready to poison you, taking into account that I would also be poisoned? When everything means nothing to me and death is better than having to live with you.

Who knows what will happen when I am alone with you again, without the people who want to help me. Maybe you will bring me to the point where I will be forced to get rid of both of us.

Respectfully,
W.L.

13.3.7.5 Letter no. 3 to tinnitus

Mr. Tinnitus

How should I interpret your silence? I see that you don't have any arguments left. So I would like to confront you with arguments which I slowly perceive in respect to the pupils you took away from me — perhaps you are in no position to judge my position properly because you didn't even know whom you crashed into with the car:

1. I was a talented teacher. I was aware of my talent — even in difficult situations — because I liked my pupils; and I felt acknowledged, I liked myself, and felt at home with myself.

2. Most pupils liked me, and those who didn't respected me, as well as the pupils' parents (where there were conflicts we mutually found solutions, for which they were very thankful — with very few exceptions), and my colleagues who regularly elected me as representative of the teachers' union.

3. I also won conflicts with the school board. And, instead of deteriorating, my relationship with the school board improved. After my accident I noticed genuine sympathy from those who once opposed me, as if they were upset by having lost a respected opponent by unfair means.

The following were essential for me: to like my pupils and be liked by them, a feeling of close contact, to be respected and liked by the pupils' parents and my colleagues and the experience of success in conflicts. I was grateful to the school for all of this.

By taking this away from me you have stolen an essential part of my life. The opposite feeling increasingly crops up: to be untalented, disliked and a loser.

It would be very unfair if you did not even answer me now, considering that you now know more of my personal situation.

Respectfully,

13.3.7.6 Letter no. 2 from tinnitus

Dear W.,

Don't you also find it absurd that we write only because you don't want to speak to me directly? We could have it much easier, but, as you wish.

In one of your letters you said you were my enemy. Why? Because you see me as your enemy? I want to tell you: because you suffer, that is why you have this hostile relationship which I did not intend.

But, as you wish. Actually I did not really know who you were before I, as you correctly say, crashed into your head with the car.

But am I some kind of a god? I became a part of you just as involuntarily as you entered into this world. Now we are together without having chosen each other. This is how it is sometimes. Do we want to get along with each other? I believe we have no other choice.

My first letter was an attempt to comfort you. What can we do? I think we should get things arranged and settle down comfortably. We should decide how we can tolerate each other best. I acknowledge that you have suffered a great loss because of me. But please don't blame me. I also have to cry when you despair. It really hurts and you feel that too. So let's consider the positive aspects.

First of all it is positive fact that you are not a pile of shit. You (better yet, we) are not yet the vegetable you fear you are. Just look, you are not bound to a wheelchair — no-one has to wipe your rear several times a day, etc. Certainly more such agreeable thoughts will occur to you if you contemplate this. The accident, which brought us together, could also have resulted in paralysis. So I must say, I am quite content to lodge in a comparatively athletic person whose rear does not have to be wiped. And if you should never have any friends who tell you this, I am with you and I will tell you this constantly.

Yes, what you wrote in your last letter is terrible. That is almost like losing your identity, so you have my complete sympathy. I also want everything to turn out differently, but neither I nor you can change the situation.

Many people are actually happy when they are rid of their professional stress. Shouldn't you be able to do this, even if you can't now? To be happy about what other people are happy about. You could actually be able to do that, or?

As far as flying is concerned, you have already acknowledged the point that not having to cope with difficult and dangerous situations is at least also positive. And at school? There was also a lot of stress, trouble and other unpleasant things. Be happy that you are now rid of all that, and then you may continue to be sad about what you lost. See the positive aspects, there are several more:

More time: you can do what you want, what you really enjoy.

More freedom of movement: you can drive wherever you like, you can stay wherever you like and, in fact, not only at quiet places, places you may travel to (thanks to me and your sensitivity to noise), but also at places that you enjoy for various other reasons.

Unencumbered you can pursue what is most important to you: Esperanto. Could you do that otherwise?

So think about it again and write. We'll stay in touch, OK?

Your tinnitus

13.4 References

Goebel, G. (1989): Verhaltensmedizinisches Behandlungskonzept psychosomatischer Erkrankungen am Beispiel des chronischen Schmerzsyndroms. Ärztezeitschrift f. Nat. v. Reg. 8: 587-599.

Moreno, J. L. (1959): Gruppenpsychotherapie und Psychodrama. Stuttgart, Thieme.

Perls, F. (1976): Grundlagen der Gestalt-Therapie. Einführung und Sitzungsprotokolle. Pfeiffer, München.

Petzold, H. G. (1978): Das Psychodrama als Methode der klinischen Psychotherapie. In: *Pongratz, L. J.* (Ed.): Handbuch der Psychologie. Bd. 8 Hogrefe, Göttingen S. 2751-2795.

Wimmer, J. (1983): Hilfe zur Selbsthilfe. Ein Therapie- und Übungsprogramm für Patienten mit sujektiven Ohrgeräuschen. Inang.-Diss., Med. Fakultät der Ludwigs-Maximilians-Universität München.

Yablonsky, Lewis (1978): Psychodrama: Die Lösung emotionaler Probleme durch das Rollenspiel. (Übersetzung *W. Krege.*) Klett-Cotta, Stuttgart.

Chapter 14

Does anxiety impair hearing? Body-oriented therapy in complex chronic tinnitus

Helmut Milz and Gerhard Goebel

14.1 Summary

Using a modified body-awareness test based on eutony according to G. Alexander (1983), phenomenological and biographical data of 26 patients with complex chronic tinnitus from the Roseneck Clinic are discussed from a holistic point of view. Our initial hypothesis was that the subjective experience of tinnitus leads to compensatory protective mechanisms of the entire body. After evaluating the body-awareness test it appears, however, that a revision of the original hypothesis is necessary. Instead, a detailed biographical case history of the patient is necessary with regard to earlier experiences of anxiety including unconsciously habitualized body posture.

Three case studies are a good description of the body-awareness test selected by us. In addition, this chapter contains brief references to the colloquial use of words and expressions related to hearing in the German language. References to the understanding of chronic tinnitus in traditional Chinese medicine supplement the perspective of a holistic view of tinnitus (Milz, 1989, 1992).

14.2 Introduction

The number of persons who suffer from occasional, intermittent or continuously disturbing sounds in their ears is much larger than the number of those who undergo medical and therapeutic treatment for tinnitus. In this respect the patients of this study belong to a specific subgroup of a larger group of acute or chronic tinnitus patients. Chronic tinnitus has changed their perceptions to such an extent that they are considerably impaired in their daily lives (complex chronic tinnitus). Seen from a holistic perspective, an individual symptom modifies the entire person, it impairs his awareness as well as his body because the body reorganizes itself around the symptom. The initial question we asked was how and in what manner does this occur in the case of chronic tinnitus.

It is a well known fact that tinnitus patients often complain about problems of the cervical spine as well as the lumbar spine. Our original assumption was that these tensions and problems were an expression of an acquired and compensatory protective mechanism, i.e. a result of tormenting tinnitus problems. Because only a few systematic investigations in respect to body-oriented therapeutic approaches in chronic tinnitus have been published, our interest was directed to the following question: initially are there similar "typical patterns" of body-awareness and body posture in patients with chronic tinnitus?

14.3 Our approach

The approach we selected to investigate body awareness of tinnitus patients had to satisfy two conditions:

1. It should rely on subjective body-awareness and perception.
2. Its proprioceptive and kinesthetic basis should not be influenced by cognitive and aesthetic considerations.

Our experimental procedure was based on a model which Gerda Alexander (1983) developed in eutony therapy. Eutony is based on a conscious perception and experience of proprioception with the goal of finding a flexible and appropriate degree of body tension.

14.3.1 Awareness exercise

In the first part of the exercise patients lie comfortably on their backs and listen to the therapist who guides them on a "voyage" through their body. The therapist concentrates on the skeletal system because it is the part of the body which allows us to stand upright. With the help of precise instructions, the individual parts of the skeletal system, from the toes to the foot, the calves to the thighs, from the pelvic area to the entire spine, from the chest and ribs to the collar bone and shoulder blades, from the arms to the hands and fingers and finally from the neck to the head are consciously perceived. The patient also concentrates on how his body is in contact with the floor. This unusual form of awareness exercise absorbs and focuses the attention of the patient in a particular way.

14.3.2 Modelling a putty figure

The patient remains lying on the floor, does not talk with other participants and receives four sticks of putty. The second part of the exercise consists of forming a human body with closed eyes using the putty for the next 20 minutes. The patients are instructed to make a model of a human body in general and not of their own body.

At the end of the exercise the patients discuss their observations, without interpreting them (phenomenological observation).

14.3.3 Phenomenological observation of the putty models

All models are observed using the following approaches and without any previous information concerning the patients' biographies:

— Were the models formed using one big piece of putty or were the four pieces of putty stuck together to form the model (analytic approach)?

— Was the head formed continuously as an extension of the torso or was the head given special attention, formed separately and then placed on the torso? (This may indicate that particular attention was given to the head.)

— Was all the putty used or was any left over?

— How are the proportions in relation to the size of the head and the rest of the body?

— Does the model tilt its head to one side and perhaps indicate an acquired body posture due to unilateral tinnitus?

— Does the posture of the arms indicate subjective dizziness often described by patients?

— Does the patient neglect certain body parts and in which way does this perhaps indicate existing "physical" memories of prior illness, traumas, operations or correspond with parts of the body which the patient has rejected entirely or perceives as problematical (synthetic approach)?

14.3.4 Results

Table 1 is an evaluation of the putty models. We used the chi-square test with continuous proof correction as a statistical instrument.

We found that about half of the 26 patients made their model in one piece ($n=12$).

In 7 of 9 patients whose models did *not* make a fragile impression, anxiety or phobic events were conspicuous in their biographies ($p < 0.1$; not significant). All figures which lost their head after modeling ($n = 6$) were also figures whose extremities were added to the body ($p < 0.05$; significant), and were also part of a group of figures ($n = 13$) in which the head had also been added to the body ($n = 12$; $p < 0.01$; significant).

With regard to the proportions between head and body, a normal relationship between head and body size was found in only four models. In five cases the head was estimated as being too small. The 17 models with a head that was too large came from patients who, in addition to the models' outstretched arms, also complained of severe dizziness ($p < 0.05$; significant). There were, however, no correlations between outstretched arms and symptoms of dizziness.

We were not able to find a correlation between the tilt of the head and the laterality of the tinnitus (Fig. 14.1). It was also noteworthy that no secondary sex characteristics were added in any of the models.

Considering the patients' case histories and biographical data, we found a direct relationship between damaged areas of the body of the model and specific physical symptoms of the patient. The damaged areas

Table 14.1 Details about the patients and their figures

Details about the patients:	n/entire random sample	Details in %
Age; average age 44 (±9.6)		
Sex: 18 men, 8 women		
Duration of tinnitus: average 7 (±6.6) years		
Subjective tinnitus volume (0-100) 66 (±14)		
Tinnitus discomfort (0-100) 60 (±12)		
Bilateral tinnitus	17/26	65%
Left-sided tinnitus	7/26	27%
Right-sided tinnitus	2/26	8%
Tonsillectomy: performed 24 years previously on average (±11)	16/28	62%
Dizziness	17/26	65%
Biography (childhood):		
Violence	14/26	54%
Phobia	17/26	65%
Isolation (e.g. institutionalization, divorce of parents)	9/26	35%
Details about the modelling of the figures:		
Formed from one piece	12/26	46%
Fragile structure	13/26	59%
Extremities formed separately	13/26	50%
Relationship of head to body:		
Head formed separately	12/26	46%
Head too large	17/26	65%
Head too small	5/26	19%
Head adequate	4/26	15%
Head tilting towards tinnitus	4/26	15%
Head tilting away from tinnitus	5/26	19%
Head tilting away from tinnitus:		
Left-sided tinnitus	5/7	71%
Right-sided tinnitus	0/2	0%
Head tilting towards tinnitus:		
Left-sided tinnitus	2/7	29%
Right-sided tinnitus	2/2	100%
Tilted head in bilateral tinnitus:		
Towards the left	6/17	35%
Towards the right	7/17	41%
Form of the neck:		
Neck too short	17/26	65%
Adequate neck	3/26	12%
Neck too long	6/26	23%
Neck too thick	9/26	35%
Neck broken off	6/26	23%
Other characteristics of the figure:		
Flat chest	14/26	54%
Impression of "inhibited breathing"	18/26	69%
Impression of "anxiety"	24/26	92%
Outstretched arms	19/26	73%
Correlation between dizziness/outstretched arms	16/26	62%
No correlation between dizziness/outstretched arms	9/26	35%
Signs of "body damage":		
Cervical spine syndrome	19/26	73%
Chest	14/54	54%
Arms	20/26	77%
Lumbar spine	15/26	58%
Pelvis	18/26	69%

related to prior injuries, diseases or abdominal and pelvic surgery.

Physical aspects of anxiety were present in 24 models. This was indicated by a narrow chest, raised shoulders, a missing neck and the frequent lack of feet or the inability to stand properly. No correlation between the models' narrow chest and the occurrence of anxiety/phobic episodes was found.

About half the patients had experienced early childhood violence or abuse. In 17 there were indications of phobic episodes and 9 experienced severe isolation due to the early death of a parent (often during World War II) or to divorce.

To explain the high number of "episodes of anxiety" in this group of patients, specific biographical details follow:

— Often intimidated by the mother during childhood; often received a "good and proper" beating; constant fear of being unloved; first attack of migraine at age 4; shyness during adolescence.

— Father was an alcoholic, was frequently beaten by him, stuttering and shyness during childhood, was forced to be right-handed.

— Father was an alcoholic, patient was beaten often, sexual abuse by the father, divorce, again repeated sexual abuse by the stepfather.

— Father was a prisoner of war for 8 years; mother beat him often; often afraid of air raids, general anxiety during childhood and adolescence.

— The patient reacted aggressively and unpredictably after his father was released from a P.O.W. camp when he was age 9, was always afraid to rebel, was very concerned with fulfilling obligations and being obedient.

— Seriously disturbed sleep (frequent nightmares) since childhood, afraid of father, who was an alcoholic and unpredictable. Shyness, blushing, running away from home and frequent digestive problems during adolescence.

— Only child, raised by grandmother, father was an alcoholic and had a violent temper, often had nightmares.

— Only child, father was killed in WWII,

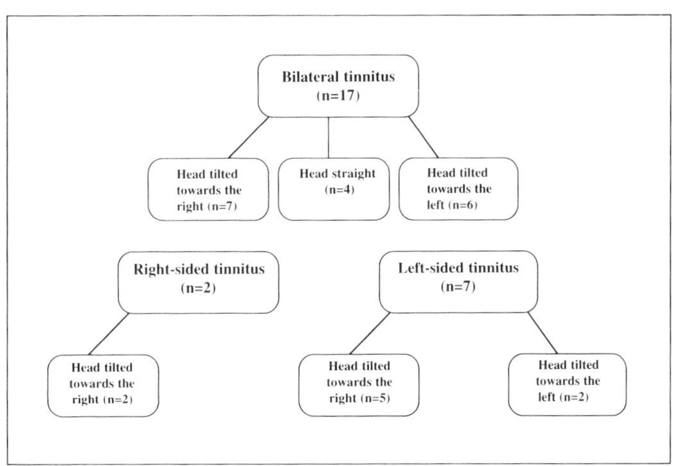

Fig. 14.1 Tilting of the head in the putty figures and tinnitus localization.

frequent beating with a whip, frequent corporal punishment at school, claims that he stuffed his ears for several years.

— Mother suffered from cardiac phobia with sensations of constriction, shortness of breath, fear of dying. Initial tinnitus problems after the daughter's birth, later chronic back problems, frequent dizziness and sleeping disturbances.

— Severe shyness and blushing during childhood, mother was very ambitious and dominant, "I avoid her as much as possible", believes that she only deserves to be loved for what she has achieved, has always had severe fear of punishment.

— Patient was sent to an orphanage at age 6 because the mother often abandoned her family which resulted in separation of the parents. Patient often suffers from dizziness, restlessness, anxiety and nightmares.

— Only child, was raised by the mother and a foster mother up to age 6, father returned from a P.O.W. camp in 1949, had a violent temper and beat him often. Complains of frequent sleep disturbances as well as social phobia.

— Family violence and traumatic war experiences.

— Had diphtheria as a child.

— The father was an alcoholic and frequently beat the patient, patient later witnessed his father's suicide using a pesticide (E605).

— Fell into a cellar during an air raid at age 5, since then repeated claustrophobic symptoms. Recurring dizziness.

— Suffered severely from whooping cough with danger of suffocation as a little child.

— Suffered a concussion with loss of consciousness at age 4, had 100–150 bee stings of the head and neck at age 7, remembers frequent nose bleeding, frequent anxiety as a child concerning brother's serious asthma, now frequent panic attacks with considerable subjective chest pain and fear of suffocation.

— Father died as a soldier during World War II, frequent blushing and stuttering since childhood, which led to hospitalization. Birth of a seriously handicapped son, since then severe anxiety concerning his son.

These are only brief biographical aspects. However, they all indicate obvious trauma and in some cases development of phobic symptoms. Most patients had chosen a so-called contra-phobic profession, which requires courage and responsibility (control). Our patients were, for example, a sailor, a nurse, an insurance salesman, an army officer, a safety engineer, a utilities engineer, a physician's assistant and a stewardess. This choice of profession could, on one hand, be coincidental, but it may also be interpreted as a means to repress and control perceived signs of weakness. It may be the case that these patients conceal their fears by fulfilling their professional obligations courageously. Frequent incidents of excessive independence and overexertion may be the result of overcompensation (e.g. trying to dissociate oneself from one's anxiety and fear).

An interesting fact is also that 62% of the patients had had a tonsillectomy.

14.4 Case reports

14.4.1 Case 1

14.4.1.1 Audiological data

The patient, a 50 year-old male, developed tinnitus due to occupational exposure to noise and a rheumatic disease. The tinnitus was bilateral and tonal with a frequency of 6000 Hz, and could be masked by narrow band noise. The supraliminal measurements indicated tinnitus of cochlear origin. A bilateral sensorineural hearing impairment existed starting at 6000 Hz of up to 60 dB. A hearing aid and masker were unsatisfactory. The tinnitus loudness was continuously rated as 80 on a visual analog scale (0-100), tinnitus discomfort was approximately 70 at the time of admission, control over tinnitus (coping) was rated as very low on the scale (10 at the beginning of therapy).

14.4.1.2 Medical history

The diagnosis at the time of admission was: bilateral complex chronic tinnitus. Additional diagnoses were ankylosing spondylitis (Marrie-Struempell Disease) and abdominal pain of unclear origin. Pyloric surgery as an infant, at age 14 concussion with loss of consciousness, at age 15 appendectomy and fracture of left wrist, at age 16 fractures of the second to fifth toes of the right foot, with amputation of the 5th toe. At age 24, pain in the lower back radiating to both legs as well as pain of the thoracic spine, shoulders, neck and upper arms as well as diagnosis of ankylosing spondylitis. The family history showed that father and brother also suffered from this disease. The patient observed that the whistling sound in both ears increased when moving the jaw muscles. At age 30, double surgery of the left elbow because of epicondylitis, at age 31 increased pain in both shoulder joints. During the initial physical examination, pain in the area of the 6th and 7th thoracic vertebrae as well as muscle tension of the entire vertebral column was present.

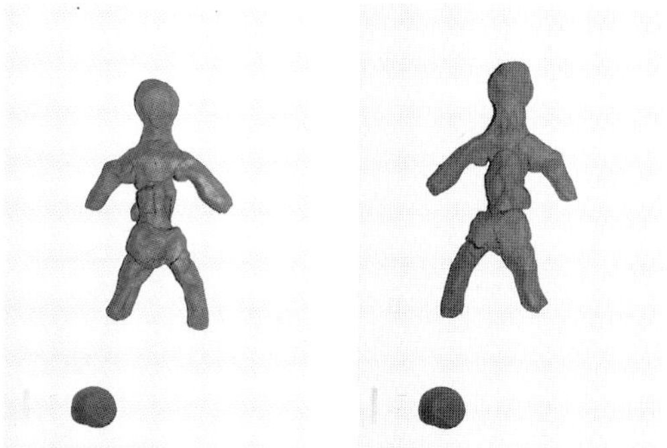

Fig. 14.2 Figure 1 (left figure = anterior position; right figure = posterior position).

14.4.1.3 Description of the putty figure

The relationship between the head and the rest of the body is clearly in favor of the head (Fig. 14.2). Even though all extremities are formed, the hands and feet are missing. The model appears to be subdivided into three parts: head/neck region, abdominal region and pelvis/leg region. There is an additionally formed plate-like layer on the abdomen. One can see that the neck is very thick. Seen from the front one sees how weakly the right leg is attached to the right hip with a great risk of breaking off. Seen from behind the body is also subdivided. The left leg is shorter than the right. The back is extremely fragile, especially the left half of the thorax where the figure seems to break apart. The patient had pieced the figure together.

The photographs of the model show that the fragile parts of the figure correspond with the patient's biography and medical history.

14.4.2 Case 2

14.4.2.1 Audiological data

The 42 year-old male patient suffered his first attack of sudden deafness of the right ear 10 years ago and recovered completely. For four years he had considerable problems with his cervical spine and suspected cervical disc prolapse leading to neurological defects in the left arm due to compression of the left median nerve. After a second attack of sudden deafness a hearing impairment of 50 dB and a predominantly tonal tinnitus of the left ear developed which could be masked with a narrow band noise of a loudness of 25 dB. The right ear had a hearing impairment of 30 dB at a frequency of 2000 Hz and the tinnitus could be masked with a narrow band noise of 5 dB. Alternating left-sided hearing loss was registered in repeated audiograms (fluctuating between 30 and 60 dB in lower frequencies). No hearing aid, no masker. The tinnitus loudness fluctuated between 40 and 80 on a visual analog scale (0-100), tinnitus discomfort between 30 and 70. Independent control over tinnitus on average 50 at the time of admission.

14.4.2.2 Medical history

Professional development: the patient was first a sailor, then a craftsman, and is now a male-nurse in an intensive care unit. Scarlet fever at age 5, at age 6 appendectomy and injury to the ligaments of his right leg. Pneumonia and gastritis at age 13. Also fracture of the lower arm as a child and bilateral double kidneys. Removal of the right meniscus as well as joint- and limb-pain at age 30. During the initial physical examination, limited mobility of the head/neck region, especially to the right, as well as hyperlordosis of the lumbar spine and vertebral kyphosis. The patient complained of disturbances of the sense of touch in the left hand with recurrent numb fingers. Bruxism was also present. In the MMPI (Minnesota Multiphase Personality Inventory), the patient indicated that he occasionally had obsessive-compulsive thoughts.

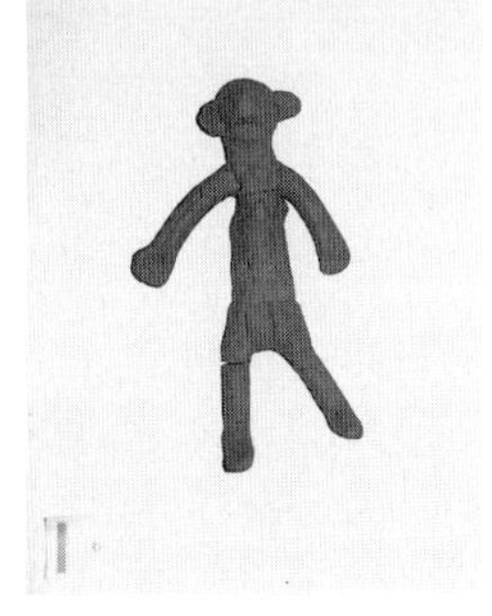
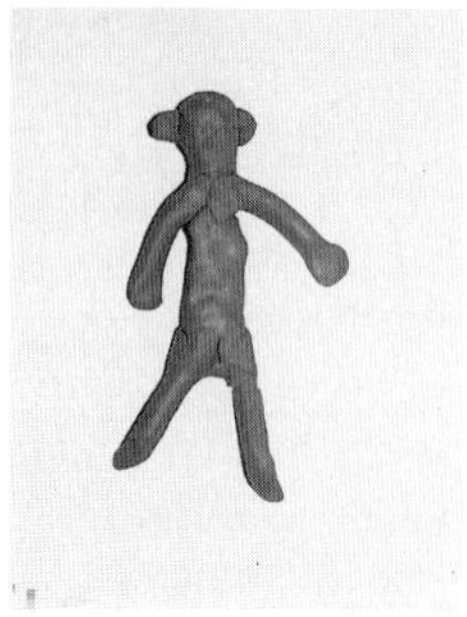

Fig. 14.3 Figure 2 (left figure = anterior position; right figure = posterior position).

14.4.2.3 Description of the putty figure

The model has an overproportioned head with very large ears and nose as well as a collar-like neck which overlaps with the shoulders (Fig. 14.3). The entire left side of the body is smaller than the right and the head tilts slightly to the right. The model consists of several fragments. There are weak points, especially the left shoulder with a somewhat shorter left arm and right hip which has the tendency to break off. The upper thoracic region is also weak and a plate-like reinforcement (as seen from behind) has been added to the right upper thorax. In the pelvic region the left pelvis is situated higher and the left leg is obviously shorter; the pelvic region consists of several parts. The right thigh is very fragile. The extremities are large and the shoulder region is so weak that the arms appear to grow straight from the neck.

Here, the model also coincides with the patient's biography and medical history.

14.4.3 Case 3

14.4.3.1 Audiological data

A 38 year-old male patient with normal bilateral hearing developed bilateral tonal tinnitus one year ago which fluctuated in its intensity and was caused by a cervical syndrome. Tinnitus frequency was ca. 6000 Hz masked by 20-30 dB HL. Tinnitus volume fluctuated between 50 and 90 on a visual analog scale (1-100), tinnitus discomfort between 40 and 90. Independent control over tinnitus (coping) had an average rating of 45 at the time of admission.

14.4.3.2 Medical history

Concussion with loss of consciousness at age 4. Suffered 100-150 bee stings of the head and neck at age 7. Frequent nose-bleeding. Frequent anxiety as a child due to his brother's serious asthma. Hospitalization because he had great difficulty swallowing and serious eating problems at age 13. First panic attacks with considerable subjective chest pain and fear of suffocation at age 21. His father died of a heart attack. He was always afraid of "going crazy". Appendectomy and orchitis. The patient's hobby was reading horror-novels, of which he had already read 350. Increased value for hostility in the SCL-test.

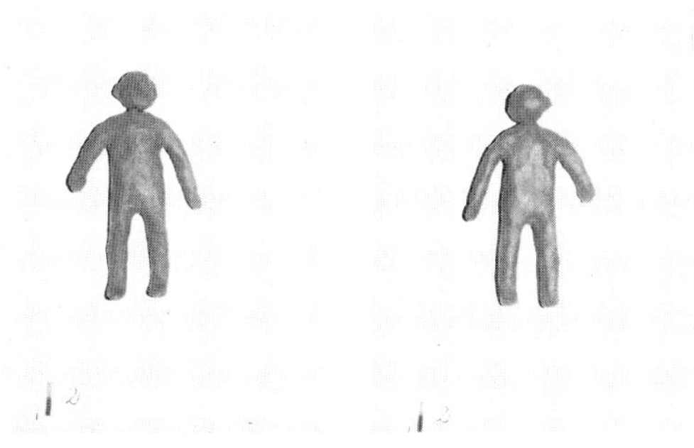

Fig. 14.4 Figure 3 (left figure = anterior position; right figure = posterior position).

14.4.3.3 Description of the putty figure

A very stocky torso with a very fragile head which was joined to the torso without a defined neck. The head tilts slightly to the left and both ears are large. The shoulders are stiff and tilt to the left, the arms rotate. The thorax, abdomen and pelvis are made from a single piece. The left leg is slightly shorter and not as developed. Seen from behind the right shoulder is weaker and the right half of the thorax is indented. The right leg is also less developed. All in all, the model makes a very compact and agile impression.

14.5 Conclusion

The development of body-oriented therapy for patients with chronic tinitus is only in the initial stage. Currently, relaxation training such as autogenic trailing and Jacobson's progressive muscle relaxation are used in particular. We know from our own experience and from corresponding research results that patients with chronic anxiety symptoms or anxiety disorders have considerable difficulties in learning relaxation training, because they have difficulties closing their eyes and "allowing themselves to relax". Here a technique such as eutony can help to improve relaxation. An interesting "side-effect" of the described eutony exercise is that it leads to increased relaxation by focusing the patients' attention on the forming of a putty figure.

Our original hypothesis was that momentary body posture and body awareness are essentially results of the experienced tinnitus. This hypothesis must be questioned following the evaluation of the figures and the patients' biographies as well as medical histories. According to our analysis, an accumulation of the patients' experiences of fear and loss, especially during early childhood, is apparent. This situation was often caused by the loss of one parent or divorce during early childhood. Frequent shyness and anxiety during adolescence are a continuation of this biographical development. As adults, the selection of a profession with increased personal risk or a high degree of responsibility is noteworthy.

Following characteristic posture reflects chronic anxiety: the tendency to pull the head between the shoulders, and to breathe flatly, which leads to a decreased movement of the diaphragm and decreased peristalsis, increased heart rate, a frequent feeling of constriction of the heart as well as the feeling of weightlessness or dizziness.

The putty figures also indicate this. Patients without anxiety were much more at ease when forming their figures. This appears to be similar to the physical phenomenon of "letting go".

An additional consequence of an anxious body posture is the inability to stand properly and, together with restricted breathing and lack of contact with the floor, dizziness and a tendency to fall.

A question which remains to be answered is to what extent increased neural activity influences equilibrium. Hypothetical guesses afford more accurate neurophysiological research. Another question is whether, as a result of chronic muscle tension of the neck due to anxiety, the circulation of the inner ear is disturbed and therefore contributes to the development of sudden deafness and tinnitus.

Disproportionately large heads with completely outstretched arms in the putty figures may correlate with symptoms of dizziness but further research is necessary.

Traditional Chinese medicine concerning tinnitus has two aspects of particular significance. The selected acupuncture points for tinnitus lie on the so-called "triple-warming-meridian". This meridian runs from the index finger to the arm and the shoulder, up to the neck and from the retroauricular region to the mandibular joint (Essentials of Chinese Acupuncture, 1980).

In traditional Chinese medicine, anxiety is assigned to the kidney meridian which embodies the inherent life energy. In traditional Chinese medicine the ear is assigned to the kidney meridian and to anxiety (Essentials of Chinese Acupuncture, 1980).

In the German language there are many etymological references which relate hearing to situations of repression, oppression and anxiety. J.-E. Behrendt also noted this (1990). The expression "those who don't want to *listen* must feel" indicates that a child must learn to "hear" what is required of him, or otherwise expect punishment, such as a "good and proper" spanking. Here Behrendt quotes Martin Heidegger, who was concerned that hearing was closely connected with a longing for security. Increased anxiety therefore emerges when this longing is not "heard" adequately and may promote the attempt to look for an inappropriate substitute such as dependent behaviour and an authoritarian society (in German: *hören* = to hear, *Hörigkeit* = bondage). Of interest is the fact that the Greek expression "hypakoein", the root of the term hypakusis (hearing impairment) also means to "subjugate" as well as to "oppress".

Could it be that our patients' search for security was only accomplished by exaggerated obedience? Could it be that the strong desire to "belong to" or of being "heard" is the root of anxiety and conceals itself behind a persistent symptom? Could it be that instead of the original anxiety only physical and psychological equivalents are now apparent? Could it be that anxiety and aggression have been internalized, and "stored" in the body? Could it be that "physically-embedded" memories and fears lead to anatomic changes and localised pathology? To what extent is it accurate that the constant defence against experienced anxiety leads to a defiant, and overtly courageous behavior as seen in the selection of "contraphobic professions"?

Could it be that tinnitus patients are afraid to give up their "physical substitute" symptom?

Our observations of a small and selected group of patients may only serve as a reference to possible directions of research from a psychosomatic viewpoint. Our results are not scientific evidence. They only intend to induce a better understanding of tinnitus in those involved in tinnitus research and therapy, as well as in the patients themselves. We have observed that many tinnitus patients are very sceptical of psychotherapy. Is this due to their being afraid of confronting the originally experienced anxiety?

14.6 References

Alexander, G. (1983): Eutonie. Kösel, München.

Behrendt, J. E. (1990): Das Dritte Ohr. Vom Hören der Welt. Rowohlt, Frankfurt a. M.

Essentials of Chinese acupuncture (1980); Foreign Language Press, Beijing.

Milz, H. (1989): Ganzheitliche Medizin. Heyne, München.

Milz, H. (1992): Der wiederentdeckte Körper. Artemis und Winkler, München, Zürich.

14.7 Appendix Instructions for self-treatment of muscle tension of the neck and jaw

Dean Marson developed these exercises and we would like to thank him for his efforts when he worked as a guest therapist at the Roseneck Clinic.

Relaxation of the neck and jaw

Please lie on your back on a firm surface during the following four exercises and take a break between the individual steps.

Step 1

Body position

The head rests on both hands with the palms facing up. The finger tips meet at the center of the back of the neck and the middle fingers are situated at the base of your skull.

Movement 1

Slowly lift your head using both your ring fingers and your little fingers so that your chin slowly moves in the direction of your chest. This stretches your neck. Your jaw should be slightly open and the stretching can be slightly increased during inhalation and relaxed during exhalation. Please repeat this movement 3-4 times and then rest.

Movement 2

The hands are in the same position. This time, move all fingers of your right hand so that your head passively rolls to the left without leaving the floor. Your jaw is slightly open while you breath through your mouth. Then repeat the same movement using the fingers of the left hand — and let your head roll to the right. Slowly repeat rolling your head back and forth about 5-6 times and be careful that your hands remain active while your head and neck are moved passively.

Take a break.

Step 2

Body position A

Gently hold your chin between the thumb and index finger of both hands.

Movement 1

Please breathe through your mouth and carefully move your chin up and down with both hands, then from side to side. Again be careful that your hands are active while your chin remains as passive as possible.

Body position B
Please put the finger tips of both hands to both sides of your jaw at the level of the joint, (in front of the right and left ear). Place your thumbs under the jaw bone on both sides.

Movement 1
Please breathe through your mouth and press your finger tips lightly on the muscles of your jaw and lightly pull your jaw forward. Then, with your finger tips and thumb, slowly stroke the entire jaw muscle with a downward motion and apply a gentle but clearly noticeable pressure, with the fingers moving slowly downward.

Movement 2
Repeat the same movement, this time, however, using one hand only each time and again allow the head to roll away from the active hand. This time be especially aware of the stretching which you feel in your neck.

Allow yourself enough time to repeat this exercise 5–6 times. Take a break.

Step 3

Body position
The left arm lies beside your body or rests on your stomach while the right arm rests on the upper left side of your chest with the right thumb over the left collar bone.

Movement 1
Now allow your head to actively roll to the right while it remains on the floor. Open your jaw and at the same time gently press your left shoulder with your right hand. This time notice the stretching reaching from jaw to shoulder along the front of your neck. Breathe through your mouth and exhale while you make the stretching movements. Repeat this exercise on the other side.

Repeat this exercise several times on each side; once with your jaw open and the next time with your jaw closed. Notice the difference in the ability to move your head between movements with a closed and open jaw while stretching.

Step 4

Body position
Lock your hands together so that the back of your hands face each other and place them under your head with the back of the hands to the floor so that the fingers face up and your neck rests on a small "cavity" formed by your fingers.

Movement 1
Slowly press all fingers together so that both the head and chin tilt somewhat in the direction of your chest causing a slight stretching of the neck. Slowly repeat this exercise several times.

Movement 2
Move your finger tips and thumbs back and forth along your neck muscles from the base of the head down to your shoulders and massage the muscles.

Movement 3
Apply pressure with the finger tips of one hand at a time and at the same time allow your head to roll from one side to the other. This time the jaw is also slightly open and you breathe through your mouth. Slowly repeat all these steps several times and notice where you feel the sensation of stretching. (For additional exercises see appendix in Chapter 15.)

Chapter 15

Tinnitus as a dental problem Effects of the temporomandibular joint and bruxism Diagnostic and therapeutic possibilities

Werner Neuhauser

15.1 Summary

Tinnitus can also be a dental problem. This chapter is concerned with pathological changes of the jaw and facial region which trigger tinnitus. We intend to describe the interrelationship between the stomatognathic system and hearing-research results, diagnostic measures, and the possibilities available to the experienced dentist to carry out a promising, effective treatment.

15.2 Introduction

The close association of the temporomandibular joint with tinnitus is demonstrated by the fact that the majority of tinnitus patients suddenly — if usually only temporarily — experiences increased tinnitus loudness while biting or notices a change in the quality of the tinnitus when moving the temporomandibular joint.

Furthermore, tinnitus can be improved or eliminated by dental measures such as eliminating premature occlusal contact, prosthetic replacement of missing teeth, occlusal overlays, splinting for programmed condyle repositioning after functional analysis, extraction of third molars, eliminating bruxism and other measures. On the other hand, it is also reported that after a difficult extraction or mandibular surgery requiring application of great force, hearing problems may occur.

Whether tinnitus is present or not is a question which is always asked and documented during a clinical functional analysis (see appendix 1). The fact that the author himself suffers from tinnitus is ironical, as dentistry was not able to eliminate the tinnitus, only the problems connected with the temporomandibular joint.

Myrhaug (1969), on the other hand, determined in his patients with disorders of mastication, that every third or fourth patient also had problems with hearing and the vestibular system. How many of these had tinnitus was not determined. No percentages are given by either Schulte (1983), who pays detailed attention to tinnitus, or Rubinstein et al (1987) or Erlandsson (1987), although all four research groups treated a relatively large number of patients with tinnitus successfully by treating existing dental problems.

15.3 Epidemiology

No definite statistics are available regarding the percentage of patients with a stomatognathic system disorder who also suffer from tinnitus. Hupfauf (1963) could only find three patients with tinnitus among 133. Graber (1987) also rarely observed the symptoms as described by Costen.

15.4 Etiopathogenesis of tinnitus in association with diseases caused by dysfunction

Disorders caused by dysfunction of the jaw and facial muscles are complex and difficult to comprehend. Graber (1987) gives

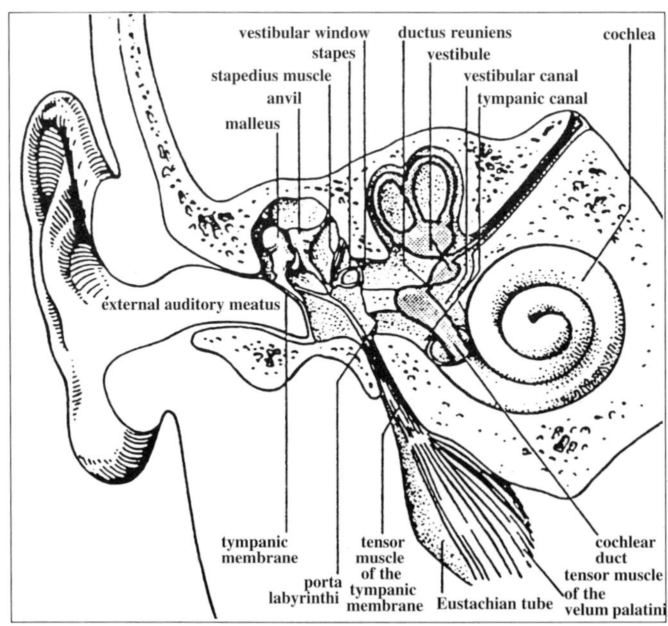

Fig. 15.1 The anatomy of the soft palate and the inner ear. The tensor muscle of the tympanic membrane and the tensor muscle of the velum palatini run parallel to each other and are directly connected. Both muscles are innervated by the trigeminal nerve (from Drumm, W., 1972).

the following explanation for tinnitus as described by Costen:

Tinnitus and vertigo are caused by hyperactivity of the middle ear musculature (tensor muscle of the tympanic membrane, stapedius muscle via the stirrup bone) in association with stimulation of the autonomic fibers (tympanic plexus, tympanic nerve, chorda tympani). In evolution the tensor muscle of the tympanic membrane stems from the same pharyngeal arch segments as the masticatory muscles and is supplied by the same nerve (Fig. 15.1). The reptilian temporomandibular joint evolved as a part of the hearing system: the former articular bone became the malleus, the quadratum bone became the anvil and a part of the masticatory musculature is now the tensor muscle of the tympanic membrane, modulating tension of the ear drum. In other words: we hear using structures which were part of the temporomandibular joint originally.

Ear pain is triggered by joint pain and by muscle spasms of the lateral pterygoid muscle and the middle ear musculature as well.

According to Borner (1987) patients (quoted from Graber, 1987) with this disorder can be subdivided into four groups:

Group 1: Primarily Occlusal factors.
Occlusal disorders in association with stress or other factors lead to bruxism and tendomyopathy and disorders of the joint.

Group 2: Primarily psychological factors.
Psychological conditions of tension and continuous stress cause muscular hypertension. The teeth become the emotional outlet.

Group 3: Primarily abnormal psychology/ psychiatric illness
A true psychological disorder is the underlying disorder. The patients either suffer from an occlusal neurosis or a psychosomatic pain disorder.

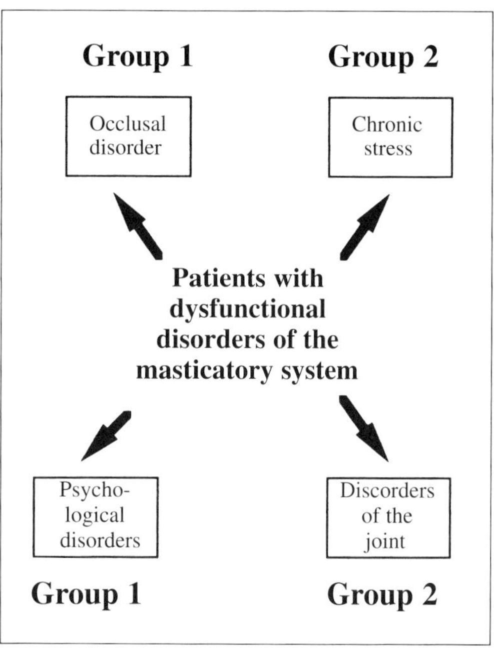

Fig. 15.2 Classification of patients according to Jäger et al. In addition to the primary etiologic factors, others may be available in any combination (in all groups): situational stress, posture disorders, spondylarthrosis, stress due to chronic pain (Jäger et al., 1990).

Group 4: Primarily articular factors
Patients who have polyarthritis or polyarthrosis also often have disorders of the temporomandibular joint. Resulting from proprioceptive and autonomous reflexes, the musculature becomes tense and thus spastic (splinting effect!).

Jäger et al (1990) attempt to classify four groups (Fig. 15.2) in a similar way.

These four groups are the starting point for diagnosis and therapy. The patient must feel sure of the dentist's empathy. Consultation with the aim of establishing the patient's confidence is the first step in the direction of medical and dental diagnosis.

15.4.1 Bruxism, parafunctions, excentric occlusions, muscular hypertension and tinnitus

If modern man only used his teeth for chewing, they would be used for only 15–20 minutes each day for food (that has been prepared in most cases). Wearing down would be extremely slight, because, while chewing, the protruberances of the teeth, which are covered with the hardest known substance of the body — tooth enamel, barely come in contact with each other. The fact is, however, that about 90% of our population show more or less severe abrasion on the chewing surfaces of the molars and premolars, and excentric, sometimes very individual patterns of abrasion in the region of the incisors and especially in the canines. This means that the teeth contact each other more often and will move with more force due to psychomotor activity than due to chewing. The pathogenetic implications of this malfunction have been to a great extent underestimated. Most myoarthropathy is the result of centric and excentric mastication and therefore can be responsible for the development of tinnitus. Bruxism puts great demands on the masticatory musculature — including the double-hinged temporomandibular joint, which is responsible for facial expression and speech — leading to damage.

Because Glavos (1980) investigated this phenomenon, we know the following details: 30.7% of the American population grind their teeth. The nocturnal grinders comprise 15.7%. Those who predominantly grind their teeth during the day are predominantly "pressers" and account for 63.2% of the population with parafunctions. Those who press and grind their teeth during the day and at night compose 21.1%. Somewhat fewer women (48.3%) do this than men (51.7%). The investigation found a clear dependence on various stress factors. Over and above that, higher coincidence exists within families. A disadvantage which I see in this investigation is that the average age was 19 years. I can say from my own experience that the percentage of central Europeans who grind their teeth, especially at night, is considerably higher (Table 15.1).

Details about this are provided by Schulte (1983) who for many years examined patients with impaired hearing for functional disturbances at the ENT clinic in Tübingen. In the vast majority of cases he found an obvious correlation. In unilateral sudden deafness and tinnitus, in unilateral palatal nystagmus and various subjective hearing impairments, excentric parafunctions existed on the contralateral side, conspicuously often on the right side. He also found a statistically more frequent left laterotrusive parafunctional tendency. He observed increased centric parafunctions in bilateral tinnitus. He diagnosed glossodynia, which often occurs simultaneously, almost exclusively in excentric parafunctions. He found a functional explanation because in most cases the mandible and the tongue, or only the tongue, are pushed forward and against the inner surfaces of the front teeth and the hard palate. He also discussed stress as a trigger of the parafunctions and mentioned neuromuscular causes.*

Miltner et al (1986) discussed behavioral therapy in this context, including EMG-biofeedback methods and so-called negative exercises and came to the conclusion that sufficient criteria did not exist to decide whether behavioral therapy of bruxism is indicated or not.

* The leaflets and instructions which *Schulte* gave to his patients are listed in the Appendix.

Table 15.1 Incidence and Stress

	Total N	Nervousness (%)	Anger (%)	Frustration (%)	Distress (%)
Total	1 052	14.9	26.0	16.9	37.5
Without bruxism	729	6.6	20.3	9.1	26.2
With bruxism	323	33.7	38.7	34.7	62.8
During the day only					
At present	141	48.9	50.4	48.2	78.7
Previously	126	38.1	46.0	42.1	71.4
Present and previously	182	41.2	46.2	41.8	73.6
At night only					
At present	35	14.3	5.7	14.3	25.7
Previously	69	8.7	13.0	10.1	24.6
Present and previously	79	10.1	12.7	10.1	25.3
Both day and night					
At present	47	51.1	57.4	48.9	89.4
Previously	51	45.1	51.0	49.0	80.4
Present and previously	62	41.9	50.0	45.2	79.0

Family incidence

	Total N	Family (%)	Parents (%)	Siblings (%)
Total	1 052	29.0	11.8	18.2
Without bruxism	729	24.7	9.5	14.8
With bruxism	323	38.7	17.0	25.7
During the day only	182	37.4	19.2	22.0
At night only	79	38.0	12.7	29.1
Both day and night	62	43.5	16.1	32.3

15.5 Symptom complexes caused by dysfunction of the jaw/facial muscles and tinnitus

15.5.1 The so-called Costen syndrome

The entire complex of periauricular problems and pain is called the "Costen-syndrome" because it was described by Costen (1934), even though this syndrome was previously described by Prentiss (1918), Monson (1920) and Wright (1920). The symptoms described at that time were periauricular pain, hearing impairment, vertigo, tinnitus, headache, glossopyrosis, herpes of the external auditory canal, and dryness of the mouth. All authors indicated that the early loss of molars caused these problems and their hypothesis was that the loss of molars caused a dorsal shift of the condyles of the temporomandibular joint leading to pressure on the auriculotemporal nerve, the chorda tympani as well as on the structure of the inner ear. Figure 15.3 documents the anatomical proximity of the temporomandibular

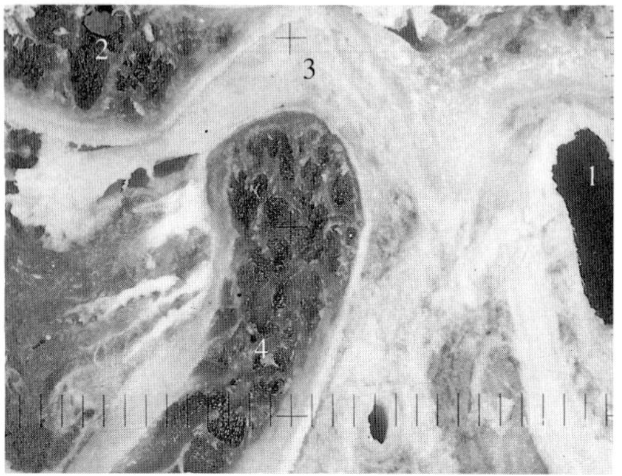

Fig. 15.3 Sagittal section of the middle third of a left temporomandibular joint: close topographical relationship between the external auditory canal and the dorsal edge of the temporomandibular joint. (1) external auditory canal; (2) eminentia articularis of the mastoid process; (3) articular disc; (4) head of the temporomandibular joint (condyle).

joint and the auricular region. The immunohistochemical sample (Fig. 15.4) shows the high degree of ennervation of this region.

In the following period a controversy concerning the entire subject developed,

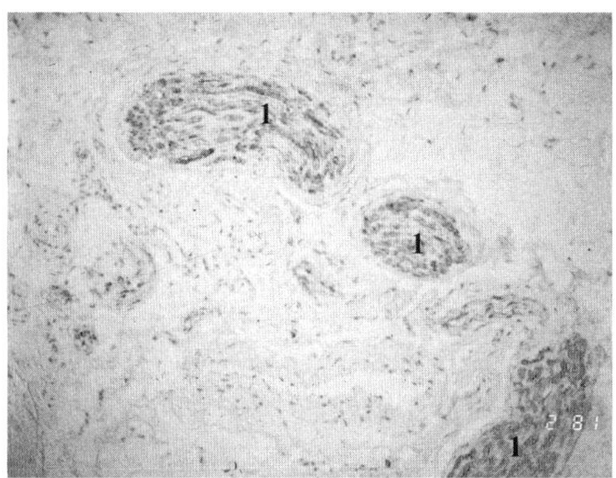

Fig. 15.4 Immunohistochemical depiction of nerve structures (1) of the dorsal region of a temporomandibular joint: abundant innervation of the region adjacent to the hearing region (enlargement 1000 ×; antiprotein S-100 staining). For the kind use of Figs. 15.3 and 15.4 we thank Dr J. Müller of the Dental Clinic, of the Ludwig Maximilian University in Munich.

not only for the reason that only a maximum of four of the eight described symptoms of the syndrome could be verified (Motsch, 1980).

These conflicting views, however, slowly led to feasible diagnostic and therapeutic results with regard to the entire syndrome as well as symptoms pertaining to the ear. Myrhaug (1969) examined 1986 patients with temporomandibular joint disorders whose symptoms correspond with the Costen syndrome and made an important discovery. It is important to know beforehand that these problem-patients had temporomandibular joint disorders due to bruxism i.e. parafunction of the masticatory muscles caused by pressing and grinding the teeth against each other. Myrhaug found that these patients jerk or flick their soft palate repeatedly and spontaneously in an upward direction without discernable reasons. This caused a cracking or clapping noise. He was able to show electromyographically and acoustically that a parafunction of the tensor muscle of the veli palatini existed. This muscle is in direct contact with the tensor muscle of the tympanic membrane, a muscle which stretches the ear drum (Fig. 15.1) and both are innervated by the trigeminal nerve. Drum (1972) notes: "Now it is easy to understand that the chain of the hearing ossicles is displaced by pulling and vibration due to rhythmic parafunctional contractions of the tensor muscle of the tympanic membrane. In the course of time, this causes damage to hearing ability and could cause tinnitus. If the chorda tympani which is situated between the malleus and the anvil, is compressed and stimulated, glossalgia (a burning tongue) can also occur."

For this reason it is evident that tinnitus must also be seen as being associated with parafunctional disorders of the jaw and facial region. A development took place in dentistry which enables clinicians to record and analyse complex functional interrelationships today. One speaks of clinical and instrumental functional analysis and therapy,

Table 15.2 Disorders caused by dysfunction of the jaw and facial regions:

- *Costen* syndrome (*Costen*, 1934)
- Temporomandibular joint dysfunction syndrome (*Lupton*, 1969; *Shore*, 1959)
- Myoarthropathies (*Graber*, 1972; *Schulte*, 1972)
- Pain dysfunction syndrome (*Laskin*, 1969; *Voss*, 1964)
- Temporomandibular joint pain dysfunction syndrome (*Schwartz et al*, 1959)
- Tendomyotic syndrome of the jaw and facial region (*Graber*, 1980)
- Occlusomandibular disorders (*Gerber*, 1971)

Symptoms (*De Boever*, 1979; *Graber*, 1972):
- Noises of the joint such as crepitus and cracking
- Movement limitations of the mandible: limitation, deviation sideways while opening, impaction of the disc and blockage of mandibular movements
- Subluxation
- Pain in the joint area
- Spasms of the masticatory musculature associated with fatigue and pain
- Pain projected to other muscle groups (chain tendomyosis) e.g. eye region, crown of the head, cervical area, neck, shoulders and upper arm
- Globus hystericus in the neck and problems with swallowing
- Pain projected to individual teeth or groups of teeth
- Ear symptoms such as decreased hearing, tinnitus, vertigo
- Saliva secretion disorders
- Disorders of the sense of taste

as the term "gnathology" is no longer used in Europe. The early loss of molars, which was the only cause for parafunction according to Costen and his predecessors, can no longer be accepted as the only cause. This is expressed by the fact that, instead of the "Costen syndrome", numerous other terms have been used by subsequent authors (Table 15.2).

According to Graber (1987), of principal importance for the course of the disease are: pain, muscle tension and functional limitation.

Pain, largely myogenic, is elicited by functional diseases of the tendon–muscle complex (tendomyopathy).

Some clinicians indicate occlusal disorders and muscular hypertension resulting from it as causes of muscle tension. Even an abnormal position of the mandible caused by malocclusion is listed as a triggering factor (Gerber, 1971; Mongini, 1985; Palla, 1985; Ramfjord, 1971; Shore, 1959; Yemm, 1979).

Other authors (Graber, 1972, 1980, 1983; Kydd, 1959; Pilling, 1977; Rugh and Solberg, 1979, 1985) see a considerable etiologic factor in emotional conditions of tension, or even in psychological disorders.

Psychologically stimulated hypertension, especially in the masticatory musculature, leads to increased long-term tooth contact. Grinding and pressing (bruxism) results in a traumatizing potential sufficient for joint and muscle disorders. This results in reactive muscle tension (tendomyosis) of the jaw, face and neck regions.

Muscle tension and limitations of movement of the mandible have a secondary effect on the temporomandibular joint; deforming arthropathies can develop.

Graber et al (1980), a research

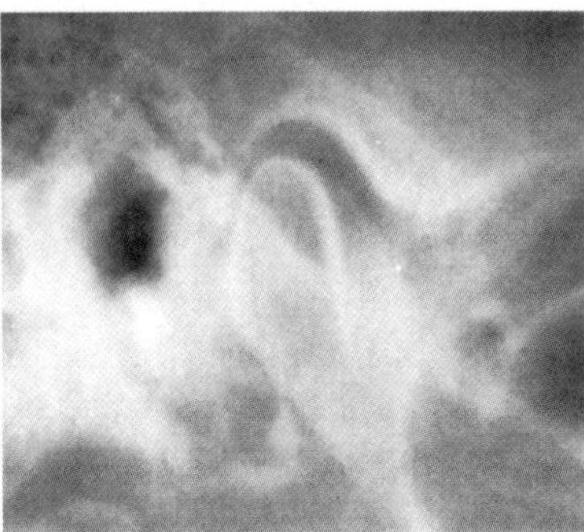

Fig. 15.5 The dorsal joint cavity, leading to the ear, is narrow and compressed. Example of dislocated posterior compression joint.

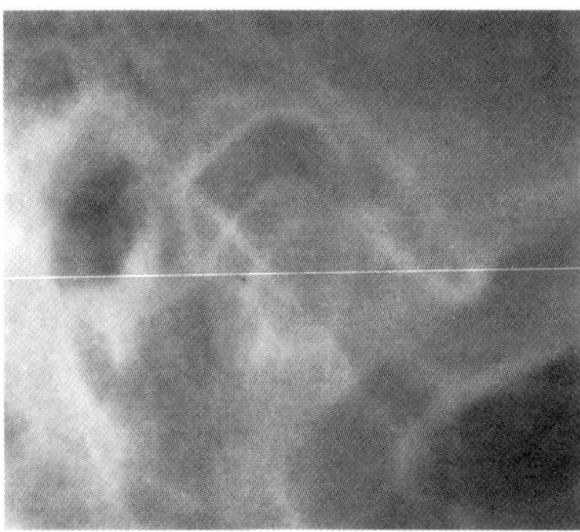

Fig. 15.6 The condyle is shifted in a mesial direction. Example of a mesial compression joint.

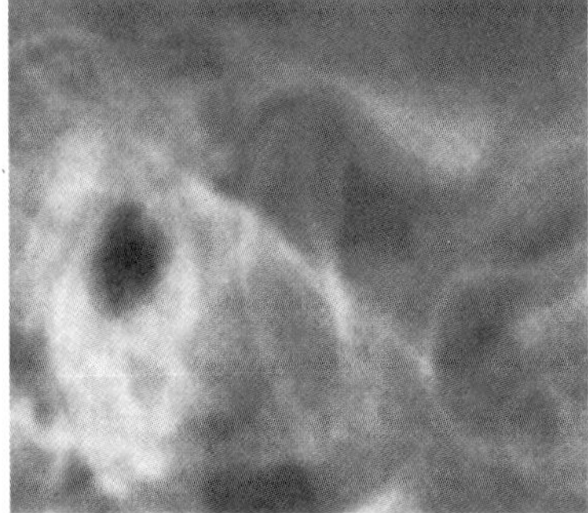

Fig. 15.7 The condyle is dislocated and is situated directly over the external auditory canal. Example of a compression at the peak of the joint cavity. Example of a superior compression joint (Motsch).

group consisting of dentists and rheumatologists, found that these symptoms are often localized symptoms of generalized tendomyopathy. In these cases neither the malocclusion nor displacement of the temporomandibular joint were primary triggering factors.

"Even primary disorders of the temporomandibular joints such as, for example, polyarthrosis and polyarthritis can lead to muscle tension by means of proprioceptive and autonomous reflexes" (quoted from Graber, 1987).

Motsch (1980) and Bumann et al (1989) suggested replacing the term "Costen syndrome" with the diagnosis "compression joint", a diagnosis which can be documented radiographically (Figs. 15.5, 15.6, 15.7).

Above-mentioned research and the comprehensive review shown in Table 15.2, are a brief as well as precise description of our present state of knowledge about the pathological mechanisms of the stomatognathic system. This summary also serves as a basic starting point for a more differentiated and extensive approach but this would, however, exceed the scope of this chapter.

15.6 Diagnosis

Diagnosis relies on three methods:

I. Detailed *clinical functional analysis* with the help of a questionnaire (functional status, see Appendix) which summarizes all objective parameters of the dysfunctional problems as well as the subjective details of the patients.

II. The *instrumental functional analysis* summarizes the results of the clinical examination. Jaw models are fabricated and mounted in an articulator. Thus, all centric and habitual functions can be simulated. The SAM-2 articulator provides an indicator analysis of the mandibular position (Mack, 1980). The deviation of the condyle positions of both temporomandibular joints from the normal (mounted) centric position can thus be obtained in three dimensions. If the resulting values do not agree, a dysfunctional disorder can be assumed. Whether the temporomandibular joint is the cause of hearing impairment or not cannot be established using this method.

III. Radiographic methods:
A transcranial, excentric x-ray according to Schüller (1911) in the modified version of Lanffs and Evans (1988) enables a sufficient localization of the condyles (decentralization). In 90% of the cases the radiographic result agrees with the intermittent functional analyzing according to Bumann (1989) (Figs. 15.5, 15.6, 15.7).

These three methods are the starting point for future therapy.

15.7 Therapy

15.7.1 The medical consultation

One of the first steps is to discuss all the examination results with the patient, especially regarding possible causes. Tinnitus is always only a part of, for example, existing generalized muscle tension and/or changes in the temporomandibular joint. Uneconomic muscle functions are always associated with parafunctions and frequently also with stress and psychiatric illness as well. The patient must be taught to observe himself more closely: improper posture at work and other habits are the starting point for individual self-treatment. I recommend "visual reminders", a method recommended by Schulte (1983). Whenever the patient, for example, sits at his typewriter at work he is reminded by a visual symbol stuck to the typewriter ("Japanese flag" — a red dot on a white background) to observe whether he is grinding his teeth or clenching them in a parafunctional position. If stress is present, stress reduction in the form of sensible changes of life-style is important. The dentist is definitely able to guide the patient properly. Schulte (1983) developed a detailed and reliable self-massage technique for the masticatory muscles, together with isometric and isotonic exercises. Finally, considerable discipline on the patient's part is required in out-patient treatment (see Appendix 3).

15.7.2 Initial treatment of pain

A myofacial pain syndrome occurs often in association with acute tinnitus as well as with chronic tinnitus. Schulte (1983) noted that the best success is achieved in patients with a brief case history. In addition to his retraction exercises — he described an impressive example in one of his case histories (a medical colleague's bilateral tinnitus disappeared after a 14-day treatment) — he recommended local anesthesia of the lateral pterygoid muscle for tinnitus and sudden deafness. With so-called objective ticking of the ear caused by tympanic nystagmus (with or without palatal nystagmus), he recommended local anesthesia of the medial pterygoid muscle. Even a placebo effect justifies these measures.

He also recommended the extraction of impacted third molars (retained wisdom teeth) and mentioned eight cases in which tinnitus disappeared after all previous measures had failed.

15.7.3 Further therapy

If occlusal disorders can be established as the primary cause by clinical and instrumental functional analysis, occlusal therapy is necessary.

> **Caution:**
> All occlusal changes should be tested with occlusal splints before irreversible changes are made by tooth reduction or insertion of prostheses (*Graber*, 1983; *Easler*, 1983; *Morsch*, 1987; *Renggli et al.*, 1984; *Rateitshak et al.*, 1984).
> However, obviously, premature contacts that lead to clear deviation should be eliminated

The choice of splints depends on the treatment goals as described by Grötsch (1983).

— occlusal splint and capping of the crowns for treatment of bruxism,

— occlusal overlays and splints for joint relief and widening of the joint cavity (see compression joint),

— relaxation plate and anterior occlusal overlay (especially in the case of stress),

— occlusal guidance and stabilization splints,

— splints for condyle positioning.

If bridges are necessary, occlusal surfaces made of ceramic should not be used. This material is even harder than enamel and can provoke bruxism, especially following exact occlusal equilibration and articular centering.

Using occlusal overlays and splints, Bumann et al. (1989) reduced the incidence of symptoms caused by compression joints to such a degree that 68% of the patients had no pain or other problems at the time of the follow-up examination (Fig. 15.8).

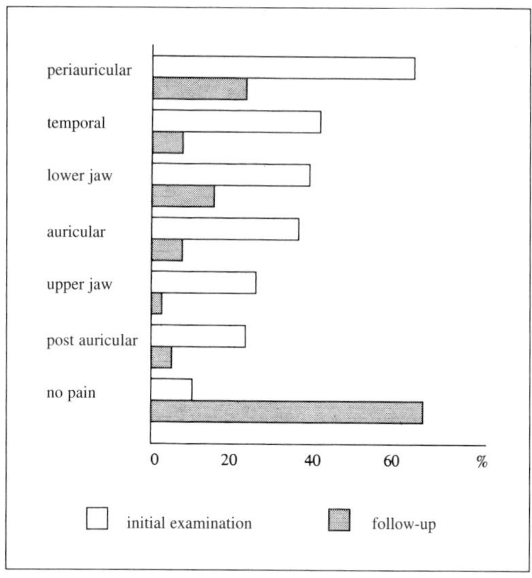

Fig. 15.8 Distribution of pain zones or regions of pain radiation according to statements made by patients (N = 50). Sixty-eight percent of the patients examined after treatment were free of pain at the time of the follow-up examination (according to *Bumann et al.*, 1989).

Rubinstein (1987) found a clear improvement in 46% of his tinnitus patients after a few months, which in most cases persisted over a two-year period, and recommended additional investigation. In several cases muscle exercises were also included in occlusal therapy. Even the latest studies by Erlandsson et al. (1989, 1991) and Rubinstein et al. (1991) recommended stomatognathic treatment including biofeedback techniques which had positive effects in the subgroup of tinnitus patients which suffered from disorders caused by dysfunction of the stomatognathic system (classified as craniomandibular disorders — CMD).

A rather less frequent cause of tinnitus is the styloid syndrome (Riediger and Ehrenfeld, 1989). The styloid process of the temporal process can grow into a megastyloid. Surgical removal has a success rate of 50–90%.

Recommendations made by Kielholz et al. (1981) should be heeded when psychological problems, especially a psychiatric disorder, are involved:

What one **should** do:

— Accept the patient and his disorder

— Discuss possible triggers and the history of the disorder

— Emphasize a favorable prognosis of the disorder

— Explain the planned therapeutic measures

— Inform about possible side-effects of medications

— Prepare for occasional changes in mood

— Step by step therapy so that the patient continuously experiences success

— Include the family and consider environmental conditions

What one **should not** do

— Instruct the patient to "pull himself together"

— Send the patient on vacation or to a spa

— Allow the patient to make important decisions

— Question the patient's fantasies

— Maintain that the patient's condition is improving when it is not the case

Schulte (1983) found that rapid treatment of sudden deafness and tinnitus is most successful, and that therapy was unsuccessful, almost without exception, when tinnitus existed for 5–7 years. This contradicts the findings of Rubinstein et al. (1987) which indicated that 29% of the patients clearly had the same chances of success despite tinnitus of a duration of more than 10 years.

15.7.4 Symptomatic treatment

The muscles of the neck, shoulder and upper arms always participate in hypertension of the masticatory musculature. In order to restore neuromuscular harmony, accompanying measures, which have proven very worthwhile in my practice, are necessary.

— Physical therapy (fango treatment – warm mud packs – of the cervical spine, massage and physiotherapy) (Sander et al., 1990)

— Chirotherapy of the atlanto-occipital joints, if need be with therapeutic blockages. One should not forget to consider a previous whiplash injury (Kopp et al., 1989; Heers et al., 1989; also see Chapter 16)!

— Lymphatic drainage

— Muscle exercises according to Schulte (1983) (see appendix), Garliner (1982), Feldenkrais-method

— Acupuncture

15.7.5 Psychosomatic therapy

- Relaxation therapy (Wiehl, 1983; Jacobson, 1929). Autogenic training
- Biofeedback techniques (Grossan, 1985; Erlandsson et al., 1991; Rubinstein et al., 1991)
- Psychotherapy (Jones, 1985)

*15.7.5.1 Case report**

A 50-year-old male patient had a cold before the first occurrence of high frequency tinnitus of whistling character. At that time he was under a lot of pressure, trying to meet deadlines at work. He tried to distract himself by listening to loud music using earphones. The ENT examination, which took place immediately, resulted in no obvious finding. However, he noticed that the tinnitus became louder and had a higher frequency when he clenched his teeth. The volume of the tinnitus fluctuated greatly.

Bilateral muscular hypertrophy of the masseter, impressions along the sides of the tongue indicating parafunctions, temporomandibular joint noises, disorders of occlusion and articulation were found. Furthermore, it was apparent that he habitually pulled his shoulders upward and held his head backward as well as downward.

Therapy consisted of modified NLP (neurolinguistic programming), a short-term psychotherapy stressing communication techniques developed by Bandler and Grinder (ca. 1970). NLP, which may lead to fundamental changes, considers each developmental step in particular and has established itself as an effective treatment of chronic pain syndromes (Besser-Siegmund, 1989). Prior case reports about its use in complex chronic tinnitus are unknown to us.

NLP assumes that changes in posture and behavior (including parafunction tendencies) are achieved by controlling specific situations with the help of a particular behavior. One patient said: "If I want to achieve something in a difficult situation, I clench my teeth in order to manage the situation better. I simply have to bite myself through it." This implies that the basic intention of this behavior is to cope successuflly with the situation or at least to remain as relaxed as possible. The intention or the reason for this behavior can easily be differentiated from the behavior itself. This should always be determined on an individual basis.

With the help of "six-step reframing", a familiar NLP technique, the "intentions" of his tinnitus were determined: the patient found out that he should look forward to his future and have more trust in himself ("I should listen to my inner voice again").

The goal of behavioral change was to find new, additional possibilities of behavior which were not restricted to only one possible body posture or behavior in a given situation simply because other possibilities were unknown. In this way the patient developed alternatives as well as the feeling of increased freedom to find the most effective and useful behavior for each given situation.

Recognition and acceptance of the previously concealed "message" of the tinnitus was an important step leading to reconciliation between the patient and his tinnitus. It was possible to modify the behavior and to maintain the good intentions of the "message" of the tinnitus on the basis of this understanding.

New behavioral possibilities consisted of finding a balance between work and recreation, improving working conditions and being satisfied with the achievable,

* We would like to thank Dr. *I. Staehle*, Prosthetic Department, Klinik und Poliklinik für Zahn-, Mund- und Kieferkrankheiten, Erlangen-Nürnberg University (Director Prof. Dr. *M. Hofmann*) for authorizing the publication of his case report in this book.

expecting less of oneself and allowing oneself more latitude, managing future tasks "in harmony with himself and his environment". The new or additional behavioral alternatives agreed with the original intentions of the tinnitus.

Several weeks after these changes, the patient reported that, even though the tinnitus itself had not changed, he often had not noticed it. He was also able to sleep better and was not disturbed as much by it in many activities. Two weeks later he reported that he was no longer aware of any tinnitus, but was still afraid that it could return. Following additional treatment he succeeded to stabilize new alternative behavior patterns and integrated these into his daily activities. This was attained by analyzing individual assumptions and convictions which were the product of his personal history.

15.8 Summary

The cumulative changes of the stomatognathic system, and individual factors derived from a series of dysfunctional disorders can trigger changes as described by the "Costen syndrome". Undoubtedly tinnitus is also a part of this.

If tinnitus exists, the case history, together with the clinical and instrumental functional diagnosis, should be determined at the earliest possible opportunity. There is a real chance to improve or eliminate tinnitus if the described possibilities are implemented.

Amalgam fillings are once again a controversial subject, but it is very unlikely that there is a close relationship between tinnitus and amalgam, unless there is premature contact caused by uncorrected fillings.

I have 25 years of experience in dentistry and dental research and would like to recommend to all ontolaryngologists, who are the specialists who are primarily concerned with tinnitus patients, to co-operate with a dentist, especially a dentist who is experienced in the fields of functional analysis and therapy as well as versed in basic psychosomatic concepts, as soon as periauricular symptoms are involved. A dentist with this experience and training can then help to set guidelines for further successful treatment.

Behavioral therapy should not neglect necessary dental treatment.

15.9 References

Bandler, R. & J. Grindler (1984): Neue Wege der Kurzzeit-Therapie. Neurolinguist. Programmieren. Junfermann, Paderborn.

Bandler, R. (1987): Veränderung des subjektiven Erlebens: Fortgeschrittene Methoden des NLP. Junfermann, Paderborn.

Besser-Siegmund, C. (1989): Die sanfte Schmerztherapie mit mentalen Methoden. Econ-Verlag, Stuttgart.

Borner, A. (1987): Epidemiologische Untersuchungen über die Ätiologiefaktoren dysfunktioneller Erkrankungen im stomatognathen System. Med. Diss., Basel.

Bumann, A.; S. Kopp; R. Ewers (1989): Das Kompressionsgelenk als Differentialdiagnose bei chronischen Gesichtsschmerzen. Deutsche Zahnärztl. Z., 12: 962-963.

Costen, J. B. (1934): A syndrome of ear and sinus symptoms dependent upon disturbed function of the temporomandibular joint. Ann. Otol. Rhinol., 43: 1.

de Boever, J. A. (1979): Functional disturbances of the temporomandibular joint. In: *Zarb, G. A., G. E. Carlsson* (eds.): Temporomandibular joint — function and dysfunction, pp. 193-214. Munksgaard, Kopenhagen.

Drum, W. (1972): Zahnmedizin für Ärzte. Quintessence, Berlin.

DuBrul, E. L. (1964): Embryological development of the temporomandibular joint. In: *Sarnat, B. G.* (eds.): The temporomandibular joint. C.C. Thomas, Springfield.

Erlandsson, S.; B. Rubinstein; S. G. Carlsson; A. Ringdahl (1987): Biofeedback and stomatognathic treatment. A prospective study of tinnitus patients. In: *Feldmann, H.* (ed.): Proceedings III International Tinnitus Seminar Münster pp. 389-392. Harsch, Karlsruhe.

Erlandsson, S. I.; B. Rubinstein; A. Axelsson; S. G. Carlsson (1991): Psychological dimensions in patients with disabling tinnitus and craniomandibular disorders. British Journal of Audiology, 25: 15-24.

Erlandsson, S.I; B. Rubinstein; S. G. Carlsson (1991): Tinnitus: evaluation of biofeedback and stomatognathic treatment. British Journal of Audiology, 25: 151-161.

Garliner, D. (1982): Myofunktionelle Therapie in der Praxis. Verlag Zahnärztlich-medizinisches Schrifttum, München.

Gerber, A. (1971): Kiefergelenke und Zahnokklusion. Dtsch. Zahnärztl. Z., 26: 119.

Gerber, W.-D. (1986): Bruxismus. In: *Miltner, W.; N. Birbaumer; W.-D. Gerber* (eds.): Verhaltensmedizin. pp. 345-354. Springer, Berlin, Heidelberg, New York, Tokyo.

Glaros, A. (1981): Incidence of diurnal and nocturnal bruxism. The Journal of Prosthetic Dentistry, 45: 545.

Graber, G. (1971): Neurologische und psychosomatische Aspekte der Myoarthropathien des Kauorganes. Zahnärztl. Welt/Reform, 21: 80.

Graber, G. (1972): Myoarthropathien des Kauorganes. Med. Habil. Schr., Basel.

Graber, G. (1989): Psychomotorik und fronot-lateraler Bruxismus — Myofunktionelle Aspekte der Therapie. Deutsche Zahnärztl. Z., 35: 592.

Graber, G.; H.P. Vogt; W. Müller J. Bahous (1980): Weichteilrheumatismus und Myoarthropathien des Kieferund Gesichtsbereiches. Schweiz. Mschr. Zahnheilk., 90, Nr. 7.

Graber, G. (1983): Psychosomatische Faktoren bei Kiefergelenkerkrankungen. Schweiz. Mschr. Zahnheilk., 93: 880.

Graber, G. (1984): The influence of psychoemotional aspects on the cybernetics of occlusion. The Journal of Gnathology, Vol. 3.

Graber, G. (1987): Die dysfunktionsbedingten Erkrankungen im stomatognathen System (Myoarthropathie). Ätiopathogenese, Diagnostik und Therapie: Monographie. Eigenverlag Univ. Klinik, Basel.

Grötsch, H. (1983): Die Behandlung des funktionsgestörten stomatognathen Systems mit Aufbeßbehelfen und Okklusionsschienen — Grundlagen, Entwicklung und Perspektiven. Inaugural dissertation, Erlangen.

Grossan, M. (1985): Biofeedback. In: *D. H. Morgan; L. R. House; W. P. Hall; S. V. Vamvas* (eds.): Das Kiefergelenk und seine Erkrankungen. Eine interdisziplinäre Betrachtung, pp. 435-446. Quintessenz, Berlin, Chicago, London, São Paulo, Tokyo

Haensler, U. (1983): Das Einschleifen. Dental Revue, Vol. 5.

Heers, H.; E. Reuter (1989): Gesichtsschmerz — Dysfunktion der Kopfgelenke. Deutsche Zahnärztl. Z., 12: 964-965.

Hupfauf, L. (1963): Symptomatik und Genese chronischer Kiefergelenkserkrankungen. Deutsche Zahnärztl. Z., 5.

Jacobson, E. (1929): Progressive relaxation. The University of Chicago Press.

Jäger, K.; G. Graber; U. Humar (1990): Die Therapie der dysfunktionellen Erkrankung des Kausystems. Deutsche Zahnärztl. Z., 1: 9-13.

Jones, W. L. (1985): Psychologische Behandlung. In: *Morgan, D. H.; House, L. R.; Hall, W. P.; Vamvas, S. V.* (eds.): Das Kiefergelenk und seine Erkrankungen. Eine interdisziplinäre Betrachtung. pp. 639-652. Quintessenz, Berlin, Chicago, London, São Paulo, Tokyo.

Kielholz, P.; W. Pöldinger; C. Adams (1981): Die larvierte Depression. Dtsch. Ärzte Verlag, Köln.

Kopp, S.; G. Plato; A. Bumann (1989): Die Bedeutung der oberen Kopfgelenke bei der Ätiologie von Schmerzen im Kopf-, Hals-, Nackenbereich. Deutsche Zahnärztl. Z., 12: 966-967.

Kydd, W. L. (1959): Psychosomatic aspects of temporomandibular joint disfunction. J. Am. Dent. Assoc., 59: 31.

Laskin, D. M. (1969): Etiology of the pain dysfunction syndrome. J. Am. Dent. Assoc., 79: 147.

Lauffs, H.-J.; R. Ewers (1988): Schräglateral-transkranielle Kiefergelenkaufnahmen im Vergleich mit ihrem histologischen Korrelat. Deutsche Zahnärztl. Z., 792.

Lupton, D. E. (1969): Psychological aspects of temporomandibular joint dysfunction. J. Amer. Dent. Ass., 79: 131.

Mack, H. (1980): Instrumentelle Voraussetzungen zur Erfassung des okklusoartikulären Systems. In: *W. Drücke; B. Klemt* (eds.): Kiefergelenk und Okklusion, pp. 67-80. Quintessenz, Berlin.

Manson, G. S. (1920): Occlusion as applied to crown and bridge work. J. Am. Dent. Ass., 7: 399.

Mongini, F. (1985): Lageanomalien von Kondyle und Okklusion. In: *W.K. Solberg; G.T. Clark* (eds.): Kieferfunktion-Diagnostik und Therapie. pp. 25-53. Quintessenz, Berlin.

Morgan, D.H. (1975): Surgical correction of temporomandibular arthritis. J. Oral. Surg., 33: 766.

Motsch, A. (1978): Funktionsorientierte Einschleiftechnik für das natürliche Gebiß. Carl Hanser Verlag, München.

Motsch, A. (1980): Das sogenannte Costen-Syndrom. In: *W. Drücke; B. Klemt* (eds.): Kiefergelenk und Okklusion. pp. 99-110. Quintessenz, Berlin.

Myrhaug, H. (1969): Parafunktionen im Kauapparat als Ursache eines otodentalen Syndroms. Quintessenz-Journal 6 und 7, Ref. 3876.

Neuhauser, W. (1990): Probleme der Diagnostik, Überweisung und Behandlungseinleitung aus zahnärztlicher Sicht, 19-23. In: *M. Ermann & W. Neuhauser* (eds.): Der orofaziale Schmerz. Perspektiven für eine Zusammenarbeit zwischen Zahnmedizin und Psychosomatik.

Palla, S. (1985): Determinanten und Röntgenanalyse der Kondylenposition. In: *W.K. Solberg; G.T. Clark* (eds.): Kieferfunktion — Diagnostik und Therapie. pp. 55-80. Quintessenz, Berlin.

Pilling, L.F. (1977): Psychosomatic aspects of facial pain. In: *C.C. Alling; P.E. Mahan* (eds.): Facial pain. pp. 213-226.

Prentiss, H.A. (1918): A preliminary report upon the temporomandibular articulation in the human type. Dent. Cosmos, 60: 505.

Ramfjord, S.P. & M.M. Ash (1971): Occlusion. *W.B. Saunders Co.*, Philadelphia.

Rateitschak, K.H.; H.F. Wolf (1984): Parodontologie — Farbatlanten der Zahnmedizin, Band 1. Thieme, Stuttgart.

Renggli, H.H.; H.R. Mühlemann; K.H. Rateitschak (1984): Parodontologie. Thieme, Stuttgart.

Riediger, D. & M. Ehrenfeld (1989): Zur Pathogenese und Klinik des Styloidsyndroms. Deutsche Zahnärztl. Z., 12: 968-970.

Rubinstein, B. (1987): Effects of stomatognathic treament of tinnitus. A retrospective study (summary). In: *Feldmann, H.* (ed.): Proceedings III International Tinnitus Seminar Münster, pp. 385-388. Harsch, Karlsruhe.

Rubinstein, B. & S.I. Erlandsson (1991): A stomatognathic analysis of patients with disabling tinnitus and craniomandibular disorders (CMD). British Journal of Audiology, 25: 77-83.

Rugh, J.B. & W.K. Solberg (1979): Psychological implications in temporomandibular pain and dysfunction. In: *G.H. Zarb & G.E. Carlsson* (eds.): Temporomandibular joint function and dysfunction. 239-268. Munksgaard, Kopenhagen.

Sander, M.; R. Siegert; K.K.H. Gundlach (1990): Erfahrungen mit der krankengymnastischen Behandlung von Patienten mit kaumuskulären Funktionsstörungen. Krankengymnastik, 42: 662-667.

Schüller, A. (1905): Die Schädelaufnahme im Röntgenbild. Archiv und Atlas der normalen und pathologischen Anatomie in typischen Röntgenbildern. Gräge & Sillem, Hamburg.

Schulte, W. (1970): Zur funktionellen Behandlung der Myoarthropathien des Kauorgans: ein diagnostisches und physiotherapeutisches Programm. Deutsche Zahnärztl. Z., 25: 422-449.

Schulte, W. (1972): Gezielte Funktionsanalyse und Physio-Therapie — Erfahrungen bei 442 Patienten mit Myoarthropathien. Deutsche Zahnärztl. Z., 27: 779-795.

Schulte, W. (1983): Die exzentrische Okklusion. Quintessenz, Berlin.

Shore, N.A. (1959): Occlusal equilibration and temporomandibular joint dysfunction. J.B. Lippincott Co., Philadelphia.

Solberg, W.K.; R.T. Flint; J.P. Brantner (1972): Temporomandibular joint pain and dysfunction: A clinical study of emotional and occlusal components. J. prost. Dent., 28: 412-422.

Voss, R. (1964): Die Behandlung von Beschwerden des Kiefergelenks mit Aufbißplatten. Deutsche Zahnärztl. Z., 19: 545-XXX.

Wiehl, P. (1983): Orale Physiotherapie — eine zusätzliche Hilfe für Myoarthropathie-Patienten. Schweiz. Mschr. Zahnheilk., 93: 235.

Wright, W.H. (1920): Deafness as influenced by malposition of the jaws. J. Nat. Dent. Ass., 7: 979.

Yemm, R. (1979): Neurophysiologic studies of temporomandibular joint dysfunction. In: *G.A. Zarb & G.E. Carlsson* (eds.): Temporomandibular joint-function and dysfunction. pp. 214-237. Munksgaard, Kopenhagen.

Appendix 1 Clinical functional status according to *Neuhauser*, 1990

CLINICAL FUNCTIONAL STATUS

Name, Surname ____________ Date of birth ____________

1. Case history

2. Previous medical history

	YES	NO
1. Do you have any other illnesses?	☐	☐
2. Do you take medication?	☐	☐
3. Did you have an accident or suffer a blow	☐	☐
4. Were you treated recently by		
a dentist?	☐	☐
a doctor? (GP)	☐	☐
a specialist?	☐	☐
5. Do you have pain or problems of		
the head (in general)?	☐	☐
the neck?	☐	☐
the ears/the jaw?	☐	☐
the temples?	☐	☐
or other areas, which?	☐	☐
6. Do your problems affect your well-being or your performance?	☐	☐
7. Noises in the temperomandibular........ joints since	☐	☐
8. Are one or more teeth painful/sensitive	☐	☐
9. Was/is chewing or opening of the mouth impaired	☐	☐
10. Do you grind/clench your teeth?	☐	☐

Date ____________ Signature of the patient ____________

3. Findings/Results

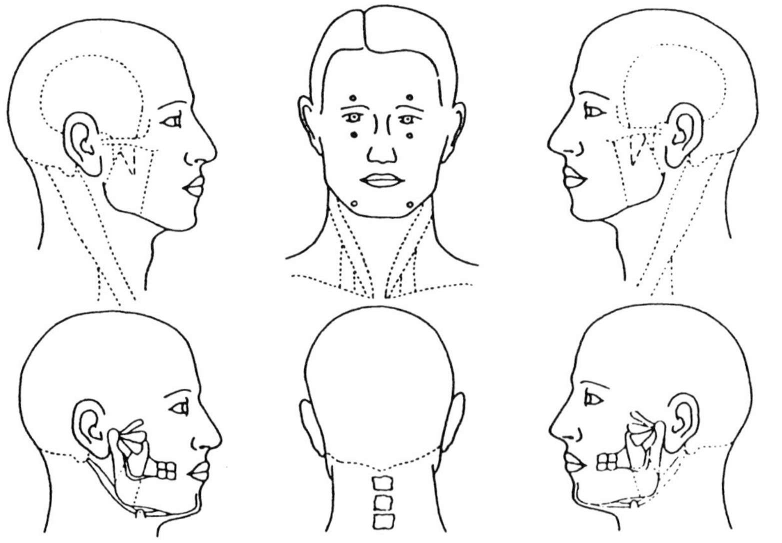

4. Palpation results

Date	R	L
Lateral temporomand. joint		
Dorsal temporomand. joint		
Masseter muscle (pars profundus)		
Masseter muscle (pars superficialis)		
Temporal muscle (pars anterior)		
Temporal muscle (pars posterior)		
Suboccipital muscle		
Digastic muscle (pars posterior)		
Sternocleidomastoid muscle		
Lateral pterygoid muscle		
Temporal tendon		
Medial pterygoid muscle		
Tongue		
Floor of the mouth		

1 = slight 2 = strong 3 = very strong

5. Special documentation

(if necessary)

6. Mobility/auscultation

Right joint

R

20 10 10 20

40

▲▼

Left joint

L

▲▼

7. Indications of parafunction

	yes	no
Clenching, grinding		
Enamel defects		
Occlusal surface defects		
Normal swallowing		
....		
	R	L
Facial symmetry		
Muscle hypertrophy		
Tongue impressions		
Biting of lips/cheeks		

	which
Psychomotor activity	
Sleeping position	

3. Molars

8. Clinical occlusion test

ICP stable	yes		no	
Gliding RCP/ICP				mm

9. Diagnosis

....

....

....

10. Treatment plan

- ☐ Physiotherapy
- ☐ Self-observation
- ☐ Physical therapy
- ☐ Relaxation splint
- ☐ Stabilization splint
- ☐ Bite regulation splint
- ☐ ____________________

11. Additional diagnostic measures

- ☐ Models
- ☐ Instrumental functional analysis (additional documentation)
- ☐ Instrumental occlusion diagnosis (additional documentation)
- ☐ X-ray of the temporomandibular joint
- ☐ Referral to specialist ____________________
- ☐ ____________________
- ☐ ____________________

12. Additional dental measures

	yes	no
Prophylactic		
Parodontal		
Prosthetic		
Orthodontic		

(Signature of examiner)

From: *Neuhauser, W.* (1990) Probleme der Diagnostik, Überweisung und Behandlungseinleitung aus zahnärztlicher Sicht, pp. 23-24. In: *Ermann, M. & Neuhauser, W. (eds): Der orofaziale Schmerz, Quintessenz, Berlin.*

Appendix 2 Case history indicating parafunction according to *W. Schulte*

Case history indicating parafunction

Occurrence of pain or increased pain	Cause of the parafunction (clenching, grinding, sucking)	Consequences (expected diagnosis)
At night and/or upon awakening →	Psychogenic during sleep (e.g. conflict situations) Sleeping position with passive tooth contact	Control of sleeping position
Increase during the day → Not during vacation/weekends ↗	Stress at work: Occupational factors (eg carpenter/ tailor holding nails/pins between the teeth; chewing on pencils, etc)	Self control using "reminders"
Especially during vacation/weekends →	Dominating psychological factors: loneliness, "Sunday neurosis"	Control using protocols/ diary
Especially in the evening →	TV-parafunctions	Self-control using "reminders"
Only during chewing	Not applicable	

Appendix 3

Pamphlet for patients with parafunctions*

> ***Please note:***
> ***For information on these exercises as well as the necessary detailed explanations, please consult your dentist before this leaflet is handed out.***

Dear Patient: Numerous dental disorders are caused by unconscious, falsely applied pressure on the teeth. This does not occur while eating; it is very common but is unknown to most people because it is unconscious and remains unnoticed.

We assume that you have this habit.

This must be diagnosed, otherwise your disorder cannot improve. For this reason please help us.

Take some cards approximately the size of a postcard, or half as large, white if possible, and on these draw clearly visible red crosses or red circles. Place these cards where you work particularly intensively during the day, or experience stress, for example next to the typewriter, under the rear view mirror in the car; but also on the television set in the evening. Fasten these cards so that you cannot avoid seeing them. Whenever you notice them, ask yourself:

What am I doing with my teeth, with my tongue or even with my lips at this moment?

Please make daily notes of your observations and next time bring your notes along.

Please do not make the following serious mistake!

Do not constantly concentrate on your teeth, tongue or lips or pay particular attention to your teeth, because then you will not notice your habit.

Please take these instructions seriously. Maybe you are inclined not to do so because you simply cannot imagine any beneficial results. Please believe that no improvement can occur if you do not follow these recommendations. We would like to help you, so please help us.

Instructions for self-treatment of your masticatory muscle disorder and your temporomandibular joint problems (basic element of the following exercises)

As was already explained to you, you suffer from a disorder of the normal chewing process which includes the teeth, the masticatory muscles and the temporomandibular joints. Even if you have more serious problems, this disorder is harmless. You must merely be aware that the aim of self-treatment is to restore the normal movement of the lower jaw as soon as possible. Please follow the medical instructions exactly. Read the *complete* leaflet before you begin the exercises.

Important: carry out the following exercises exactly! Do not lose patience! Above all, do not stop the exercises too early, especially if your problems have improved rapidly.

The goal of the exercises is flexibility, improved circulation of your masticatory muscles, normalization of the movement of your jaw and, finally, normal chewing. If this goal is reached your problems will also disappear.

Individual exercises

Sit on a chair in front of a table so that you can prop up your elbows and can comfortably support your head in both hands. Place a mirror in front of you in which you can continuously watch your head. Place a clock, if possible with a second hand, next to

* We would like to thank Dr *W. Schulte*, Medical Director of the Dental Clinic, Eberhard Karls University, Tübingen, for kindly authorizing the publication of his leaflet.

the mirror. Then perform the exercises in the following order:

Exercise A: Massage instructions for self-treatment of your masticatory muscle disorder

1. Prop up your elbows, knead both large cheek muscles with both hands simultaneously (thumbs, index and middle fingers) for 3 minutes; look for painful lumps and knead them — even if it hurts — between your fingers (Fig. 15A.1).

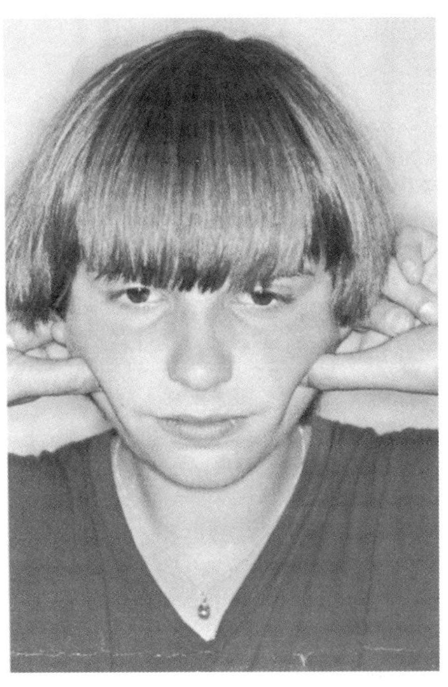

Fig. 15A.1

2. Prop up your elbows, press the balls of your thumbs against your temples on both sides and make circular movements applying strong pressure for 3 minutes. If you find painful points, massage them for another 2 minutes with your middle and index fingers (Fig. 15A.2).

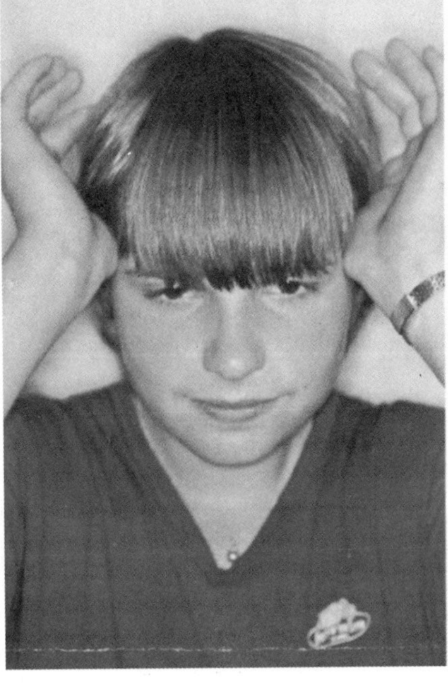

Fig. 15A.2

3. Look for very sensitive points with your index fingers, under your ear lobes. The physician showed you these points beforehand. Perhaps you will also feel a painful lump. Massage these areas with small circular movements of the tips of your index fingers, applying strong pressure for 2-3 minutes (Fig. 15A.3).

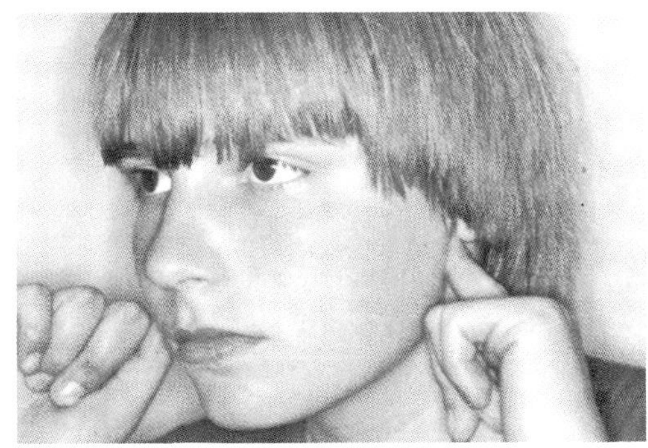

Fig. 15A.3

4. Touch the lower back edge of the lower jaw on both sides with thumbs and index fingers while your chin is lowered. The thumbs rest inside, the index fingers are bent and rest on the large cheek muscles, so you can clearly feel the lower jaw bones between your fingers. Now strongly massage the bone for 3 minutes and, while doing so, press the thumbs as much as possible into the soft tissue of the neck (Fig. 15A.4).

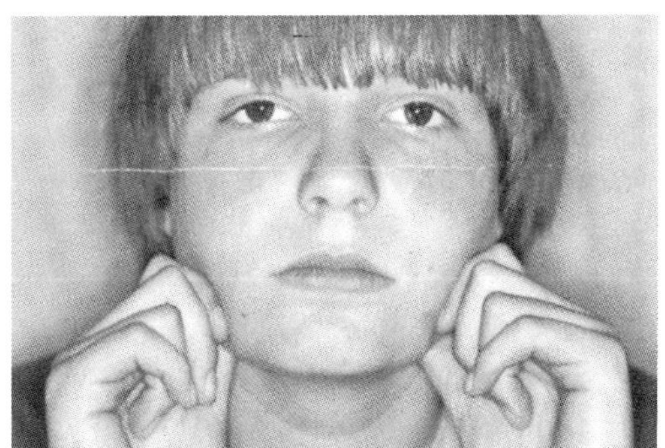

Fig. 15A.4

Exercise B for patients with limitations of movement of the jaw bilaterally

I. Prop up both elbows, put your chin in both hands, open your lips and jaw somewhat, then press your lower jaw to the front into your hands as hard as you can, as if you wanted to "shove away" your hands. While doing this, press into your right hand somewhat more strongly than into your left. The hands should never give way to the pressure, the lower jaw should not move while you press, and you should not press your hands against the lower jaw. Press for 10 seconds, then support your forehead with both hands and allow your lower jaw to hang loosely as if it did not belong to you. Then shake your head gently and try to let your lower jaw "dangle back and forth". Repeat this exercise 10 times in a row, i.e. alternating between tension and relaxation.

II. Look into the mirror. Your hands lie on the table. Open the lips so that you can see the upper and lower incisors. Now alternate between the following exercises:

a) Without closing or opening the mouth, push the lower jaw to the front as if you wanted to touch the tip of your nose with your lower incisors. Be very careful that the lower jaw does not deviate sideways when you push it to the front. You can judge this best by looking at whether the middle lines of the upper and lower incisors deviate. Allow the lower jaw to remain in this position (pushed to the front) for 10 seconds. If pain occurs in the area of the temporomandibular joint, push — always in a straight direction — only as far as you can tolerate during each exercise, but every day push the lower jaw a little more to the front.

b) Again check if the middle lines of the incisors deviate. Now open your mouth slowly and as much as possible. Again, the lower jaw must not deviate sideways, especially not to the left. If you have problems stretch a black thread vertically over the middle of the mirror. Simply fasten it to the top and bottom with tape. Now hold your head so that the thread on the mirror runs exactly through the middle line of the upper incisors. When you open your mouth you can trace the middle line of the lower jaw exactly along the thread on the mirror. First do this slowly and as soon as you can master it try — always without deviating to the side — to open your mouth quickly.

Always perform exercise a) first, then b), and each exercise 5 times. After a few days, as soon as you have mastered both exercises, combine the two. Open your mouth without deviating sideways and at the same time push the lower jaw to the front as much as possible. Do this 10 times in a row.

And now something very important: After every 5 exercises insert a flexibility exercise as described in point I.

Exercise C for patients with left-sided limitation of the movement of the jaw

I. Prop up your right elbow and place the right side of your chin in your right hand. Open your lips and jaw somewhat, then push your lower jaw hard to the right against your right hand, as if you wanted to push your hand to the side. Your hand must not give way and the lower jaw ***must not move*** when it applies pressure. Pay attention to this in the mirror! Press for 10 seconds, then support your forehead with both hands and allow the lower jaw to hang loosely as if "it did not belong to you". Then shake your head gently and try to let your lower jaw "dangle back and forth".

Repeat this exercise 10 times in a row, i.e. alternating between tension and relaxation.

II. Look into the mirror. Your hands lie on the table. Bite and open the lips so you can see the upper and lower front teeth in the mirror. Now be aware of the middle line of the upper and lower incisors and open your mouth. You will notice that the middle line of the lower jaw deviates to the left because the entire lower jaw moves to the left. Perhaps you will notice a "crackling" noise in the right temporomandibular joint while you open your mouth. This sideward movement is associated with masticatory muscle disorder and must be normalized. You will achieve this with the following exercise (10 times in a row):

First close your mouth again and open your lips so that the middle lines are visible again. Press the tip of your tongue strongly against the last upper molar on the right. Now, with the tongue remaining in this position (this is difficult!) open your mouth slowly. During this movement the lower middle line should not deviate to the left of the upper one. There should also be no more crackling noise coming from the right joint while opening your mouth. At first you will barely achieve this, but it will get easier from one exercise to the next. At the beginning open your mouth only as wide as you can achieve without deviation to the left side, but do not forget your tongue.

From one exercise to the next and each day open your mouth a little more. Your aim is to open your mouth wide, rapidly, without deviating sideways or causing a crackling noise in the right joint. If you have problems doing so, stretch a black thread vertically over the middle of the mirror. Simply fasten it to the top and bottom with tape. Now hold your head so that the thread on the mirror runs exactly through the middle line of the upper incisors. Now, when you open your mouth, you can trace the middle line of the lower jaw exactly along the thread in the mirror. If you have problems and the lower jaw continues to deviate to the left or opens with an S-shaped movement, practise — also 10 times in a row — opening your mouth only to the right. The middle line of the lower incisors always remains to the right of the thread.

Exercise D for patients with right-sided limitation

I. Prop up your left elbow and place the left side of your chin in your left hand. Open your lips and jaw somewhat, then push your lower jaw hard to the left against your left hand, as if you wanted to push your hand to the side. Your hand must not give way and the lower jaw must not move when it applies pressure. Pay attention to this in the mirror! Press for 10 seconds, then support your forehead with both hands and allow the lower jaw to hang loosely as if "it did not belong to you". Then shake your head gently and try to let your lower jaw "dangle back and forth". Repeat this exercise 10 times in a row, i.e. alternating between tension and relaxation.

II. Look into the mirror. Your hands lie on the table. Bite and open the lips so you can see the upper and lower front teeth in the mirror. Now be aware of the middle lines of the upper and lower incisors and open your mouth. You will notice that the middle line of the lower jaw deviates to the right because the entire lower jaw moves to the right. Perhaps you will notice a crackling noise in the left temporomandibular joint when you open your mouth. This sideways movement is associated with masticatory muscle disorder and must be normalized. You will achieve this with the following exercise (10 times in a row):

First close your mouth again and open your lips so that the middle lines are visible again. Press the tip of your tongue strongly against the last lower molar on the left. Now with the tongue remaining in this position (this is difficult!) open your mouth slowly. During this movement the lower middle line should not deviate to the right of the upper one. There should also be no more crackling noise coming from the left joint while opening your mouth. If you have problems, simply fasten a black thread to the middle of the mirror. Now hold your head so that the thread on the mirror runs exactly through the middle line of the upper incisors. Now when you open your mouth you can trace the middle line of the lower jaw exactly along the thread in the mirror, but do not forget the position of the tongue (see above). In the beginning open your mouth slowly, especially if you are uncertain and the joint deviates. If pain occurs in the right temporomandibular joint during the exercise, first open your mouth only as wide as you can tolerate. With every exercise and each day open your mouth a little more. Your aim is to open your mouth quickly without deviating sideways!

Please perform exercises 1-4 or I-II 3 times a day, once in the morning, once at noon, and once in the evening, and if time allows also more often. Do not worry that this is too complicated. In only a few days you will know the exercises by heart, so you will no longer need these instructions. Finally, you will not necessarily have to sit at a table or in front of a mirror. You can practise whenever and wherever you like — during a short break at work, in the evening in front of the television, etc.

To change your chewing habits please buy chewing gum. Keep on chewing it during the day for a longer period of time ***exclusively*** on the side opposite the side of the disorder (so with right-sided limitation predominantly on the left side, with left-sided limitation predominantly on the right side; in the case of limitation of both sides, alternating between the left and right sides). Even while eating, for the next 10-14 days, chew exclusively on the side opposite the side of the disorder. As soon as you notice that you can open your mouth normally again, stop chewing gum or chew it as if you are eating, ***consciously on both sides.*** (For additional exercises see Appendix to Chapter 14.)

Chapter 16

Chronic tinnitus associated with functional disorders of the cervical spine

Eberhard Biesinger

16.1 Summary

Treatment of cervical functional disorders will improve certain types of tinnitus, especially unilateral tinnitus, when hearing impairment is not present, as well as tinnitus suffered by children and adolescents and tinnitus which is modified by movements of the head. In several cases it was also possible to eliminate tinnitus. Thus the tinnitus patient, meeting these criteria, should undergo examination of the cervical spine. For this examination, in addition to the usual orthopedic measures, a thorough functional diagnosis of the small spinal joints is essential. The pathophysiologic interrelationships between the cervical spine and the inner ear are not clear; but a neural interrelationship is probable. The therapeutic principle consists of the use of functional treatment which considers the complex biomechanics of the upper cervical spine and the cranial joint. Fundamental components of this treatment are physical therapy and manual therapy by a physician trained as an orthopedist.

16.2 Introduction

Particularly the upper cervical spine is treated by many contemporary authors not only as a specific segment, responsible for movement of the spine, but also as an independent "organ" which, on the one hand has a stable structure, on the other is very susceptible to acute or chronic trauma leading to disturbances of adjacent structures (e.g. Gutmann, 1982; Hohmann et al., 1983; Hulse, 1981; Kügelgen, 1989; Wolff, 1988). Because of the variety of the resulting symptoms, this part of the body is occasionally experienced as being overpowering and omnipotent.

The great difficulty in giving the existing symptoms a plausible explanation based on pathological changes of the cervical spine is reflected in the great number of court cases dealing with whiplash injuries (deceleration trauma), a development which has frustrated many specialists who were responsible for an expert's opinion.

Subjective tinnitus, the entire spectrum of functional complaints and various forms of dizziness are clinical manifestations which, at best, can only be indirectly identified using the current diagnostic methods. After all attempts to explain the patient's symptoms using directly accessible and objective parameters have been futile, only the patient's and the therapist's actual experiences remain to show when treatment of the cervical spine can help in individual cases.

Whereas the patient is satisfied with the help he has received, the therapist is obliged to document his findings and the course of treatment thoroughly and cannot evade an analysis of the success or failure of his treatment. Only the therapist can find criteria based on empirical data which clarify the course of the chosen treatment and avoid a random and unscientific approach.

16.3 Therapeutic modalities

Three significant effects play an important role regarding the treatment of the cervical spine and its effect on tinnitus:

16.3.1 The placebo effect or the "doctor as a drug"

The conscious or unconscious psychological intervention of the physician sometimes leads to a favorable influence on the symptoms. The physician's care and empathy reduces the patient's anxiety (see Chapter 5).

16.3.2 The relaxation effect

Many of the treatment methods described lead to muscular relaxation and as a result relaxation of the body and the psyche, thus initiating a healing process (see Chapter 5 and Chapter 10).

16.3.3 The "organic" effect

This is the direct elimination of the disorder which triggers the symptoms.

This effect, the goal of somatic medicine, means, in respect to tinnitus and the cervical spine, the prompt alleviation of tinnitus by chiropractic manipulation.

In the individual case, it is difficult to find out which effect leads to a successful treatment.

Taking the complexity of the patient's tinnitus and the lack of reproducibility into consideration, only careful documentation of conclusions and results leads to parameters which allow a valid assessment of the chosen therapy.

This means recording the results of the tinnitus patient's functional and radiological examinations of the cervical spine as well as documenting audiologic findings.

If treatment of the cervical spine is indicated, based on limited function or pathological changes, the audiological parameters and the subjective tinnitus must be checked at the conclusion of treatment.

This fundamental approach is missing in existing references (Aubry, 1968; Decher, 1969; Domnick, 1965; Feinmesser, 1987; Hülse, 1983; Moritz, 1953).

A disturbed function of the small joints of the cervical spine, leading to increased nociceptive stimulation, must always be present to justify treatment of the cervical spine. This disturbed function manifests itself in the form of hypo- or hypermobility.

A lack of function resulting from degenerative changes is not equivalent to the activation of nociceptor stimuli and the corresponding disturbances. The opposite is true: here the body, with the help of "repair" mechanisms, has been successful in immobilizing a static or even traumatically changed joint. The pain stimuli caused by movement of the damaged joint subside when the damaged segment is immobilized.

The approach to a causal treatment of the spinal column is to re-establish normal function as much as possible while taking the pathophysiologic changes of the affected segment of the spinal column into consideration. If normal function cannot be re-established, the segment must be integrated into the entire movement by strengthening the shortened musculature, and by correcting the altered architecture so that ordinary movements are possible without pain.

16.4 Pathophysiology

A conclusive and scientifically based model which explains the pathophysiology of vertebral tinnitus is not yet available. The existing ones, predominantly of a more mechanistic nature, must be evaluated critically.

16.4.1 Disturbed circulation resulting from degenerative changes

Circulatory disorders of the cranial region caused by degenerative changes in the cervical spine are very rare (Decher, 1969; Feinmesser et al., 1987; Kehr, 1985). Even with massive degenerative changes in the cervical spine and after serious trauma, the vessels carrying blood to the cervical spine are not, as a rule, impaired enough to cause a decreased circulation of the cochlea with corresponding damage. An insufficiency of the vertebral artery with the development of hearing impairment and tinnitus is extremely rare (Kehr, 1985) and can easily be ruled out using Doppler-sonography.

Tinnitus, which is synchronous with the pulse, can occasionally be caused by existing stenosis of the blood vessels. This is, however, a tinnitus resulting from the vessels of the neck, which cannot be influenced by treatment of the cervical spine.

16.4.2 The neural theory

According to the (so-called) neural theory, a reactive vasoconstriction and thus reduced perfusion of the cochlear structures and, under certain conditions, even damaged cochlear function are the result of nociceptor stimuli from the receptors of the articular and periarticular structures of the cervical spine.

These considerations are based on the sympathetic innervation of the cochlea (Spoendlin et al., 1965, 1967) and the influence on cochlear function by stimulation or dissection of the cervical sympathetic nerves (Beausang-Linder et al., 1980; Maass et al., 1978).

According to Spoendlin, two adrenergic systems can be found in the cochlea:

1. a perivascular network of sympathetic fibers stemming from the superior cervical ganglion and the central nervous system which reaches the periphery of the cochlea together with the cochlear nerve.

2. interaction with the cervical spine is conceivable due to the connection between the cochlea and the cervical sympathetic trunk.

Various attempts with stellate blocks, medication or sympathectomies (Lempert, 1946) have been undertaken for the treatment of tinnitus to prevent the sympathetic influence on the cochlea. Unfortunately the success of such methods remained unsatisfactory. Because of their risks, these invasive measures have now been largely abandoned.

16.4.3 The neuronal theory

The neuronal theory is based on a still hypothetical connection between peripheral afferent nerve structures of the cervical spine and efferent or afferent neurons of the inner ear or the central auditory path (Fig. 16.1).

The following clinical phenomena may be explained with this theory:

16.4.3.1 Example 1

The triggering of and influence on tinnitus by certain movements of the head:

We treated a 17-year-old girl who developed a tinnitus at age 13, which occurred only when she held her head in certain positions (especially while playing the flute) and when she sat or stood; it could be masked with 50 dB and had a frequency of 6 kHz.

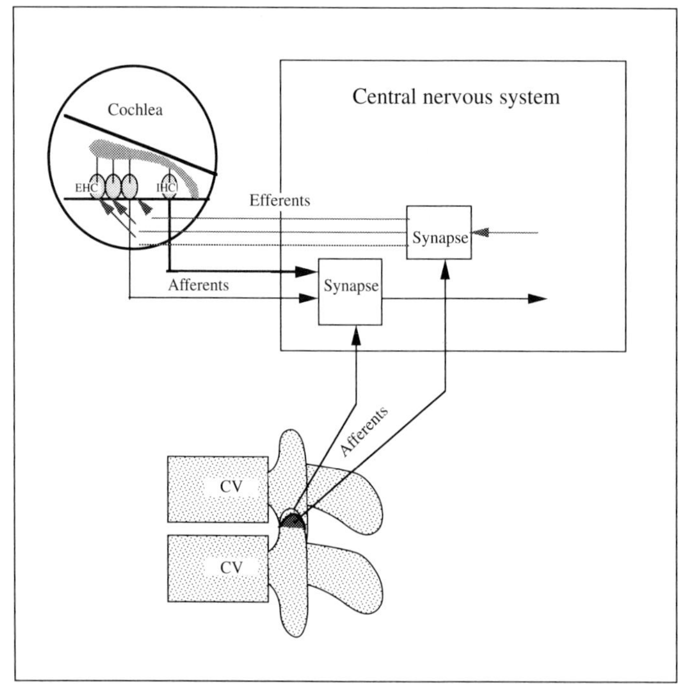

Fig. 16.1 Model of the neuronal theory (IHC = internal hair cells; EHC = external hair cells; CV = cervical vertebra).

Careful functional examination of the cervical spine showed a hypermobile segment C2/C3 and a relative shortening of the right levator muscle of the scapula. Isolated contraction of the right levator muscle of the scapula in a lying position also produced the tinnitus.

Local anesthesia of the insertion of the muscle at the level of C2/C3 regularly eliminated the tinnitus for short periods of time.

16.4.3.2 Example 2

The emergence of hearing impairment and tinnitus caused by movements of the head:

Example: The so-called "acoustic trauma" is a special form of sudden deafness which typically occurs when the head makes an unphysiological movement or is positioned abnormally while listening to a moderately loud noise.

This most often results in a pancochlear loss of hearing and not infrequently in deafness of one ear, often associated with tinnitus.

The etiologic mechanism is not clear, but, because of the triggering factors, an association with the cervical spine is probable.

16.4.3.3 Example 3

Tinnitus due to trauma of the cervical spine:

Tinnitus is unfortunately also related to improper treatment of the cervical spine.

A 36-year-old female patient had regular orthopedic treatment and manual therapy for 11 years because of recurring problems of the cervical spine. In October 1990, this resulted in a tinnitus after a series of five manipulations of the cervical spine. The tinnitus disappeared almost completely within 1 week. Because of the residual tinnitus a further manual therapy was initiated, after which the tinnitus immediately increased and persisted. On October 16, 1990 hospital admission to an ENT clinic followed. In the audiogram there was slight left-sided hearing impairment of high frequency starting with a decrease in hearing of 30 dB at 6 kHz and a maximum of hearing loss of 50 dB at 12 kHz. The tinnitus could be masked with 50 dB at 12 kHz.

16.4.3.4 Example 4

Therapeutic success due to infiltration of the cervical spine region with a local anesthetic:

Occasionally the tinnitus can be influenced and, rarely, even eliminated by the injection of a local anesthetic at certain points of the neck musculature:

A 47-year-old female patient had left-sided tinnitus after a whiplash injury of the cervical spine. The tinnitus could be masked with 40 dB at 4 kHz, and hearing was normal. Initial treatment began 6 weeks after the occurrence of the ear noise by infiltrating the insertion of the ipsilateral sternocleidomastoid muscle. Twenty minutes after the injection the loudness of the tinnitus was assessed at only about 20 dB and as subjectively considerably improved. After two additional injections in intervals of 3 days the tinnitus disappeared.

16.4.3.5 Example 5

Therapeutic success due to manual therapy of the cervical spine:

A 56-year-old male patient had right-sided tinnitus masked with 70 dB at 6 kHz, left-sided tinnitus masked with 30 dB at 4 kHz. Slight levels of high frequency hearing loss were observed in the audiogram. A functional disorder of the segments C0/C1 and C2/C3 was present. Following manual therapy, which restored the normal function of these joints, the left-sided tinnitus disappeared and the right-sided tinnitus improved considerably (masked with 40 dB). Identical findings were observed 3 months later.

16.4.3.6 Example 6

Disappearance or improvement of tinnitus after surgery of the cervical spine:

Kehr (1985) described a complete remission of tinnitus following surgery to the cervical spine (uncoforaminectomy).

This operation is (rarely) performed when life-threatening stenosis of the vertebral artery is present. A few patients (26%) had tinnitus prior to operation which, depending on the type of surgery, improved post-operatively in up to 44%.

No therapy can however be derived from these results alone.

16.5 Indications for treatment and prognosis of tinnitus and functional disorders of the cervical spine

Because of the described observations and the successful treatment results, the cervical spine must be included in the differential diagnosis of tinnitus.

Under certain conditions it can be assumed that, at best, tinnitus is favorably influenced in 12% following therapy of the cervical spine (Biesinger, 1989).

These conditions are:

1. Normal hearing. Tinnitus with normal hearing in general has a better prognosis. If there is also cochlear damage (e.g. with hearing impairment from noise trauma), experience tells us not to expect that treatment of the cervical spine relieves or alleviates tinnitus. It is assumed that in these cases the cause of the tinnitus is located exclusively in the cochlea.

2. A more favorable prognosis exists when the tinnitus exists unilaterally.

3. With fluctuating tinnitus, it must be determined whether it is perceived only in quiet surroundings or if it actually fluctuates.

4. Age: the younger the patient, the sooner success can be achieved following treatment of the existing functional disorder of the cervical spine. This applies especially to children.

5. Influence on tinnitus due to movement of the head.

   If the case history and palpation prove that the existing tinnitus increases or decreases by applying pressure on specific pressure points in certain body and head positions this indicates that an initial step in the direction of treatment can be made by analyzing these movements with the aim of integrating the results into physiotherapy.

6. When tinnitus follows trauma of the cervical spine.

If one or more of these criteria are fulfilled, the cervical spine should be thoroughly examined. The complicated biomechanics of the cervical spine, including the special importance of the cranial joints (Wolff, 1988) as well as interrelationships with the rest of the body, requires an experienced physician.

As a rule, this ought to be an orthopedist who has completed training in diagnosis and therapy according to the guide-

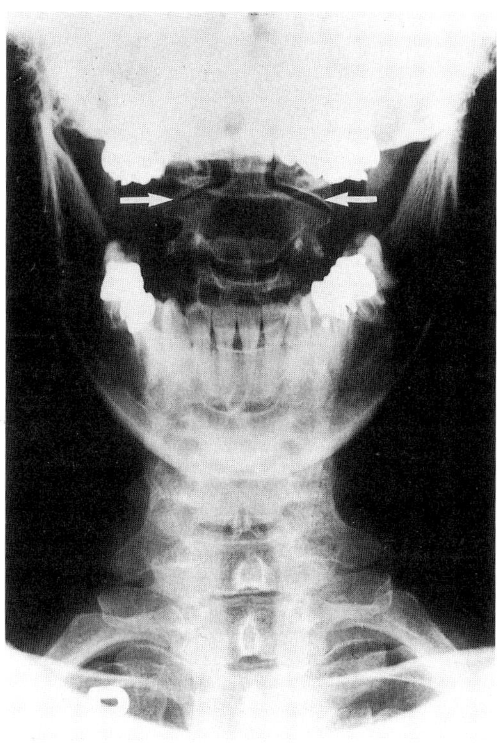

Fig. 16.2 In the absence of pathological anatomical changes the atlas rotation can be a radiological indication of a functional disorder of the cranial joints.

lines of the German Society for Manual Medicine with an additional degree in *"chirotherapy"*.

Only a few otolaryngologists have such training or have the necessary experience in the treatment of the cervical spine.

Finally, sound knowledge of radiology of the cervical spine is necessary. It is not sufficient to be aware of only the degenerative changes; rather it is necessary to analyse the x-ray of the cervical spine with regard to its function (Gutmann, 1981; Kamieth, 1990; Wackenheim, 1974), as Fig. 16.2 indicates.

16.6 Necessary considerations in the diagnosis of cervical spine disorders

In taking the case history, specific questions pertaining to the cervical spine must be asked.

In chronic tinnitus it is often not easy for the patient to date and characterize the development of tinnitus.

Precise questions can establish the possible relationship between trauma, occasional acute problems and immobilization of the cervical spine following other afflictions or even surgery and the development of tinnitus. The questionnaire (Table 16.1) may help to indicate that the tinnitus is related to the cervical spine.

The essential components of a functional examination are shown in Table 16.2. An examination which compares the freedom of movement of the left with the right side of each cervical segment is particularly important. With precise knowledge of the biomechanics, the freedom of movement of every individual cervical segment is assessed. Results, as to whether a joint is classified as hypomobile, normal or hypermobile, are found in this examination. According to the pain noted by the patient, the exact location as well as the quality and quantity of the abnormal movement can be defined.

This thorough examination technique is taught in Germany, Switzerland and Austria in courses of the corresponding organizations for Manual Medicine* and are the method of choice for obtaining qualified findings.

A general assessment of the entire cervical spine, especially if assessed as a single

* German Society for Manual Medicine, Heerstraße 163, D-56154 Boppart. A list of names and addresses of trained physicians and physical therapists can be requested here.

Table 16.1 Questionnaire concerning tinnitus in relation to the cervical spine

- Does the tinnitus fluctuate with regard to volume?
- Does the tinnitus fluctuate with regard to the pitch of tones?
- Does the tinnitus occur only in certain positions of the head?
- Can the tinnitus be influenced with regard to intensity and frequency by movements of the head?
- Is the tinnitus influenced by posture (e.g. sitting for a long time)?
- Are there pressure points on the head or the back of the neck which can influence the tinnitus?
- Did the tinnitus ever change after massage, physical therapy or other treatment?
- Does muscle tension of the back of the neck influence the tinnitus?
- Does exercise or other physical work influence the tinnitus?

Table 16.2 Examination of the cervical spine

1. Case history
2. Inspection of body posture, the statics of the cervical spine and other parts of the body (e.g. *Brügger*, 1979; *Klein-Vogelbach*, 1976; *Frisch*, 1989)
3. Palpate the skin and inspect for possible segmental irritation, sensitivity, tension and myogelosis; palpate the shoulder girdle and register the development of the muscles of the neck and back of the neck
4. Differential functional test of the muscles of the neck and back of the neck including specific stretching tests
5. Freedom of movement test: general examination, movement of the entire cervical spine in three directions; segmental freedom of movement of each vertebra including C7, and specific tests for hypermobility
6. X-ray: cervical spine in two planes (*Gutman*, 1981): after trauma for exact documentation as well as X-ray of freedom of movement, which can be evaluated according to *Arlen* (1981). When dysplasias is present, tomography or computer tomography is necessary. For the exact assessment of adjacent soft-tissue, suspected tumor or after trauma: nuclear resonance tomography. Assessment of the X-rays also considering functional aspects
7. Results: Signs of infection, consultation with a specialist in internal medicine

functional unit, is inadequate in view of the complexity of the biomechanical and neurological interrelationships.

16.7 Therapeutic principles

16.7.1 Indications

The goal of treatment is to re-establish a balanced function of the individual cervical joints as well as the paravertebral muscles.

An examination which compares the freedom of movement of the left with the right side of each cervical segment is particularly important.

The individual measures concentrate on the actual situation. An acute disorder of the cervical spine with tinnitus requires a relaxed position, for example, with a neck support. For serious muscle tension, relaxation can be achieved temporarily with benzodiazepines, perhaps combined with anti-inflammatory drugs or analgesics (refrain from aspirin, because it may cause tinnitus in high doses).

After trauma of the cervical spine, the time to commence physical therapy must be chosen carefully and in accordance with an orthopedist.

The premature commencement of physical therapy can contribute to chronic problems; however, stabilizing exercises must be initiated at the right time to re-establish the active protective function of the musculature.

16.7.2 Functional treatment

With a disorder which is not acute and with proof of functional disorders, functional treatment begins with physical therapy or manual therapy performed by an experienced physician. Massage alone should be rejected.

In physical therapy, active exercises are taught, corresponding with the clinical findings. This includes precise and differentiated exercises for certain muscles and joints; contracted muscles must be stretched.

It is almost always necessary to show the patient which exercises he has to learn to do by himself. This exercise program is developed individually, according to the anatomical and muscular findings. For this reason it makes sense that no general exercise program can be suggested.

16.7.2.1 Conditions for functional treatment using physical therapy

A thorough medical examination is the starting point for physical therapy.

The prescription for physical therapy should include the location and type of functional disorder. The physiotherapist must also be informed of pathological changes in the x-ray if it is relevant (eg degenerative changes, dysplasias, trauma, hypermobility of movement).

An example for a precise prescription follows:

6 × physical therapy with application of ice packs

Diagnosis:
Tinnitus with functional disorder of C0/C1 right > left, degenerative changes of C5-C7, hyperlordosis of the cervical spine

The physiotherapist must have experience with the special characteristics of the cervical spine and must consider the principle of functional unity between the cervical spine, the shoulder girdle as well as the remaining spinal segments.

As a rule, the requirements are fulfilled if the physiotherapist has an appropriate degree in "Manual" therapy (also: "Brügger", "Cyriax", "McKenzie") and "Functional movement therapy according to Klein-Vogelbach".

A manual containing the names of registered physiotherapists, in which the completed additional training is also listed, can be requested in Germany from each provincial physiotherapy association.

It is important, especially in the care of the tinnitus patient, that the prescribing physician works closely with the physiotherapist. This promotes the effectiveness of the physiotherapy. The personal relationship between the patient and physiotherapist is naturally more intimate and thus the physio-

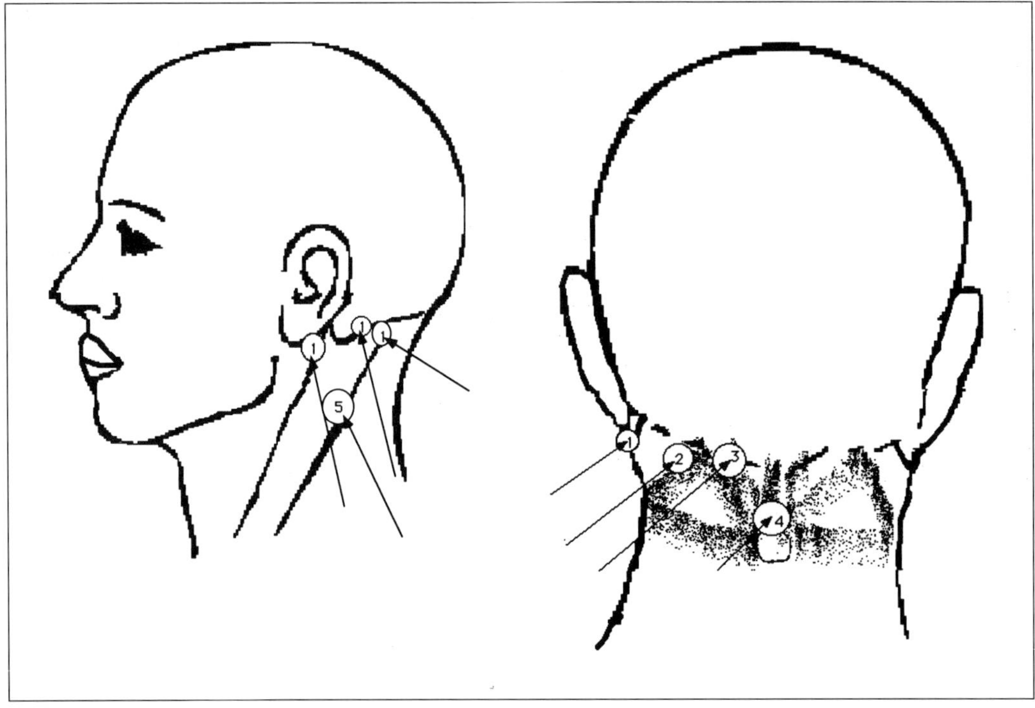

Fig. 16.3 Important points for injection of a local anesthetic in the treatment of the cervical spine.

therapist is often more informed than the physician.

16.7.3 Physiotherapy in functional treatment

For physiotherapy, the application of warmth (e.g. mud packs, fango) is suitable as well as the application of ice packs (i.e. when ice is briefly applied during muscle contraction.) In no case should ice be applied while the patient is at rest (Biesinger, 1988).

16.7.4 Manual therapy

When sufficient indication exists, the physician trained and experienced in manual therapy can control functional disorders of the small spinal joints by controlled manipulation (so-called manipulation of the joint) or also by special treatment of the muscles (e.g. "muscle energy technique"). The success of such manual techniques is immediate and can be detected in an improvement in freedom of movement of the treated joint and the relaxed patient. The effect on the tinnitus can also be expected immediately or at least within hours.

16.7.5 Injection techniques with local anesthetics

Occasionally tinnitus can be influenced by the injection of a local anesthetic at certain points of the cervical spine. Here the following points, which are seen as "trigger points" (Figs 16.3 and 16.4) have special significance:

1 The insertion of the sternocleidomastoid muscle at the mastoid
2 The insertion of the superior oblique muscle of the head and major rectus posterior muscle of the head directly below the nuchal line
3 The insertion of the minor rectus posterior muscle of the head
4 The spinal process of the axis
5 Insertion of the levator muscle of the scapula at the level of C2–C3, if necessary also at its insertion at the medial scapular border

For injection, 0.5–1% lidocaine solution up to 1 ml is suitable at these points. A local anesthetic (e.g. bupivacaine hydrocloride) with a long-term effect only has a temporary effect.

16.7.6 Adjunctive therapy

If tinnitus is influenced by certain positions of the head, relief can sometimes be achieved by appropriate positioning of the head (e.g. special orthopedic pillows, neck support, special seat cushions). The use of such aids should be discussed with the physician and the physiotherapist.

16.7.7 General relaxation techniques

The cervical spine is, to a certain degree, also a "barometer" of the "inner condition". Muscle tension, which can finally lead to functional disorders of the spinal joints, is maintained in many patients by "inner" tension. Relaxation techniques which contribute to re-establishing the spiritual equilibrium will also lead to a physical balance specifically with respect to muscle relaxation.

The selection of the correct relaxation exercise must also consider individual wishes of the patient (e.g. aversion toward group therapy, realistic evaluation of therapeutic opportunities and time at hand). A principal criterion should be, however, that the patient can use the technique by himself without depending on a therapist or expensive technical aids.

Autogenic training, Jakobsen's relaxation techniques, Feldenkrais methods, yoga (risk of damage to the cervical spine) and biofeedback are suitable.

16.8 Perspectives

Successful therapy of tinnitus by treatment of the cervical spine can be achieved.

This fact alone justifies the assumption that tinnitus can occur under as yet unclear conditions following functional and/or morphological pathological changes of the cervical spine.

The upper cervical spine with the cranial joints between the occiput and the second vertebra is of particular importance because of its physiological significance (Wolff, 1988). Additional scientific research is urgently needed to define more objective examination methods.

Future research into the afferent and efferent nerves of the inner ear will possibly also provide additional information.

16.9 References

Aubry, M.; P. Pialoux; P. Narcy; P. Fontelle (1968): Sindrome cervicale posttraumatique. Recenti. Prog. Med., 45: 422.

Arlen, A. (1981): Die röntgenologische Funktionsdiagnostik der Halswirbelsäule. Orthop. ihre Grenzgeb., 119: 557-582.

Beausang-Linder, M.; E. Hultcrantz (1980): Early effects of cerical stimulation on cerebral, ocular and cochlear blood flow. Acta physiol scand 109: 433-437.

Biesinger, E. (1989): Funktionelle Störungen der Halswirbelsäule in ihrer Bedeutung für die Hals-Nasen-Ohren-Heilkunde. In: *Ganz, H.; W. Schätzle* (1989): HNO-Praxis Heute. Springer, Berlin, Heidelberg, New York.

Biesinger, E. (1988): Krankengymnastik und Hals-Nasen-Ohren-Heilkunde: Von der Halswirbelsäule beeinflußte Krankheitsbilder in der Hals-Nasen-Ohren-Heilkunde. Z. Krankengymnastik, 11: 932-935.

Brügger, A. (1979): Die Erkrankungen des Bewegungsapparates und seines Nervensystems. Fischer, Stuttgart.

Decher, H. (1969): Die zervikalen Syndrome in der Hals-Nasen-Ohren-Heilkunde. Thieme, Stuttgart.

Domnick, L. (1965): Über die Beziehungen der Halswirbelsäule zu Hals-, Nasen-, Ohrenerkrankungen. Erfahrungsheilkd., 14: 585.

Feinmesser, R.; Y. Fluman (1987): Cervical tinnitus: legend or fact? The Journal of Laryngology and Otology, 101: 376-380.

Frisch, H. (1989): Programmierte Untersuchung des Bewegungsapparate 3. Aufl. Springer, Berlin, Heidelberg, New York.

Hohmann, D.; B. Kügelgen; K. Liebig; M. Schirmer (eds.) (1983): Neuroortopädie 1, Halswirbelsäulenerkrankungen mit Beteiligung des Nervensystems. Springer, Berlin, Heidelberg, New York, Tokyo.

Hülse, M. (1981): Die Gleichgewichtsstörung bei der funktionellen Kopfgelenksstörung. Man. Med., 19: 92.

Gutmann, G. (1981): Die funktionelle Pathologie und Klinik der Wirbelsäule, Bd. 1: Die Halswirbelsäule. Die funktionsanalytische Röntgendiagnostik der Halswirbelsäule und der Kopfgelenke. Fischer, Stuttgart, New York.

Gutmann, G. (1982): Die funktionelle Pathologie und Klinik der Wirbelsäule, Bd 1 und 2: Die Halswirbelsäule. Fischer, Stuttgart, New York.

Kamieth, H. (1990): Das Schleudertrauma der Halswirbelsäule. Grundlagen, Röntgenfunktionsdiagnostik. In: Die Wirbelsäule in Forschung und Praxis, Bd. 111. Hippokrates, Stuttgart.

Kehr, P. (1985): Chirurgie der Arteria vertebralis an den Bewegungssegmenten der Halswirbelsäule. In: *Gutmann, G.*: Funktionelle Pathologie und Klinik der Wirbelsäule. Bd. 1, Teil 4. G. Fischer Verlag, Stuttgart, New York.

Klein-Vogelbach, S. (1976): Funktionelle Bewegungdslehre. Springer, Berlin, Heidelberg, New York.

Kügelgen, B. & A. Hillemacher (eds.): Problem Halswirbelsäule. Springer, Berlin, Heidelberg, New York, London, Paris, Tokyo, Hong Kong.

Lempert, J. (1946): Tympanosympathektomie: A surgical technique for the relief of tinnitus aurium. Arch. Otorhinolaryngol, 43: 199.

Moritz, W. (1953): Das cervicale Sympathikussyndrom und seine praktische Bedeutung. Z. Laryngol. Rhinol., 32: 270.

Maass, B.; H. Baumgärtl; D. W. Lübbers (1978): Lokale p02- und pH2-Messungen mit Mikrokoaxialnadelelektroden an der Basalwindung der Katzencochlea nach akuter oberer zervikaler Sympathektomie. Arch. Otorhinolaryngol., 221: 269-284.

Spoendlin, H. & W. Lichtensteiger (1965): The adrenergic innervatin of the labyrinth. Acta Oto-Laryng., 61: 423-434.

Spoendlin, H. & W. Lichtensteiger (1967): The sympathetic nerve supply to the inner ear. Arch. klin. exp. Ohren-, Nasen- und Kehlkopfheilk., 189: 346-359.

Wackenheim, A. (1974): Roentgen diagnosis of the craniovertebral region. Springer, Berlin, Heidelberg, New York.

Wolff, H. D. (1988): Die Sonderstellung des Kopfgelenkbereiches. Springer, Berlin, Heidelberg, New York, Tokyo.

Chapter 17

Medical and psychosomatic glossary

Gerhard Goebel

The comprehensive interdisciplinary glossary is the "special treat" of this book. Its purpose is to facilitate the understanding of the terms used irrespective of whether the reader is psychologically or medically oriented. At first it may prove to be a bit difficult to comprehend because it is listed alphabetically and not according to the separate disciplines, but this was in accordance with the editor's underlying intentions e.g. to contribute to a mutual understanding between ENT and psychosomatic medicine. Only intense co-operation can cope with the immense problems posed by chronic tinnitus. A mutual understanding of terminology is an important precondition to which this glossary contributes.

Many terms and definitions can only be described in a simplified manner and gaps may open which can only be closed by referring to more specific literature. The glossary's intention is also to facilitate the understanding of definitions which were initially assumed to be known.

Acoustic neurinoma, eighth nerve tumor

Acoustic neurinomas are derived from Schwann cells (vestibular schwannoma). They arise twice as often from the vestibular division of the eighth nerve as from the auditory division and account for approximately 7% of all intra-cranial tumors. As the tumor increases in size, it projects from the internal auditory meatus into the cerebellopontine angle and begins to compress the cerebellum and brain stem. The fifth and later the seventh cranial nerves become involved. Hearing loss and tinnitus are early symptoms. Although the patient complains of dizziness, true vertigo is not usually present. Sensory-neural hearing loss is characterised by greater impairment of speech discrimination than would be expected with a cochlear lesion. Recruitment is absent.

Acoustics

The field in physics describing sound phenomena. In audiology only those acoustic phenomena are of interest which are within the range of (human) hearing (physiologically and psychologically).

Acoustic trauma

Acute noise trauma caused by detonation, explosion, noise or a combination of various factors together with a cerebral trauma (bone conduction), which leads to a degeneration of hair cells and stereocilia in the organ of Corti and temporary or permanent sensory hearing loss with a depression of the hearing threshold-curve at 4,000Hz or abrupt decrease at high frequencies; positive recruitment; a tinnitus of high frequency develops often.

Acting out

According to *S. Freud*, the individual experiences his unconscious wishes and fantasies in a given situation as being vivid and unique and is unaware of the fact that their origins lie in the past and are repetitious in character.

Affect

A strong, clearly perceivable emotion. According to the clinical categories of psychological phenomena, e.g. thinking, feeling and volition, feeling is identical with affect, which may also be understood as emotion or mood. According to modern classifications and usage, affect is usually an aspect of cognition (affective component). According to psychiatric terminology, affects are emotions which cause excitation and/or physical reactions.

Affective disorder

Pathological change in the reactivity of and expression of affects. DSM-III-R: major depression, dysthymia, bipolar disorder, cyclothymia.

Afferent

Neurophysiological definition of nerves (afferents) that relay an impulse from a peripheral sensory organ centripetally to an associated central structure (central nervous system). Equivalent of sensory nervous system.

Aggravation

Conscious and goal-oriented exaggeration of actual symptoms and subjective feelings concerning an illness. Contrary to simulation, actual symptoms are present.

Agoraphobia

Fear of places or situations which seem to be difficult to escape from or in which help does not seem to be available (large squares, elevators). According to DSM-III-R classification, the pathological fear of certain places and situations in which the sudden outbreak of physical symptoms is expected and a tendency toward increasing avoidance behaviour develops.

Air conduction

Transmission of sound via the eardrum/tympanic membrane and the hearing ossicles (ossicular chain). Decrease due to compacted cerumen (ear wax) in the outer ear, perforation of the tympanic membrane or otosclerosis.

Ambivalence

Simultaneous presence of two opposing impulses, urges attitudes or emotions.

Analogue scale

See tinnitus loudness.

Anamnesis

Case history.

Antidepressants

Psychopharmaceuticals of various chemical structure, which decrease depression, reduce anxiety and improve drive. Contrary to tranquillisers, dependency risk is not present.

Anxiety

A state of emotional arousal, which arises when external stimuli (for example, a loud noise) or internal stimuli (for example, fantasies and body perceptions) are perceived as being dangerous.

Anxiety management training

Technique of behavioral therapy in which the patient practises coping skills (for example, relaxation, confrontation etc.) in anxiety-inducing situations.

Appraisal

The process of intuitive evaluation of situations. Appraisal has become a principal term in cognitive psychology which presumes that the individual evaluation of a given situation is the guideline for its experience and the resulting behavior.

Art therapy

Special form of occupational therapy based on depth psychology (*C. G. Jung*). Emphasis on the creative potential, using different material (clay, paint, paper, music), different aspects of life are expressed and reflected upon.

Association

Description of the interrelationships between two or more elements which then form a chain of association. For example, psychotherapy is concerned with associations concerning a dream with the aim of analysing the words chosen by the patient with respect to thoughts, memories or feelings which are associated with a dream.

Attention

State of increased vigilance, tension, selective orientation. Older theories describe a conscious process of selection. At the centre of attention, the impression appears to be clear, distinct and graphic (apperception); in the periphery of attention the impressions are at the most unclear and therefore less conscious. Modern theories of cognitive psychology describe attention as the more or less conscious adjustment of a filter regulating a stream of data of a specific kind or origin. Changes of adjustment lead to a change of attention.

Attitude, change of)

A general term describing changes of the assessment of symptoms, situations, etc.

Attribution

The process of attributing a confusing and therefore unexplainable experience to one or more preconceived explanations which may then lead either to relaxation or arousal.

Audiology

The scientific field concerned with hearing, a sub-discipline of acoustics.

Audiometry

Method of investigating hearing ability with the help of electronic devices, for example, psycho-acoustic measurement of the hearing threshold, the tinnitus intensity and frequency using an audiometer, objective audiometry using BERA, reflex-audiometry etc. Tone audiometry: the measurement of the hearing threshold with sine tones via air or bone conduction differentiates between sound conduction and sound perception hearing impairment. Speech audiometry: words and numbers are spoken with increasing loudness and the number of correct/ false answers are registered so as to evaluate the degree of speech perception.

Auditory system

All anatomical structures which participate in hearing.

Autogenic training

A relaxation method developed by *J.H. Schultz* with the aim of influencing certain body functions, states of tension, pain, sleep disturbances etc. by auto-suggestion.

Awareness

In the classical psychological approach to thinking and consciousness, this term describes a form of awareness which does not refer to specific perceptions or specific aims, for example the intention to accomplish a task in which the specific details are not yet known or perceived as well as possible with a minimum of mistakes and without being distracted. Gestalt therapy concentrates on the development of awareness (self-awareness). This term does not coincide with the term "state of consciousness" e.g. knowledge of contextual interrelationships.

Barotrauma

See decompression sickness.

Baseline

Curve which describes the natural and spontaneous course of the observed phenomenon.

Behavioral analysis

Important diagnostic procedure in behavioral therapy, analysis of the following inter-related dimensions (S-O-R-C-Co):

S: Triggering stimulus (social, physiological, internal — for example, thoughts) of tinnitus reactions.

O: Organic and psychological variables (for example, personality factors or genetic determinants) which mediate between the stimulus (S) and the reaction (R).

R: The detailed description and registration of the reactions even on the level of physiological subjective and psychosocial components (tinnitus behavior).

C: Consequence — the direct or delayed positive or negative consequence of a reaction which either reinforces the reaction or prohibits alternative reactions or behavior.

Co: Contingency — the liability for the consequence (C) to occur following a reaction (R), for example intermittent or continuous reinforcement, risk of behavioral deficits (for example, lack of social competence) and behavioral extremes (for example, complete isolation, lamenting). These factors are registered in relation to the controlling stimuli. Further analysis of triggering stimuli in the family and at work as well as a thorough history of the disturbance ("noise history") + hypotheses of the patient concerning the development (analysis of attribution). Considerations concerning the relationships to others (partner, parents), who may participate in reinforcing tinnitus behavior, are also considered.

Behavioral medicine

(W. D. Gentry.) Implementation of behavioral therapy in somatic medicine, partially in combination with somatic treatment; management of somatic illnesses according to guidelines of behavioral therapy (for example, with tinnitus).

Behavioral therapy

Term introduced by *H. J. Eysenck* to describe all therapeutic techniques and procedures which concentrate primarily on behavioral change instead of an analysis of concealed psychic conflicts. Contemporary definitions stress the scientific validity of behavioral therapy: learning theory, classical and operant conditioning, desensitization, cognitive therapy, etc.).

Behaviorism

(J. B. Watson, 1878-1958). Psychological theory with the aim of attaining the most objective observation of human and animal behavior possible. This theory led to decisive achievements in the research of the conditions for and forms of behavioral change (etc.) (*Skinner*).

BERA

Abbreviation for Brain-stem Electric Response Audiometry; method of registering early acoustic evoked potentials which allows the differentiation of the origins of sound perception hearing impairment between a cochlear (sensory), retrocochlear (neural) and central origin (objective audiometry).

Binaural hearing

The capability of hearing with both ears, allowing spatial localisation of the sound sources and detection of the direction of sound; the impulses coming from other sensory organs (for example, the sense of sight, muscle contraction) are integrated with hearing impulses in the brain.

Bioenergetics

Psychotherapy based on *W. Reich* (1933) and developed by *A. Lowen* (1972) according to which psychic trauma leads to blockage of energy-flow in a system (the body, for example, in the form of muscle tension). Therapy concentrates on the musculature, body expression and structure, posture and breathing, leading to a discharge of "blocked" emotions which are then treated.

Biofeedback

Method of behavioral therapy which gives the patient the opportunity to observe processes of the body with the help of technical devices either by visual or acoustic means (pulse, muscle tension, skin-resistance, breathing frequency). By applying this method, the patient can experience to what extent autonomous processes can be influenced by psychological or therapeutic interventions.

Biography

Personal account of one's life.

Body awareness

Psychological focussing with the aim of becoming aware of the body.

Bone conduction

Direct transmission of sound via the bones of the skull (tuning fork or other sound source with direct contact to the mastoid bone) circumventing direct air-conduction through the ear to the inner ear.

Camera silencia

Soundproofed room in which the physiological tinnitus can be heard due to total silence.

Catharsis

Discharge of emotional tension in a psychotherapeutic setting, for example sudden outbreak of previously suppressed anger or sadness.

Central auditory pathway

The segment of the auditory system which follows the eighth nerve and is responsible for the analysis of the neurally-conducted electrical impulses up to the point of conscious hearing.

Cerebral trauma, head injury

Concussion of the cochlea with or without basilar skull fracture, often together with central (neural) or peripheral (sensory) functional disturbance; direct damage due to acute noise trauma (direct concussion).

Cerumen obturans

Impacted ear wax.

Cervical

Term pertaining to the neck.

Cholesteatoma

During the healing of acute necrotising otitis media, the remaining tissue of the mucous membrane and the stratified squamous epithelium of the ear-canal migrate to cover the denuded areas. Once the stratified squamous epithelium is in the middle ear, it begins to desquamate and accumulate and a cholesteatoma results. Other origins are also known such as ventilation disturbance of the Eustachian tube or as the result of peripheral defects of the ear-drum/tympanic membrane. Cholesteatomas may be recognised on otoscopic examination by the white debris in the middle ear and the destruction of the external auditory canal bone above the perforation. The presence of cholesteatoma increases the probability of a serious complication (e.g. purulent labyrinthitis, facial paralysis or intracranial suppurations), also leads to sound-conduction hearing loss. Therapy: surgery.

CNS

Abbreviation for central nervous system which includes all anatomical structures of the brain.

Cochlea

Inner ear. The inner ear is subdivided into three compartments: the scala vestibuli and scala tympani as well as the cochlear duct which is situated between the scalas. Acoustic stimuli, after having passed through the middle ear and through the scala vestibuli and scala tympani impinge upon Corti's organ, which is situated in the cochlear duct. In Corti's organ, hair cells, embedded within a scaffold of phalangeal and pillar cells, are rubbed against the tectorial membrane. In the cochlea, low tones are picked up near the tip, high tones near the oval window. The hearing organ transduces the soundwave, which was transmitted by the middle ear to the inner ear via a liquid-wave into neural action potentials.

Cognitive therapy

Psychotherapeutic interventions with the aim of improving psychological disorders by changing attitudes and assessments concerning certain situations and symptoms (behavioral therapy). This includes changing the perception or attitude toward the tinnitus and oneself, developing alternatives concerning one's own personal future and learning from other patients, who participate in a process of change. The fundamental hypothesis is that dysfunctional moods are caused by conscious and unconscious assumptions, opinions and thoughts.

Conditioning, classical

Regulating principle of reflex-reactions by means of initially neutral external stimuli (*J. P. Pawlow*).

Conditioning, operant

Specific type of conditioning, "operant" describes the fact that the subject has to perform a certain task (operation) to receive a reinforcing stimulus (for example, a reward).

Conflict, psychic

A conflict arises when two opposing impulses are present simultaneously. The conflict can be apparent or manifest (for example, between a certain desire and a moral command) or latent, appearing in an altered pattern during a manifest conflict, or in the form of symptoms, disturbed behavior or personality disorders.

Conversion

Psychic mechanism leading to the development of symptoms in hysteria or conversion disorder (see hysteria). It consists of the transformation of a psychic conflict into somatic, motor (for example, paralysis) or sensory (for example, anaesthesia or pain) symptoms with the aim of resolving the conflict.

Consciousness

In a descriptive sense: the momentary quality which characterises the internal and external perception of psychic phenomena. Topically speaking: the system of perception-consciousness is situated at the surface of the psyche; it receives information simultaneously originating from external as well as internal sources (sensations which belong to the pleasure/pain category and revived memories). Consciousness plays an important role in conflict-dynamics (conscious avoidance of pain-inducing situations, regulation of the pleasure-principle) and in psychotherapy.

Coping

A technique, based on research by *R. S. Lazarus* using consciously implemented behavioral and appraisal strategies which are employed in potentially stressful and dangerous situations to reduce possible reactions such as anxiety (anxiety-coping, stress-coping).

Counselling

Psychological technique with the aim of improving insight into a problem, changing behavioral attitudes, informing the patient with respect to psychological models of disease, supporting self-help groups, industrial counselling.

Countertransference

The conscious and unconscious reactions of the analyst concerning the patient especially with respect to the patient's transference concerning the analyst.

Courageous behavior

Acquiring courageous behavior is clearly related to an increased perception of self-efficacy (*A. Bandura*). Frequent confrontation with anxiety-inducing stimuli, development of coping-behavior, capabilities, positive reinforcement, high motivational level and model-learning (for example, from other tinnitus patients) are important elements of this behavioral repertoire.

dB

See decibel.

Decibel

Unit used in audiology to measure sound-intensity defined as the logorithmic relationship between baseline-sound-intensity (0dB) and the measured sound-intensity. An increase of intensity of 10dB doubles the loudness.

dB HL (hearing level) is the sound-intensity derived from the average human hearing-threshold (0dB). Tinnitus with the intensity of 80dB HL is a tinnitus which can be masked by a comparative tone of the same intensity.

dB SL (sensational level) is the sound-intensity derived from the individual hearing threshold. If the tinnitus is measured in dB SL it is measured in relation to the individual hearing-threshold, for example, given a hearing loss of 70dB HL and a maskability of the tinnitus of 80dB HL, the tinnitus intensity equals 10dB SL.

Sound	**Intensity in decibel**
Water dropping from a leaking faucet	40
Refrigerator	45
Normal rain	50
Chirping of birds	60
Washing machine	65
Dishwasher	65
Vacuum cleaner	70 to 85
Mixer	70
Cocktail party (100 guests)	70 to 85
Heavy traffic	70 to 85
Window ventilator	80
Alarm clock	80
Diesel truck or lorry	80
Electric razor	85
Screaming child	90 to 115
Compression hammer	100
Chain-saw	100
Subway/underground (measured inside)	100
Motorcycle	100
Generator motor (combustion engine for generating electricity)	100 to 105
Rock music (live, amplified)	90 to 130
Spectators at an ice-hockey game	120
Loud thunder	120
Air-raid siren	130
Jet engine (at take-off)	120 to 140

Decompression sickness

Equivalent to caisson disease or the bends; decompression sickness of the ear is a barotitis media (aerotitis), a disorder resulting from reduction of the surrounding pressure, as in ascent from a dive, exit from a caisson or hyperbaric chamber, or ascent to altitude, attributed to formation of gas bubbles in tissues or blood vessels and characterised most commonly by pain, less frequently by neurologic symptoms and rarely by pulmonary complications. This may also cause damage to the middle ear, leading to vertigo, loss of hearing, tinnitus. Therapy: recompression chamber with subsequent slow decompression.

Defence

(Sigmund Freud.) All psychological mechanisms whose intentions are to suppress modifications which may potentially endanger the integrity and consistency of the biopsychological entity of the individual. Generally speaking, defence mechanisms confront internal stimuli (urges) and specifically stimuli related to ideas (memories, fantasies), a specific situation, which can set the stimuli free, given the fact that these stimuli disturb the inner equilibrium and are therefore aversive to the ego. This takes place partially on an unconscious level. Different forms: sublimation, regression, reaction-formation, denial, rationalisation, suppression.

Depression

In the depressive syndrome, the mood typically is depressed, irritable or anxious, or a combination thereof. However, in masked depressions, consciously experienced depression may be paradoxically absent. Instead, the patient complains of being somatically ill and may even wear a defensive mask of smiling. Others complain of various aches and pains, fears of calamity to themselves or their loved ones, and fears of going insane. Finally in some the morbid effect is of such depth that tears dry up; here, return of ability to cry is usually a sign of improvement. It is in such severe depressions that morbid states of depersonalisation and derealisation occur, with loss of a capability to experience usual emotions, and a feeling that the world has become colorless, lifeless and dead. The morbid mood is accompanied by preoccupation with guilt, self-denigrating ideas, decreased ability to concentrate, indecisiveness, diminished interest in usual activities, social withdrawal, helplessness and hopelessness, diminished sexual drive and recurrent thoughts of death and suicide. DSM-III-R: major depression, dysthymia etc.

Depth psychology

Psychoanalytically-oriented psychology/psychotherapy.

Desensitization

Technique of behavioral therapy which is effective in the therapy of phobias. The therapist initially confronts the patient with a conception of or a symbolic representation of the lowest level of anxiety-producing stimuli (anxiety hierarchy). The patient then learns to employ anxiety-incompatible reactions (for example, relaxation techniques).

Detonation

Sound in the form of an acoustic impulse.

Digital analogue scale

A line is sub-divided into equal intervals (like a thermometer) and the tinnitus loudness can be assessed directly (for example, 0 = no tinnitus, 10 = extremely loud tinnitus).

Distraction

To divert attention, for example away from the tinnitus in the direction of an external stimulus. Technique of behavioral therapy.

To Double

Technique of psychodrama in which one member of a therapy group identifies himself with another and tries to describe the unexpressed thoughts or feelings of the other member of the therapy group.

DSM-III-R

Abbreviation for Diagnostic and Statistical Manual of Mental Disorders, Third and Revised Version. Classification of pyschiatric disorders introduced by the APA (American Psychiatric Association).

Dualism

Term describing the philosophical thinking which assumes the existence of two independent substances, e.g. the mind and the body (*René Descartes*).

Dynamic

Definition for psychic phenomena as a result of a conflict and the interrelationship between opposing psychic "energies" which result in a specific impulse which initially originates in instincts or urges.

EEG

Abbreviation for Electro-encephalogram, a method of measuring the changes of biochemical potentials of the brain with the aim of ascertaining the presence of brain tumors or epilepsy.

Efferent

Neurophysiological term describing those nerves (efferents) which transport a neuronal impulse from the central nervous system (centrifugally) to the corresponding peripheral organ (muscles, glands, external hair cells, etc.).

Ego

The core structure of personality which *Sigmund Freud* differentiates from the id and super-ego and depends on the desires and impulses of the id and the commands of the super-ego as well as the demands of reality. Even though it functions as a mediator of the complete personality structure, it is only relatively autonomous. Psychodynamically speaking, the ego is the psychic defence in a neurotic conflict and uses a range of defence mechanisms which are perceived as being aversive (ego-pain, "unpleasure", anxiety, "unlust").

Egotism

Self-interest.

Electrostimulation

Therapeutical method with the aim of influencing tinnitus by stimulating the inner ear or the eighth nerve with an electrode placed in the vicinity of the tympanic membrane or the inner ear.

Emotion

General term describing psychophysiological change of state, which is produced by an external stimulus (sensory perception) or an internal stimulus (body perception) and/or cognitive processes (assessment, conception, expectation/anticipation). The perceived quality of this experience, which more or less transcends cognitive and motivational experience, is equivalent to the term "feelings". Intense feelings of short duration with disorganising or constricting effects on perception and behavior are called affects.

Empirical

General term describing knowledge based on experience.

Endogenous

General term for a phenomenon which evolves out of a system or structure: in relation to psychoses, a description of suspected (genetically) determinated causes.

Epidemiology

General term describing the research of the frequency of diseases, disorders or customs.

Etiology

Term describing the specific causes of medical or psychological phenomena.

Etymology

The discipline which deals with the origin of words and usage.

Evaluation

Assessment.

Exploration

A psychiatric term used also in clinical psychology; interview of a patient with the aim of clarifying the presented symptoms and problems.

Exposition

See desensitization, a technique of behavioral therapy, confrontation with aversive stimuli, for example annoying or anxiety-provoking sound stimuli.

Extroversion

Term originally defined by *C. G. Jung* describing a fundamental attitude concerning perception and behavior which is principally oriented to the surrounding environment. Personality variable, the degree of extroversion, can be evaluated using questionnaires (see FPI, MMPI, Eysenck Personality Questionnaire).

Fantasy

Imagined scene in which the subject is present, indirectly due to the effects of defence-mechanisms.

Fear

A feeling of tension and involvement in the face of or in expectation of an actual or potential danger or comparable feelings without actual objects or situations which evoke fear or anxiety. Uncontrollable fear is called phobia. An anxiety state includes both anxiety and fear (*W. D. Fröhlich*).

Feedback

Term used in psychotherapy to denote a remark given in response to a specific behavior or statement.

Flight into disease or illness

Term which describes the fact that

a patient uses his neurotic mechanisms to evade his psychic conflicts (primary gain). This term became popular in psychoanalysis. Today it is not restricted to neuroses but is used for all somatic illnesses which also have a psychic component.

Flooding

Technique of behavioral therapy. Patients are confronted with stimuli related to anxiety or phobia in full intensity and rapid succession as opposed to desensitization or anxiety-hierarchy-therapy, which then leads to anxiety-stimulus-extinction.

Fowler test

Measurement of recruitment in unilateral hearing impairment, see also SISI test.

FPI

Abbreviation for the Freiburger Personality Inventory, a personality test developed by *J. Fahrenberg* et al for German-speaking countries consisting of 138 questions and 10 standard scales (contentment, social orientation, competitiveness, inhibition, hostility, etc.) and 2 secondary scales (extroversion, emotionality). Comparable with the Eysenck Personality Inventory (EPI) and the Minnesota Multiphasic Personality Inventory (MMPI). Stanine-value between 1 and 9, norm between 4 and 6.

Gain from illness

Every general (direct or indirect) form of satisfaction an individual derives from being ill.

Gain from illness, primary

The prime motivational force of a neurosis: achieving satisfaction by means of a symptom, flight into illness, change of relationship to one's surroundings.

Gain from illness, secondary

The following differences exist between primary and secondary gain from illness. Secondary gain: 1) takes advantage of pre-existing illness; 2) has features which are different from the initial determinating factors of an illness and the initial purpose of the presented symptoms; 3) deals primarily with the satisfaction of narcissistic tendencies and self-preservation, not direct satisfaction of libidinous needs.

Gestalt therapy

Psychotherapy developed by *F. S. Perls* (1940) and related to depth psychology. Emphasis on the "here and now"; goal of therapy: resolution of fixated reactions and behavior, improvement of self-perception.

Globus hystericus or globus feeling

Functional disorder with the subjective sensation of a lump or mass in the throat which may lead to fear of strangulation.

Glomus tumor, paraganglioma

Non-chromaffian paragangliomas (chemodectomas) which arise in the middle ear from glomus bodies in the jugular bulb (glomus jugulare), the carotis (glomus caroticum) or the medial wall of the middle ear (glomus tympanicum). They produce a pulsating red mass in the middle ear. The first symptom is often tinnitus which is synchronous with the pulse (objective tinnitus). Hearing loss and later vertigo develop. Tympanometry: seldom changes of impedence which are synchronous with the pulse. Therapy: excision, radiation therapy.

Group dynamics

Research discipline, founded by *H. Lewin*, which is concerned with the types and forms of the development and functions of social groups considering the causes, the motivational aspects and effects.

Group therapy

Recently developed form of psychotherapy in which small groups of patients and a therapist come into mutual contact with each other, allowing increased therapeutic possibilities of influencing the individual group member beneficially.

Guilt feelings

Global term used in psychoanalysis. It can describe an affective/ emotional state which follows a behavior or a committed act which the perpetrator perceives as punishable for more or less sound or adequate reasons (feeling of guilt in a criminal on the one hand, absurd self-reproach on the other hand) or a mixed feeling of personal worthlessness which is not related to any specific behavior or committed act. Psychoanalysis also postulates that guilt feelings are a system of unconscious motivations which describe behavior which leads to delinquent behavior or suffering. The term feeling may only be used with caution in the latter definition because the individual does not feel consciously guilty.

Habituation

General term for decrease or inhibition of a behavioral reaction by means of becoming accustomed to the acoustic stimulus.

Hair cell

Sensory neuro-epithelial cell of the inner ear which transforms acoustically-generated liquid-waves into neurally-conducted electrical impulses; inner hair cell (IHC): the actual sensory neuro-epithelial cell, outer hair cell (OHC): modulates hearing by means of an active contraction via efferent nerves.

Hardiness

American term in pain research for a lack of influence on well-being through disease, stress and pain; high feeling of control concerning aims and goals in life, unreserved attitude towards social changes, ability to devote oneself optimistically to one's profession and family, to confront challenges and believe in oneself.

Hearing limit

See Hz (Hertz).

Hearing ossicles

Little, interconnected bones with the purpose of transmitting sound from the tympanic membrane to the inner ear (malleus, incus and stapes) situated in the middle ear.

Hearing threshold

In dB HL, a threshold at which sine tones are initially perceived.

Helplessness, learned/acquired helplessness

A state of negative and pessimistic expectations together with the conviction that problems cannot be solved with the cognitive and behavioral possibilities at hand; similar to depression; develops after continual experience of the fact that a certain behavior does not lead to the desired positive or negative reinforcement; feeling of lack of control, risk of generalisation.

Hypnosis

Diversion of the focus of attention in the direction of the source of induction of hypnosis. Decrease of the perception of reality, loss of initiative, highest degree of susceptibility for induced thoughts and perceptions (see below).

Hypnotherapy

Combination of cognitive therapy and hypnosis. In an extremely relaxed, "hypnotic" state (trance) the patient is induced to, for example, transform the tinnitus into a more acceptable visual/acoustic impression or to change the existing attitudes towards the tinnitus. Tape recordings of the individual sessions help the patient to improve the effectiveness of hypnotherapy at home.

Hypochondriasis, hypochondriacal neurosis, atypical somatoform disorder

A neurotic disorder characterised by a preoccupation with bodily functions and a morbid fear that one is suffering from a serious disease. Etiology is unknown but clinical evidence suggests that, like somatisation disorder, hypochondriasis is related to a narcissistic character organisation marked by excessive self-observation and concern with self and with the gratification of dependency needs. High scores in the MMPI indicate an unfavourable prognosis for patients with a chronic pain syndrome without evident organic origin. Research results concerning tinnitus have not been published to date.

Hysteria, hysterical neurosis, conversion reaction, dissociative reaction, histrionic personality

Is sub-divided into a conversion and dissociative disorder of consciousness and results either in the loss of bodily function (e.g. conversion disorder) or the loss of conscious awareness/loss of voluntary recall of specific internal mental contents (memories, ideas, feelings, perceptions) (e.g. dissociation) and the integrating function of self-identity. An hysterical (e.g. histrionic) personality is characterised by conspicious egocentricity. Winning the esteem and admiration of others is of paramount importance, attention-seeking and theatrical behavior is prominent. Symptoms: globus feeling, paralysis, anaesthesia, etc.

Hz or Hertz

Abbreviation for Hertz, the unit of frequency or number of sound oscillations per second. Human sound perception range: hearing threshold 16Hz, hearing limit 20,000Hz (*H. Hertz* 1857-1894).

Ideal ego

The controlling element of personality, which is the result of the convergence of narcism (idealisation of the ego) and identification with the parents, their surrogates and collective ideals. As an individual personal structure, the ideal ego is the model of an ideal which the individual tries to attain (*Sigmund Freud*).

Identification

Psychological mechanism in which the individual assimilates an aspect or capability or trait of another individual and thereby experiences a complete or partial change of behavior or attitude.

Incidence rate

This term refers to the frequency with which new occurrences of an event are noted as a group is observed during a defined period of time.

Incus

Hearing ossicle, a bone of the ossicular chain, which is connected to the malleus and stapes via joints, phylogenetically the equivalent of the os quadratum, which is responsible for mandibular joint function in reptiles.

Inferiority complex, sense or feeling of inferiority

A feeling which arises due to an actual or suspected psychic or somatic defect. An inferiority complex is the result of the individual's attempts to compensate his defect.

Interpretation

To uncover the latent meaning of words or behavior of the patient by means of the analytical approach. In the actual therapeutic context the cue given by the therapist which enables the patient to realise and analyse the latent meaning.

Introversion

Term introduced by *C.G. Jung* which describes fundamental attitudes of an individual who orients his perception and behavior according to his inner-self. A personality variable which is assessed by questionnaires (see FPI, Eysenck Personality Questionnaire).

Item

Specific single question or task in a psychological test/questionnaire.

Labyrinth or cochlea

Consists of the organ responsible for equilibrium and the inner ear.

Limbic system

Sub-cortical structures of the brain extending along the hippocampal formation of the medial temporal lobes, fornix, mammillary bodies to the anterior nuclei of the thalamus, singulum, septal area and the orbital surface of the frontal lobes. Probably responsible for memories and the development and duration of emotional reactions.

Loudness

Subjective perception of the intensity of an acoustic event, which is determined by comparing it with predetermined sound-producing sources or psychometrically with visual analogue scales (see tinnitus loudness). Although the unit Sone exists (for example, twice the loudness of a sound equals an increase of 10 Phon, half the loudness of a sound equals a decrease 10 Phon; one sone equals 40 Phon, 2 Sone equals circa 50 Phon, 4 Sone equals circa 60 Phon, etc.), this unit has not become established.

Malleus

Hammer-shaped hearing ossicle with a handle and a protuberance which is connected to the tympanic membrane and is joined to the incus, phylogenetically the equivalent of the os articulare (part of the temporomandibular joint) of reptiles.

Masking

Degree to which acoustic oscillations can be cancelled by control sounds.

Menière's disease

A disorder characterised by recurrent prostating vertigo with nausea and vomiting, sensory-neural hearing loss and unilateral tinnitus, associated with generalised dilation of the membranous labyrinth (endolymphatic hydrops). Often a feeling of pressure in the ear is present. Positive recruitment (cochlear disturbance). Fluctuating low-frequency hearing loss. During an attack spontaneous nystagmus in the direction of the affected ear and later in the direction of the healthy ear is present. Tinnitus is more severe during an attack than during an interval.

Middle ear

Consists of the air spaces of the middle ear and ossicular chain. (The external ear consists of the external auditory canal and the tympanic membrane (eardrum), the inner ear consists of the cochlea, the vestibular apparatus and the eighth nerve).

MMPI

Abbreviation for Minnesota Multiphasic Personality Inventory. Popular psychological test in English-speaking countries which consists of 399 true/false questions and assesses a wide range of psychological dimensions such as hypochondriasis, hysteria, depression. The patient-score is computed as a T-score which has a mean value of 50 and a standard deviation of 10.

M. stapedius
(stapedial muscle)

The smallest human muscle, which is innervated by the facial nerve (seventh nerve), inserts at the head of the stapes (hearing ossicle); contraction is caused by acoustic stimuli (stapedial reflex, dependent on loudness and sound-intensity), is responsible for adaption to loudness of acoustic phenomena.

M. tensor tympani
(tympanic tensor muscle)

Muscle which is phylogenetically part of the masticatory musculature, is innervated by the mandibular branch of the trigeminal nerve (fifth nerve) and inserts at the handle of the malleus (hearing ossicle) and leads to a change of the tension of the tympanic membrane (impedence); only tactile stimuli (such as blowing in the eye) lead to contraction but this muscle may also take part in the adaption to acoustic phenomena.

M. tensor veli palatini
(tensor muscle of the velum palatini)

This muscle is innervated by the mandibular branch of the trigeminal nerve (fifth nerve) and opens the Eustachian tube when swallowing together with the M. levator veli palatini which is innervated by the glossopharyngeal nerve (ninth nerve) as well as the vagus nerve (tenth nerve).

Narcissism

Term based on the Greek myth of Narcissus describing an exaggerated sense of self-importance with fantasies of unlimited success and constant attention-seeking behavior (exaggerated self-love).

Narcissism, primary

Term for an early stage of development in which a child concentrates its complete libido on itself (*Sigmund Freud*).

Narcissism, secondary

Regressive behavior of an adult which becomes apparent when libido is diverted away from original object choices (*Sigmund Freud*).

Neural deafness

See sound perception hearing loss.

Neuroleptics, major tranquillizers

Psychotropic drugs used in the treatment of psychoses and states of extreme agitation leading to sedation and a decrease of hallucinations and delusions.

Neurosis

Group of disorders in which specific, usually ego-alien and distressing, neurotic symptoms occur, i.e. anxieties, phobias, obsessions, compulsions and hysterical conversion and disassociative phenomena. The symptoms are the symbolic expression of a psychic conflict which has its roots in childhood; the neurotic symptom itself represents the compromise between a desire or urge and its defence mechanism. The definition of this term has undergone changes, in the DSM-III-R it is no longer used; instead the more neutral term disorder has replaced the term neurosis.

N. facialis (facial nerve)

Motor division: lower portion of pons in recess between inferior peduncle and olive. Passes through internal acoustic meatus along facial canal and makes its exit at stylomastoid foramen. Running forward through parotid gland, it divides into many branches. Responsible for motor supply of facial muscles, scalp, auricle, buccinator, platysma, stapedius, stylohyoid, posterior belly of digastric. Sensory division (intermedius): geniculate ganglion in facial canal. Branches run by way of chorda tympani to periphery. Centrally it proceeds through acoustic meatus entering brain between inferior peduncle and olive. Taste in anterior two-thirds of tongue. Sensation to soft palate. Innervation of salivary glands. (Seventh nerve.)

N. glossopharyngeus (glossopharyngeal nerve — ninth nerve)

Passes from medulla oblongata laterally to the jugular foramen, through the petrous temporal bone, making its exit between internal carotid artery and internal jugular vein. Taste in posterior third of tongue. Sensation to fauces, tonsils, pharynx and soft palate. Motor for pharynx and stylopharyngeus muscle. Impulses to parotid gland.

Nocebo

See placebo.

Noise

A mixture of tones on a continuous spectrum or many tones of which the ratios of the frequencies are not whole numbers; our ear is specialised to a greater degree to analyse noise than to receive pure tones. Children and animals react to noise more intensely than to harmonic music (*Mehmke/Tegtmeier*).

Noise

Subjective description of a sound which disrupts the perception of a desired sound or disrupts desired stillness. Even noise which is perceived as agreeable may lead to a hearing disorder (for example, loud noise through headphones or in a discotheque).

Noise-induced hearing loss

Occupational exposition over years with a noise level greater than 85- to 90dB without ear protection (occupational disease, also damage caused by "recreational noise" such as Walkman audio-tape recorders, discotheques and rock concerts).

Noises in the ear

See tinnitus.

Numbing

Numbing of the contralateral ear to allow a separate measurement of the ipsilateral ear (for example by using noise).

N. vagus (vagus nerve — tenth nerve)

Arises in the groove between inferior peduncle and olive, passes through the jugular foramen where it is joined by the cranial portion of the spinal accessory nerve and continues down the neck and thorax into the abdomen. Sensory fibres to skin in back of auricle, posterior portion of external acoustic meatus, pharynx, larynx, thoracic and abdominal viscera. Motor fibres to pharynx, base of tongue, larynx and to autonomic ganglia innervating thoracic and abdominal viscera.

N. vestibulocochlearis (acoustic nerve — eighth nerve)

Cochlear division: spiral ganglion of cochlea; peripheral fibres to the organ of Corti; central fibres go to the internal auditory meatus and enter the inferior peduncle, responsible for hearing. Terminates in the ventral and dorsal cochlear nuclei.

Vestibular division: bipolar cells in the vestibular ganglion; superior, inferior and posterior branches end in the utricle, superior and lateral semi-circular canals, the saccule and in the ampule of posterior semi-circular canal respectively. Maintenance of equilibrium; terminates in the medial, lateral, superior and spinal vestibular nuclei and in cerebellum.

Object

This term is used in psychoanalysis and has three principal aspects:

1) As a correlative of instinct and urges. By means of the object an instinct or desire attempts to reach its aims or goals (i.e. satisfaction). The object may be another person or a partial object, an actual object or a product of fantasy.
2) As a correlative of love (or hate). The relationship is in this case between a whole person or the ego-instance and an object, that is strived for as a whole (person, unity, ideal, etc.)
3) As a correlative of the perceiving and knowledgeable subject in the traditional meaning in philosophy and psychology of consciousness. It has traits which do not undergo changes, is objectively perceivable in all subjects and is independent of the desires and opinions of an individual.

Ontogenesis

Individual development of members of a certain species, contrary to phylogenesis, which refers to the development of a certain species as a whole.

Operant behavior

Based on research by *B.F. Skinner*; behavior which arises spontaneously without being provoked by a specific stimulus and can become conditioned behavior due to reinforcement.

Organ of Corti

Consists of internal and external hair cells with supporting cells and stereocilia which are rooted in the basilar membrane of the cochlear duct and are covered by the tectorial membrane (first described by *A. G. G. Count of Corti* (1822-1876).

Otosclerosis

A disease of the labyrinth capsule and the most common cause of progressive sound conduction hearing loss in the adult with a normal tympanic membrane. The foci enlarge and cause ankylosis of the footplate of the stapes. Sound perception hearing loss may also occur. Diagnosis possible with the examination of the stapes reflex; low-frequency tinnitus occurs more often. Tendency is familial, accelerated development during pregnancy and anti-conceptives. Treatment: microsurgical techniques: stapes removal and replacement with prosthesis, hearing aid.

Perception

The first, preconscious phase of apprehension (followed by apperception).

Phobia

Abnormal, uncontrollable fear of objects or situations. See anxiety, agorophobia. DSM-III-R differentiation between: 1) agoraphobia with panic attacks; 2) agoraphobia without panic attacks; 3) social phobia; 4) simple phobia.

Phon

Unit for the psycho-physical assessment of loudness.

Phylogenesis

The development of the species as a whole due to evolution.

Placebo

Inactive substances used in controlled studies for comparison with presumed active drugs (with the intent to relieve symptoms or meet a patient's demands). A placebo may be any type of therapeutic manoeuvre including surgical or psychological techniques or medication in any form ("placebo-reactivity"). The opposite term is nocebo: consciously or unconsciously contructed study or control study in which the researcher is convinced of the ineffectiveness of the tested drug or therapy under investigation and therefore causes negative effects.

Presbycusis

Sensory neural hearing loss that occurs as a part of normal aging; stiffening of the basilar membrane and deterioration of the hair cells play a principal role in pathogenesis, binaural hearing loss especially for high frequencies. Tinnitus usually not loud. SISI test positive.

Prevalence rate

Frequency with which an event exists at a particular time in a particular group.

Psychoanalysis

Discipline founded by *Sigmund Freud* who differentiated between three aspects:

1) A method of analysis which consists predominantly of an analysis of the conscious meanings of what the patient says, does or imagines (dreams, fantasies, de-

lusions). This method is based on the "free associations" of the patient which themselves serve as the verifying factor for their interpretation. Psychoanalytical interpretation can also be used for psychic operations or forms which cannot be expressed by means of "free-association".

2) A method of psychotherapy which is based on this analysis (1) and consists of a controlled interpretation of the resistance, the transference and the desires of the patient. This method is synonymous with psychoanalytical treatment.

3) The entire complex of psychological and psychotherapeutical theories which result from analysis and treatment (1 and 2).

Psychodrama

A form of psychotherapy developed by *J. L. Moreno* (1921), in which patients role-play, allowing the therapist to analyse the patients' symptoms and their causes by deducing from the social context of the role-playing persons or group. A combination of psychoanalytical concepts and group dynamics, certain techniques are now used in the training of salesmen and self-assertiveness training.

Psychosis

Psychiatry uses this term in a broad sense including various psychic illnesses independent of the fact whether they are of organic origin or not (for example, schizophrenia); in DSM-III-R this term is restricted to schizophrenia and related disorders.

Psychotherapy

General term for all methods used to treat psychological disturbances or somatic illnesses by psychological means: hypnosis, suggestion, psychological education, etc. In this sense, psychoanalysis is a specific form of psychotherapy.

Rationalization

Psychic defence-mechanism: the emotional impetus of a specific situation is decreased by means of over-emphasis of a cognitive analysis, which leads to a logically coherent and morally acceptable resolution without having to face the actual motives.

Recruitment

Abnormal increase in the perception of loudness or the ability to hear loud sounds normally despite hearing loss. Recruitment is absent in neural/eighth nerve hearing losses (negative recruitment) and present in sensory/cochlear hearing losses (positive recruitment). Recruitment can be demonstrated by having the patient compare the loudness of sounds in the affected ear with the loudness of sounds in the normal ear. In sensory hearing losses, the sensation of loudness in the affected ear increases more with each increment in intensity than it does in the normal ear. In neural hearing losses, the sensation of loudness in the affected ear increases less with each increment in intensity than it does in the normal ear (decruitment).

Regression

In considering the nature of a psychic process, which in itself implies movement and development, regression is a relapse from a point attained back to a point situated at an earlier stage of the given develoment. Formally speaking, regression is the transition to modes of experience and behavior on a less mature level with respect to complexity, structure and differentiation.

Reinforcement

Increase, augmentation (to reinforce = to strengthen).

Relaxation training

General term for different relaxation methods (autogenic training, progressive muscle relaxation according to *Jacobson*, the hypnotic state or trance). About half of the patients suffering from chronic tinnitus profit from relaxation training which leads to increased tinnitus tolerance, change of attitudes towards tinnitus (decrease of the feeling of helplessness) and improvement of sleep disturbances. A decrease of tinnitus intensity can only be expected if the tinnitus is predominantly due to muscle tension of the temporomandibular and neck muscles.

Reliability

Term describing the statistically assessed exactness of a unit or test.

Residual inhibition

After giving a masking tone or noise over a period of 1 minute, the interval between cessation of the masking tone and reattainment of the original level of tinnitus intensity is measured. The longer the interval, the more favourable are the chances of success for a masker therapy. A long interval (more than 1 minute) is an indication for a tinnitus of cochlear origin.

Retraining therapy

Combination of behavioral therapy/counselling and masking/hearing aid therapy.

Role-play

Technique used in psychotherapy (psychodrama, self-assertiveness training, Gestalt therapy, etc.).

Rupture of the membrane of the oval window

Symptoms identical with those of sudden deafness, always in combination with vertigo, with loss of endolymphatic liquid. Therapy: rapid operation.

Scale

Statistical term for the reference system of measurement.

Schizophrenia

Mental disorders with a tendency towards chronicity which impair functioning and which are characterised by psychotic symptoms involving disturbances of thinking, feeling and behavior. Six specific criteria for the diagnosis include: 1) certain psychotic symptoms, delusions, hallucinations, formal thought disorders; 2) deterioration of a previous level of functioning; 3) continuous signs of illness for at least six months; 4) a tendency towards onset before age 45; 5) not due to affective disorders; and 6) not due to organic mental disorder or mental retardation. Syndromes which look like schizophrenia but which last less than six months are called schizophreniform. If symptoms last more than six months, a schizophrenic disorder is probable.

SCL

Abbreviation for Symptom Check list (Derogatis), a psychological test used internationally to assess different psychopathological symptoms; often also called Hopkins Symptom Check-List (HSCL). Ninety different psychological and psychosomatic symptoms are considered which are sub-divided into nine scales (somatisation, obsessive symptoms, depression, phobia, psychoticism) and three main scales (general symptoms, number of symptoms and stress index).

Self-assertiveness training

Technique of behavioral therapy, programme in which patients learn to overcome inhibitions in social situations.

Self-help organisation

Group organised by patients which is co-ordinated by a board which usually publishes pamphlets or newsletters for its members. Group members meet regularly (exchange of opinions and experiences in a group setting, without a professional helper, organisation of information meetings and invitations for health-professionals).

Sensation

Term describing aspects of basic elements of sensory perception.

Sensation of hearing

Acoustic perception.

Sensory hearing loss

See sensory hearing loss.

Simulation

Conscious fabrication of symptoms or subjective feelings of illness (contrary to aggravation).

SISI test

Abbreviation for Short Increment Sensitivity Index. Sensitivity to small increments. Intensity can be demonstrated by presenting a continuous tone of 20dB above the hearing threshold and increasing the intensity by 1dB briefly and intermittently. The percentage of small increments that the patient can detect yields the SISI. A high SISI (80-100%) is characteristic of sensory hearing loss, while a patient with a neural lesion, like a person with normal hearing, cannot detect such small changes in intensity. (Negative value: 0-15%).

Somatization

Complaints which seem to be of a somatic nature but lack clinical findings (functional symptoms). The term somatization is purely descriptive.

Sone

Unit of sound intensity.

Sound

Acoustic phenomenon consisting of different tones which are in harmony with each other.

Sound

Mechanical oscillation which leads to the perception of hearing ("the vibrations of the ear turn to sound only where there is an ear" *Lichtenberg*); see also Hz.

Sound conduction hearing loss

Due to a lesion in the external auditory canal or the middle ear (impacted ear wax, blocked movement of the tympanic membrane or otosclerosis). Audiogram: bone conduction unaffected, air conduction impaired.

Sound intensity

Sound pressure is measured in Phon, a unit which considers the physiological perception of sound intensity of the ear. The scales for dB and Phon are identical at 1,000Hz.

Sound perception hearing loss (sensorineural hearing loss)

Hearing loss due to disturbance of the eighth nerve and/or central auditory pathway (neural hearing loss, retrocochlear hearing loss = neural hearing loss or disturbance of the cochlea = sensory hearing loss). Audiogram: air conduction as well as bone conduction hearing threshold are increased; BERA differentiates between cochlear and retrocochlear disturbance.

Speech audiogram

See audiogram.

Stapes

Hearing ossicle that is joined to the incus (hearing ossicle) with its head and to the oval window with its footplate. It is part of the ossicular chain which connects the middle ear with the inner ear.

Stereocilia

Fine hairs, which are situated on top of the hair cells of the organ of Corti and are in close contact with the tectorial membrane. A shearing motion of the tectorial membrane leads to a distension of the stereocilia, which then leads to a discharge of electrical impulses in the hair cells, the actual process of hearing; dysfunction (dissection, etc.) is the cause of sensory hearing loss. Positive recruitment, deterioration of speech discrimination (speech audiogram) and tinnitus result.

Sudden hearing loss, sudden deafness

Severe sensory neural hearing loss that usually occurs in only one ear and develops over a period of a few hours or less. Hearing loss is usually profound, but fortunately the hearing returns to normal in most patients and partial recovery occurs in others. Tinnitus and vertigo may be present initially. The vertigo usually subsides in several days. Other symptoms: feeling of pressure in the ear. Neurological symptoms are not present. Common false diagnosis: cerumen obturans (impacted ear wax) or inflammation of the Eustachian tube. Treatment: (emergency situation!) vasodilators, anti-coagulants, dextrane, corticosteroids.

Temporal bone

Bone located at the base of the skull, which envelops the inner ear (cochlea) and the vestibular apparatus; hardest bond of the human skeleton.

Test of significance

Statistical technique to establish the numerical magnitudes that allow a significant difference to be regarded as statistically (or stochastically) significant.

Tinnitus aurium

Subjective noise located in the ear; term derived from the latin word tinnire = to ring.

Tinnitus cerebri

Subjective noise located in the head, most probably due to a disturbance of the central nervous system.

Tinnitus, compensated

A tinnitus which can be tolerated and does not interfere with normal daily life.

Tinnitus, complex chronic

Synonym for decompensated tinnitus, this term was introduced by *P.N. Duckro* (1984).

Tinnitus, decompensated complex

A tinnitus which influences and dominates daily life and leads to complications such as sleep disturbances, lack of concentration, depression, phobia, etc.

Tinnitus diary

Daily protocol of tinnitus-specific variables used in behavioral therapy (loudness, tinnitus disturbance or annoyance, feeling of control, tinnitus tolerance time) as well as general variables (duration of sleep, mood, stress, assessment of success of therapy). The assessment can be measured using visual analogue scales (for example, 100mm scale: 0 = nil, 100 = extreme), a verbal analogue scale (no tinnitus/slight tinnitus/moderate tinnitus/extremely disturbing tinnitus/tormenting tinnitus).

Tinnitus intensity

Psychoacoustical assessment of the volume of the tinnitus compared with defined acoustic signal measured in dB HL or dB SL (see dB).

Tinnitus loudness

Contrary to tinnitus intensity (see above), the subjective perception of tinnitus measured with analogue scales.

Tinnitus loudness scales

These scales are often incorrectly defined as tinnitus intensity scales.

Grade-scale of *Klockhoff & Lindblom* (1967) (see Chapter 2):

Grade I: Tinnitus audible only in quiet surroundings.

Grade II: Tinnitus audible at normal noise level and maskable with loud noise.

Grade III: Tinnitus is louder than all surrounding noises, causes sleep disturbances and is the dominant problem in life.

Six-Point Scale of *Schönweiler* (1986) (not mentioned in this book):

0: No tinnitus.
1: Tinnitus audible only in absolutely quiet surroundings.
2: Tinnitus barely audible (only when one concentrates on it).
3: Tinnitus permanently audible but not to distracting.
4: Tinnitus constantly audible, concentration and sleep are disturbed.
5: Tinnitus constantly audible, very disturbing, cannot be suppressed.

Six-Point Scale of *Schumann* et al (1990) (not mentioned in this book):

0: No tinnitus.
1: Slight humming — not distracting.
2: Humming — still tolerable tinnitus.
3: Loud humming or buzzing — is constantly registered, distracting.
4: Roaring, constant or oscillating noise, very disturbing, problems falling asleep.
5: Roaring like a waterfall, very disturbing, influences the psyche negatively, concentration problems, lack of incentive, cardiac arrythmia, severe sleep disturbances.
6: Roaring and rushing like a hydro-electric plant — penetrating noise of intolerable intensity, the loudness only decreases in

the evening, severe detrimental influence on the psyche, leads to complete lack of incentive, loss of interest, suicidal tendencies and severe sleep disturbances.

Tinnitus masking

(*H. Feldmann.*) Tinnitus is maskable with white noise, a broad-band noise, on the one hand or sinus tones or narrow-band noise on the other hand. A convergence curve (simultaneous masking) and maskability are typical for a tinnitus of cochlear origin (see residual inhibition).

Tinnitus matching

Assessment of tinnitus frequency and intensity using sinus tones or narrow-band noise produced by an audiometer for comparison.

Tinnitus, objective

A tinnitus caused by a source of sound situated in the body, which can be heard by the examining physician (for example, stenosis of the carotid artery, artificial heart valve, glomus tumor).

Tinnitus self-help organisations

Australia
Australian Tinnitus Association WA
29 West Parade
Perth 6000 WA

Austria
Österreichischer Schwerhörigenbund
Referat Tinnitus
Radegunderstraße 10
8045 Graz

Canada
Tinnitus Association of Canada
Co-ordinator: Mrs E. Eayrs
23 Ellis Park Road
Toronto, Ontario M6S2V4
Magazine: Newsletter (edition 1000)

Czech Republic
Ing. Bohumil Schneider
Rimska 41
12000 Prag 2

Denmark
Landforeningen For Bedre Hoerelse
Tinnitus-Udvalget
Kong Georgs Vej 13
2000 Frederiksberg

France
France Acouphènes
Président: M. Maurice Demiaz
Secrétariat et Trésorerie, La Varizelle
F-69510 Thurins

Germany
Deutsche Tinnitus-Liga e. V. (DTL)
Präsident: Hans Knör
Am Lohsiepen 18
42353 Wuppertal 21
Membership: ca. 10,000
Magazine: Tinnitus-Forum
(Edition 28,000) quarterly

Great Britain
British Tinnitus Association (BTA)
Room 6, 14-18 West Bar Green
Sheffield S1 2DA
Magazine: Quiet, earlier newsletter

Netherlands
Nederlandse Vereningen voor
Slechthorenden
Commissie Tinnitus
Verdiweg 305
3816 KJ Amersfoort

New Zealand
New Zealand Tinnitus Association
31 William Souter Street
Forrest Hill
Auckland 10

Norway
Hørselhemmedes Landsforbund (HLF)
Boks 5293 Majorstua
0303 Oslo

Sweden
Tinnitusföreningen i Göteborg
Hörselrehabilieringen
Första Länggatan 30
413 27 Göteborg

Tinnitussektionen
Norrley Tuärgata 11-13
502 64 Boras

Hörselskadakes Riksförbund
M. Anderson tinnituskonsulent
Sköldungagatan 7
114 86 Stockholm

Switzerland
Schweizer Tinnitus Liga
Postfach
CH-8052 Zürich

USA
American Tinnitus Association
P.O. Box 5
Oregon 97207-0005, Portland
Magazine: Tinnitus Today

Tone audiometry/pure tone audiometry

See audiometry.

Trance

State of consciousness similar to sleep with reduced perception of environmental stimuli, predominance of automatic behavior, lack of willed movement, which is induced by hypnosis or hysteria. Trance in a religious context is defined as ecstasy; specific EEG modifications; wide pupils.

Tranquilizer, minor tranquilizer

Sedative, pharmacologically predominantly or benzodiazepines — risk of dependency.

Transaction

Interaction with the environment (persons, objects, situations).

Trauma

A situation defined by its intensity of experience; a trauma is characterised by stimuli which overwhelm the subject's capacity to cope with them.

Tube, Eustachian

Epiphelially enclosed connection of a length of 3.5cm between the tympanic cavity and the pharynx which opens during swallowing (tensor muscle of the velum paletini, innervated by the mandibular branch of the trigeminal nerve (fifth nerve); levator muscle of the palate, innervated by the glossopharyngeal nerve (ninth nerve) and the vagus nerve (tenth nerve)), responsible for the regulation of air pressure allowing the tympanic membrane to oscillate properly.

Validity

Term for the empirically assessed correlation between a test and a relevant criterion of the examined context.

Variable

A mathematical term used in the evaluation of empirical data-characteristic dimension which is inconstant.

Vestibular

Pertaining to the vestibular organ which is responsible for equilibrium.

Visual analogue scale

A 100mm scale for tinnitus loudness; the left end of the scale is marked 0 (= no tinnitus), the right end is marked 100 (= extremely loud tinnitus); using a millimetre ruler, the score can be assessed.

White noise

Noise in which all frequencies have the same sound intensity.

Working over, psychic

Term used by *Sigmund Freud* to describe the work accomplished by the psyche in different contexts such as control of agitation or arousal which may endanger the proper functioning of the psyche. It consists of an integration of the arousal and the development of associations (compare with coping).

The definitions were partially taken from the:

DSM-III-R (APA-1987): Diagnostic and statistical manual of mental disorders, 3rd edition, revised. American Psychiatric Association, Washington DC.

Fröhlich, W. D. (1987): Wörterbuch zur Psychologie, dtv, München.

Laplanche, J., J.-B. Pontalis (1977): Das Vokabular der Psychoanalyse; Suhrkamp Verlag, Frankfurt a. M.

The Merck Manual of Diagnosis and Therapy, *Berkow, Robert*, Editor in Chief, published by Merck Sharp and Dome Research Laboratories Division of Merck & Co. Incorporated.

Rahway, N. J. (1982) and *Frank H. Netter*, The CIBA Collection of Medical Illustrations, Line 1: Nervous System.

I would like to thank *T. Lenarz*, *E. Biesinger* and *C. Kober* for their support in compiling this glossary.

Index

T

U

V

W

Y